A Colour Atlas of
VETERINARY DENTISTRY AND ORAL SURGERY

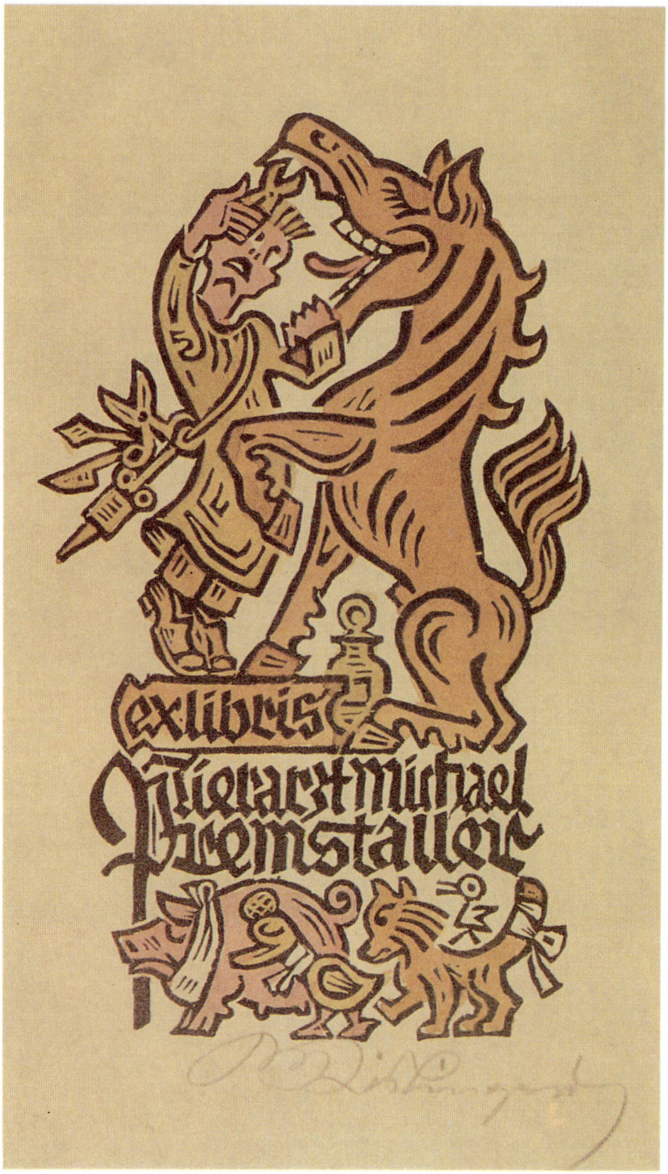

Handcoloured woodcut, by Max Kislinger c. 1949
(signed).

Bookplate — Ex-libris — of Dr Michael Premstaller
(1894–1972).

Professor Kislinger (1895–1983), a civil servant from Linz, was an authority on Austrian art. Also a keen amateur painter, his folk-art style is unmistakable in the 600 ex-libris which he designed and produced. This unique bookplate by Kislinger was inspired by seeing his veterinary friend Michael Premstaller at work.

A Colour Atlas of

VETERINARY DENTISTRY AND ORAL SURGERY

Peter Kertesz
BDS (U. Lond.), LDS RCS Eng.
Dental Surgeon
Honorary Research Fellow and Dental Consultant to the Veterinary Science Department of the Zoological Society of London
Dental Consultant to the International Zoo Veterinary Group

Wolfe Publishing

Published in 1993 by Wolfe Publishing, an imprint of Mosby-Year Book Europe Ltd
Printed by BPCC Hazells Ltd, Aylesbury, England
ISBN 0 7234 1542 0

A CIP catalogue record for this book is available from the British Library.

For full details of all Mosby-Year Book Europe Ltd titles please write to Mosby-Year Book Europe Ltd, Brook House, 2–16 Torrington Place, London WC1E 7LT, England.

Dedicated to the memory of
my parents Alice and Edgar,
for all the laughter and
happiness they generated,
even at the most
difficult times.

Contents

Contributors

Orthopaedic surgery of the mandible and maxilla
John E. F. Houlton MA, VetMB, DSAO, DVR, MRCVS
Specialist in Small Animal Surgery (Orthopaedics),
University Surgeon, Department of Clinical Veterinary Medicine,
University of Cambridge.

Oral tumours
Richard A. S. White BVetMed, PhD, DVR, FRCVS, Diplomate ACVS
Specialist in Surgery (Small Animals),
Lecturer in Small Animal Soft Tissue Surgery, Department of Clinical Veterinary Medicine, University of Cambridge.

Equine dentistry
J. Geoffrey Lane BVetMed, FRCVS
Senior Lecturer, Department of Veterinary Surgery, University of Bristol.

Preface

In the fourth century Publius Vegetius Renatus stated in his book *Mulomedicina Chironis*: 'The animal cannot speak for itself, whereas a man can describe his symptoms'. The implementation of this philosophy is highly relevant when considering the dental treatment of animals 1600 years later.

It is imperative to understand the treatment requirements from the animals' point of view; they are silent and have no say in the options available. We must think for them when it comes to planning treatment. All the factors must be weighed up — pain, neglect, acute local and resultant chronic systemic infections, surgical trauma, function, repeated anaesthetics and associated risks — as well as the insignificance of aesthetic considerations.

A Colour Atlas of Veterinary Dentistry and Oral Surgery was written with the aim of putting this rapidly expanding subject into perspective. Representing a unique, meticulous and broadly based photographic record compiled over many years, the overriding purpose of the atlas is to outline the objectives, principles and practice of a high standard, ethical approach to veterinary dental care, so that animals truly benefit from the treatment they receive.

Acknowledgements

This atlas reflects the extensive clinical work, the recording of thousands of photographs and the development of surgical techniques and instruments that have been the result of years of team effort. I am indebted and grateful to many people for their assistance, dedication and commitment, not only throughout the time I have been involved in veterinary dentistry but for the influence they have had on my life. Hence, the importance I attach to this comprehensive Acknowledgements section.

First, my thanks and appreciation are due to certain individuals for their outstanding help and support. My uncle Professor Endre Wolf has been a constant source of motivation and encouragement throughout my life in Britain. He was responsible for my education at Dartington Hall: a unique start, which I believe made it all possible. His linguistic ability has been a great help in translating some scientific texts for me. My wife Brenda has been exceptionally tolerant of my sometimes obsessive behaviour. She has been a full-time sounding board for my ideas and without the support of such a partner life would be unimaginable. A great deal of thanks goes to my dental nurses Samantha Elkington and Armelle Grunchec; working with such true professionals, often under very difficult conditions, made the tasks infinitely easier. I am especially grateful to them for sharing with me the clinical photography, which they mastered to an exceptionally high standard. Without their dedication such a detailed and comprehensive atlas could never have been produced.

I must thank Keith Loach for his advice on applied biology at Dartington Hall; Varinka and Rory Symington who have always provided tremendous support and encouragement, even in those early days. At King's College Hospital Medical and Dental School the excellent teaching of Professor John Sowray provided the groundwork in oral surgery and Mr Sam Halder the essentials of endodontics. Their coaching in the fundamentals has been invaluable; it has been so easy to build on, especially when tackling the problems and variations encountered in multispecies dentistry. Dr Richard Haskell's theory and advice on critical analysis has been one of the most important aspects of my undergraduate training.

Further acknowledgements must start with Dr Bruce Fogle, who introduced me to the world of veterinary surgery; Mike Chapman, who suggested the idea of this atlas to Wolfe Publishing Ltd and has been a help in locating some historical references during my research for this book; my contributors John Houlton, Geoffrey Lane and Dr Richard White, for their invaluable and original suggestions and for sharing their unique knowledge and photographic records with me; my desk editors David Burin and Jonathan Lewis, and designer Lara Last, who helped to transform my manuscript and slides into this magnificent atlas.

In the veterinary field I have had the privilege of working with exceptionally caring and academically stimulating people, some of whom have become close friends. I am greatly indebted to these individuals, who have shared their clinical cases with me and have showed unfailing confidence throughout the years.

Zoo veterinarians I should like to thank, in order of hours spent working together over operating tables and straw bales, are Dr John Lewis; Andrew Greenwood; Suzie Jackson; Dr Frances Gulland; Dr James Kirkwood; James Barnett; Chris Artingstall; David Taylor; Dr Barkley Hastings; Dr Motke Levison; Derek Lyon; Dr Willem Schaftenaar; Richard Kock; Peter Scott, who supplied the information and photograph for **506**; and Andrew Cunningham, for his help with the pathological specimens at the Zoological Society of London.

Small animal practitioners I would like to thank include Richard Bleckman; Keith Butt; Andrew Carmichael; Dave Cuffe; Mike Gordon; Nick Jeffrey; Charlie Johnson; Simon Meyer; Nigel Norris; Owen Pinney; Bradley Viner; Mark and Aine Weingarth; and Tom Yarrow, who introduced me to endoscopy.

A special thanks must go to the dedicated veterinary nurses and technicians without whose help none of the work recorded would have been possible, especially Alison Beasley; Jenny Berry; Sue Cottier; Christine Dean; Tony Fitzgerald; Janet Hinson; Jude Howlett; Meryl Lang; Janet Markham; Ashley McManus; Lynda Methold; Jacky Mills; Liz Nichol-Smith; Etta Ramsey; Manda Jane Topp; Cathy Thorpe; and Yvonne Wheatley. The staff of the London Zoo Hospital were a great help with many of the unique radiographs that are reproduced in the chapter on comparative odontology (Chapter 4).

In the field of captive wild animals a great deal of my appreciation goes to the keepers, curators, directors and proprietors. Their priority has always been the animals' welfare. Their help in the management of cases, the logistics of organisation and assistance in following up cases has been invaluable. Inevitably some may be missed from this important list and I apologise for any omissions. In alphabetical order: Chris Anscombe; Mick Carman; Sally Chipperfield and Jim Clubb; Igal David; Brian Harman; Mat Hennessey; Mick Jones; David Magna; Ofer and Einat Matalon; Duncan McGinnie; Jeff Nicklin; Paul O'Donaghue; Warren Pritchard; John Pullen; Doug Richardson; Michael Riotzi; Jim Robson; Lionel Rowe; Lynda Rusbridge; Lee Sambrook; Neil Spooner; Richard Spurgeon; Dominic and Anthony Tropeano; Dr Amelia Turkel; Ian Williams and Frank Wheeler.

Dentistry is a highly equipment- and technique-dependent discipline. Veterinary dental surgery would still be in its infancy were it not for the dedication and unselfish assistance so freely given by many instrument and equipment companies. Some of them had no dental background, but I was able to rely on the profound understanding they have of their field and their ability to interpret my highly specialised needs into reality. I am greatly indebted to Nigel Freeland, my friend and technical adviser; AEG Power Tools; Raymoss Air Tools: Atlas Copco; Alan Bayle and Olga Cardozo of Cardozo Dental Supplies; Bill and Peter Bolton of Bolton Surgical Services; Eric Bower of Bower Precision Engineering; David Cox of SGS Carbide Tools; Paul Fox of Desoutter; Dominic Kearney of Allscrews; Simon Cowdrey of Loctite (UK); Peter Long of Testrade; Austin Mercer of Mercer Skillcraft; Mike Pittas of Richard Wolf (UK), for his help and advice on endoscopy; Metabo Power Tools; Paul Miskovcky of Aseptico; Oscar Muller of Prima Instruments; Paul Smith of Tridac Dental Equipment; John Thompson of Associated Dental Products. Dental technicians responsible for the excellent laboratory work illustrated in the atlas were the late Lawrence Ely; Mick Kedge and Cliff Quince; and John Beardow and Paul Thompson of J.J. Thompson Orthodontic Laboratories.

I am also grateful to the staff of Graham Nash Photographic Laboratory for handling my unique films with such care and for consistently producing high-quality transparencies; Robin Clarke of Keith Johnson Photographic Ltd, for helping with my photographic supplies; Mike Allen of Fixation Ltd; and the staff of Nikon (UK) who looked after my photographic equipment which received considerable punishment over the years.

Many thanks also go to the tireless and enthusiastic dental nurses, Jo Burke, Lois Cox, Debbie Mullish, Julie Seaton, and Renee Sexton who also assisted me over the years.

I wish to show my appreciation to Andrew Davison, Roger Farbey and Julian Rowland of the British Dental Association Library; hygienists Maggie Buchsbaum and Sarah Munday, who made some valuable comments regarding the manuscript; Andrew Butterworth, for sharing the results of his research into wild elephant tusk conditions; Mrs Hilary Chung of the Needham Research Institute, Cambridge, for her help with ancient Chinese texts and **1** and **2**; Martin and Marie Clarke, who have been a great support; Dr Christopher Cullen of the School of Oriental and African Studies, London, for his advice on ancient Chinese history; the Department of Customs and Excise; Dr Erik Erikson of Copenhagen for **626**; L. R. Brightwell for **13;** David Gardner for illustrations **21, 22, 23, 24, 26** and **481**; Dr Caroline Grigson of the Odontological Museum of the Royal College of Surgeons of England, for allowing me to radiograph **50** and photograph **77**; Dr John Harrison of King's College Hospital Dental School, London, for his preparation, advice and interpretation of the histological specimens **40, 213, 214, 219, 558** and **559**; Dr David Hunt of Van Mildert College, Durham University, for his advice on the Classics; Ian Johnson of SmithKline Beecham Pharmaceutials; Richard Frost and Kostas Georgiadis, for their help with Greek terms; Professor Kanwen Ma of the Wellcome Institute for his advice and interpretation of some ancient Chinese veterinary texts; Dr Christina Lockyer of the Sea Mammal Research Unit, Cambridge, for **504** and information regarding cetacean ageing; the National Gallery of Art, Washington, DC for allowing me to reproduce **3** from their collection; Drs Juliette Clutton-Brock, Martin Sheldrick and Barry Clarke of the Natural History Museum, London, for the loan of specimens **34** and **39**; Jennifer Nuttall, for her helpful comments regarding the Glossary; Dr Walter Nuki, for being such a great source of inspiration over the years and for his philosophy on wisdom and dentistry as well as for translating some German papers for me; Jane Pickering of the Oxford University Museum, for helping to locate specimen **503;** Benita Horder, for allowing me to photograph the watercolour for **4,** and Vivien Carbines at the Royal College of Veterinary Surgeons' Wellcome Library; Dr John Scheels of Wauwatosa, for the loan of **667**, and for his encouragement and enthusiasm; Mrs Etti Schnalczer of Vienna, for the historical information relating to her father, Freddie Milne, and for allowing me to photograph the painting in **7**; Dr Ben Swanson Jr of the University of Maryland, for allowing me to photograph items from his collection for the Frontispiece, **5, 6, 10** and **18**; Aran Taylor, for illustrations **492** and **493**; Colin Tennant; Adam Thompson, for **11**; Dr Boyd Welsch of Gainsville, for sharing his knowledge and experiences; Dr H.M. Wens and the Hanover Military Veterinary Museum for **9**. At the Institute of Zoology, Zoological Society of London, thanks go to Terry Dennett, for his help with the ultra close-up photographs **37** and **52**; Dr Thijs Kuiken, for inviting me to photograph **501** and **502**; Caroline Smith, for the scanning electron micrographs in **167, 169** and **171**; Dr Geoffrey Smith, for sharing his knowledge on necrobacillosis; and the librarians of the Society, especially Frances Smyth, who obtained some important and rare scientific papers to help my research.

Finally, a big hug and thanks to my faithful dog Macko who stayed up with me through many late nights, keeping me company when the words were hard to find.

Introduction

The mouth is the gateway to existence for all creatures. At the same time, however, injury or damage to the dental apparatus can present an ideal pathway for pathogens to enter the body and cause local and major systemic repercussions.

We know from our own experiences that dental pain can be amongst the most severe, but animals do not have our complex psychological attitudes and, because of primitive instincts of survival, interpret it differently. When they do show signs of pain, these may be pawing at the mouth; rubbing the side of the face on the ground; hypersalivation; aggression; hiding; dropping food; attempting to eat, but dropping the food and running away from it; avoiding hard food; anorexia; licking the lips constantly; and masticating only on one side.

Oral and dental disease can be a threat to general health and an inspection of the mouth is part of a comprehensive physical examination. A full assessment should be made when opportunities arise through general anaesthetics or sedations performed for other procedures. In most cases, the treatment should be only concerned with the elimination of the condition and in establishing a comfortable and infection-free mouth. This must be provided through the least traumatic, most predictable and rapid procedures

To date, no publication or textbook on veterinary dentistry has analysed in detail the objectives or considered the ethical aspects of the subject. Previous texts have concentrated on procedures and treatment techniques, usually transposed directly from human dental literature, where the objectives are often quite different and come under the headings of comfort, function and aesthetics. By ignoring the prerequisites, an increasing number of operators involved in the discipline fail to appreciate that veterinary dentistry is not human dentistry practised on animals and see the treatment objectives through their own dental criteria. In an effort to satisfy the animal owners' anthropomorphic wishes and deliver the best treatment, they attempt to provide the whole range of human restorative and cosmetic techniques on their patients without fully comprehending the true clinical needs of the animals. This naive approach can be a formula for unnecessary treatment and overprescribing of anaesthetics as well as frequent failure of therapy and dental materials when crossing the species barrier.

Considerable thought has been put into the development of this atlas and its content to ensure that it is handleable, practical and fully comprehensive. It was not written as a textbook to include embryology, detailed dental and head and neck anatomy, radiography and dental materials, or as a dental operative handbook. To discuss these topics in the detail necessary would make the book unmanageable in size or so superficial as to be worthless. Such subjects are examined fully in numerous specialised books. Neither was the book written to be a review of current literature or a 'teach yourself' or 'do-it-yourself' manual of dentistry 'by numbers'.

This book has been written with specific aims in mind:

- To illustrate vividly the clinical conditions and pathology encountered in the mouth of a large range of animals, as an aid in diagnosis.
- To analyse the real dental needs of animals to assure consistent results and a predictable prognosis.
- To discuss and show in detail the most suitable treatment options and possible prognosis.
- To illustrate the correct handling procedures of some commonly used dental materials.

Many small animal veterinary surgeons work in co-operation with dentists. An important aspect of this book is to show these practitioners how they have to modify their skills, techniques and instruments in the light of the different anatomy, dimensions, patient co-operation and function, as well as the clinical requirements of the animal, so they avoid the many pitfalls an alien environment can present. By avoiding some of the learning curve, a high level of predictability can be introduced to the speciality.

Inevitably some overlap has occurred in the book. Some of the basic dental principles outlined are routine to dental surgeons as, similarly, some are to veterinary surgeons.

A great deal of effort has gone into following-up cases, demonstrating the long-term efficacy of treatment, failures and postmortem findings.

The book is broadly divided into three main sections. Chapters 1–12 cover the principles of the basic disciplines. Domestic companion animal cases are used as models to demonstrate the various techniques. Chapter 13 deals with the highly-specialised topic of equine dental treatment. The third section (Chapter 14) is unique; it covers the dental diseases and appropriate treatment lines for a wide range of wild animals. An extensive and detailed glossary is included, so the atlas can be utilised by all readers, whether familiar with veterinary, dental or medical vocabulary.

PETER KERTESZ

1 A Concise History of the Oral and Dental Treatment of Animals

Large domestic animals (equine and other hooved livestock)

Equine

Until the middle of the 19th century, procedures performed on the mouth and teeth of animals were almost exclusively limited to horses. They held a place of vital importance in transport, military and agricultural use; the word 'veterinary' originates from *veterinae*, meaning draught animals in Latin.

Ancient Chinese period

As early as 600 BC there is evidence in a Chinese didactic story of their understanding that the age of horses could be estimated through the coronal morphology of their incisors. In one of the oldest Chinese books, *Zuo Zhuan*, or *Book of Annals*, is written: 'Here are your jades and horses, the same as before, but the horses are somewhat longer in the teeth.'

The earliest Chinese book found on veterinary medicine is from the Sung period, dated 1135 AD. It is entitled *Su Mu An Chi Chi* or *The Administration and Care of Herds*. Compiled by Li Shi and others, the preface of the book indicates that it was already a revised and reprinted edition. It includes sections on ageing and judging the quality of horses through their teeth and on hypersalivation, acupuncture, herbal medicines and the relationship of teeth to the internal organs.

Ancient Chinese culture followed a holistic approach to both human and veterinary medicine. It was believed that dental symptoms were a sign of internal disease. As teeth are calcified tissues, and the roots originate from bone, they connected them with bone, which in traditional Chinese medicine was connected with the 'kidneys', their term for the reproductive organs. Usually, acupuncture and herbal medicines were the treatment of choice. Acupuncture in the treatment of animals dates back to 659 BC, the period of the warring states, where a general named Bo Le was well known for his expertise in that form of therapy for horses.

Acupuncture, an important and distinct part of traditional Chinese medicine, aims to regulate the *chi (qi)*, the life energy, or life force, of the body and the blood. This is achieved by stimulation of certain points or channels on the body,

1

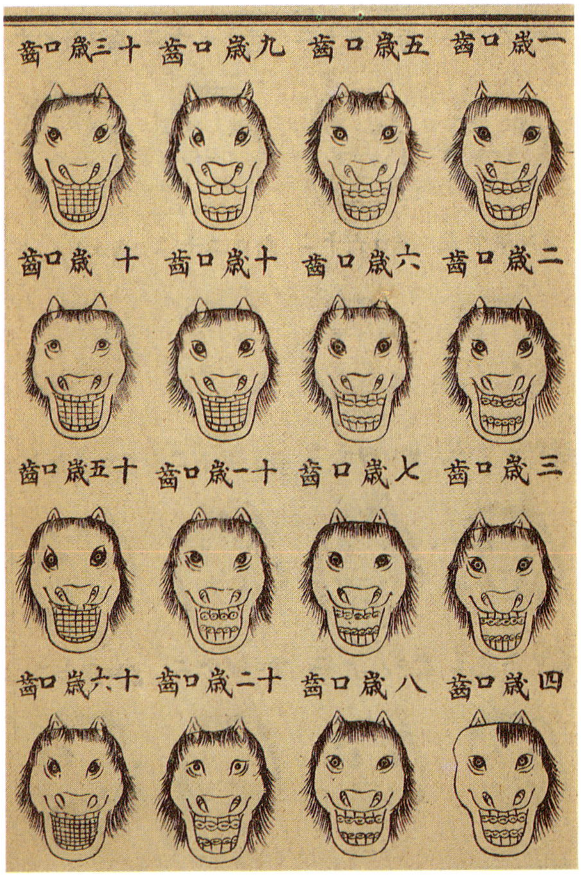

1 17th century Chinese illustrations indicating the ageing of horses through their incisors.

2

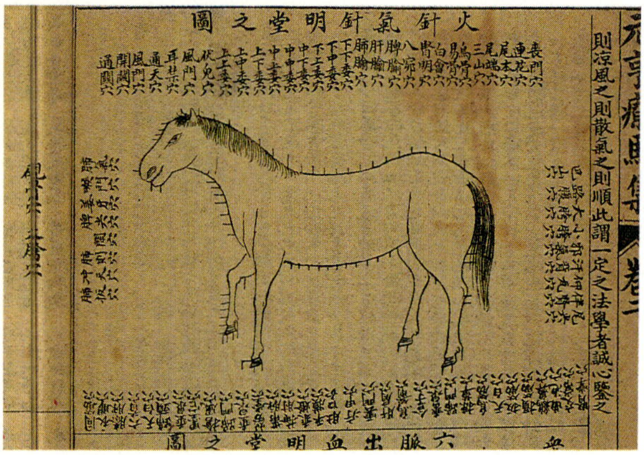

2 Acupuncture points of a horse illustrated in a 17th century book on veterinary medicine.

which are always connected with the internal organs.

One of the most influential Chinese books dealing with the treatment of animal diseases was published in 1608, in the Ming period. Entitled *Yuan Heng Liao Ma Niu Tuo Jing Quan Ji*, or *Complete Collection of Yuan Heng's Treatment for the Horse, Cattle and Camel*, it was a 'summary of all the past knowledge of veterinary treatment'. It is well illustrated with woodblock prints, including how to examine the mouth of a horse. The section also contains information on how to age horses through their teeth, to an age of 36 (**1**). The text was written in rhyme so that it could be easily memorised.

Traditional Chinese veterinary medicine attached great importance to the mouth and teeth as indicators of diseases of the internal organs. The colour of the lips, teeth, gingivae and the tongue were also understood to be signs of the health of the animal and the prognosis of treatment. Common oral and dental ailments, such as hypersalivation, dysphagia and ulceration of the buccal mucosa or tongue, were recognised and treated through acupuncture of the appropriate channels. The acupuncture instruments were either needles; fire needles, which were used red hot; or small cautery irons. Pictures of the location of acupuncture points, of which there are over 360 in the horse, also appear in the book. They are labelled with the appropriate illnesses as a guide to their use (**2**); for example, the acupuncture point to treat the swelling of the buccal mucosa was cauterisation of a point at the rostral border of the facial crest. Swelling of the tongue was treated by using fire needles on the 'root' of the tongue at a lateral and ventral point. For a 'tight mouth', which may have been tetanus, the treatment was to make the Yu Tang point in the palate bleed and rub salt into it. Quidding and dysphagia were treated through fire needles of the Kai Guan point, inside the cheek; or the Hou Men point, 'one finger width below the cheek'. Diseases of an embryo were also believed to show up in the ulceration of the mouth from the molars; the treatment prescribed was cutting the palate with a sharp knife and rubbing salt with oil into the incision. The Chinese also believed that certain body postures of the camel and horses were associated with tooth symptoms.

Traditional Chinese Medicine recognised inflammation, which was termed 'the red conditions'. One of the five such ailments in the horse occurred at the commissure of the lips, and was recognised as being the result of overzealous use of the bit. The prescribed treatments were:

- 'If the injury becomes a boil use a sharp knife to cut it'.
- 'If there is pus use a medicinal concoction to wash it'.
- 'If it is bleeding use a packing with powdered medicine applied to the injured part'.

Although traditional Chinese medicine and physiology are not related to modern Western theories, the Chinese had an understanding of the general principles of health and were conservative in their approach.

The period of Ancient Greece and the Roman Empire

The Greek philosopher Aristotle (384–322 BC) in *Historia Animalium*, described periodontal disease in horses as a symptom and not a syndrome itself. He stated that if the condition did not disappear spontaneously it was incurable.

During the period of the Roman Empire there was also an awareness of the anatomical and morphological significance of horses incisors in ageing. Some modern writers hypothesise that the falsification of horses' ages through their teeth was already performed at that time. Pelagonius, *c.* 350, compiled a treatise from his notes and letters on the medical treatment of horses. Chapter 18 was entitled *De Dentibus* ('About the Teeth'). The text was translated from Latin into Greek and published, with sections by other authors on horse medicine, under the title *Hippiatria*.

In the 4th century, Vegetius had some advanced philosophical ideas on the principles and practice of veterinary surgery. In his book *Mulomedicina Chironis*, he advocated the practice of suturing up tongues and soft tissues injured through the use of the bit in breaking-in horses, and applying poultices to encourage the pointing and drainage of extra-oral abscesses. In contrast, Hippocrates *Indicus* in the 6th century advocated the extraction of the canine teeth and the partial amputation of the tongue in horses for a more ready acceptance of the bit.

In Europe, after the fall of the Roman Empire the treatment of animal diseases was generally based on religious beliefs, superstition and folklore. In the Middle Ages even the slightest progress gained at the time of the Roman Empire was forgotten, and the oral manipulation of horses entered a dark age.

The period of the Masters of the Horse

An important period in the treatment of equine diseases in Central Europe, although sterile for its scientific advances, was at the time of the Hapsburg Empire. The commencement of the era has been taken as the publication of the first book in Europe on the subject in 1250, entitled *Medicina Equorum*, by Jordanus Ruffus, followed by *Marescallus Major*, a work of the Emperor Staufer Frederick II of the Imperial Hohenstaufen Dynasty.

This era has been termed the period of the *Stallmeisterzeit* (stablemasters or Masters of the Horse), obtaining its name from the institutionalised court office of stablemaster. Important and well-paid people, who were employed by large estates to take responsibility for the management of the horses, stablemasters were theoreticians and considered themselves above performing manipulations on the animals. Any operations were performed on their diagnosis and instructions by the *hufschmiede* (blacksmith). Although procedures were based on physical ideas rather than on superstition, they had no scientific basis and the barbaric techniques employed resulted in extreme cruelty. If animals died as a result of the treatment the operators were usually not held responsible.

The reasons for treatment of the mouth and the teeth at that period are as follows:

1. There was a lack of diagnostic knowledge of how to treat diseases that affect the digestive system and, as the mouth was the only part that was accessible, attention was concentrated on that area.

2. The breaking-in of horses was a brutal procedure, with an overemphasis on the use of the bit and the rein. More than 450 types of bits, which became sharper and more violent in their action, have been illustrated. Broken glass was also placed in the mouth in the belief it would help in the acceptance of the bit. The consequences of these measures, the injuring, stretching and paralysing of the tongue, were corrected through its partial or total amputation. The canine and wolf teeth were hammered out to make room for the bit and to make the mouth more sensitive as well as to 'break the horse's spirit'. The *laden*, the area of edentulous alveolar ridge immediately rostral to the cheek teeth, was considered of great importance in the use and effectiveness of the bit. One procedure involved opening the gingivae and implanting splinters of broken glass to increase the bulbosity of the alveolus. The idea was that the increased pain in the area through the use of the bit would encourage the horse to be more responsive. Others had opposing opinions and gouged out alveolar bone from this area to make more room for the bit.

3. Humoral pathological principles, already advocated in ancient Greek and Roman times, were another common reason for operating on the mouth and the teeth. The method of eliminating the redundant and bad fluids of the body involved the use of venesection. This was usually performed by making sagittal incisions in the palate, often on a monthly basis for prophylactic reasons. Swellings, ulcers and other intra-oral pathology, collectively called the *frosch* (frog), were excised. The term was at first confined to ulcerations of the buccal mucosa adjacent to the cheek teeth. A 15th century text describes the oral condition associated with loss of appetite and dropping of food that in the 20th century would often be suspected as buccal ulceration caused by enamel pointing of the cheek teeth. Rather than search for a cause that could be treated, the ulcers were excised.

The 'frog' was also used to describe sublingual swellings, which were probably salivary mucoceals resulting from ruptured salivary ducts through trauma: like other abnormalities, they were excised. The *lampas*, which were physiologically normal but temporarily bulbous and inflamed rostral palatal rugae and incisive papillae at the time of permanent tooth eruption, were burned with a red hot iron well into the 20th century.

The earliest European pictorial record relating to equine dental treatment originates from the Netherlands. Dated 1648, *A Farrier's Shop* (**3**), by Paul Potter (1625–1654), is part of the Widener Collection in the National Gallery of Art, Washington, DC. The painting also illustrates a twitch being used.

3

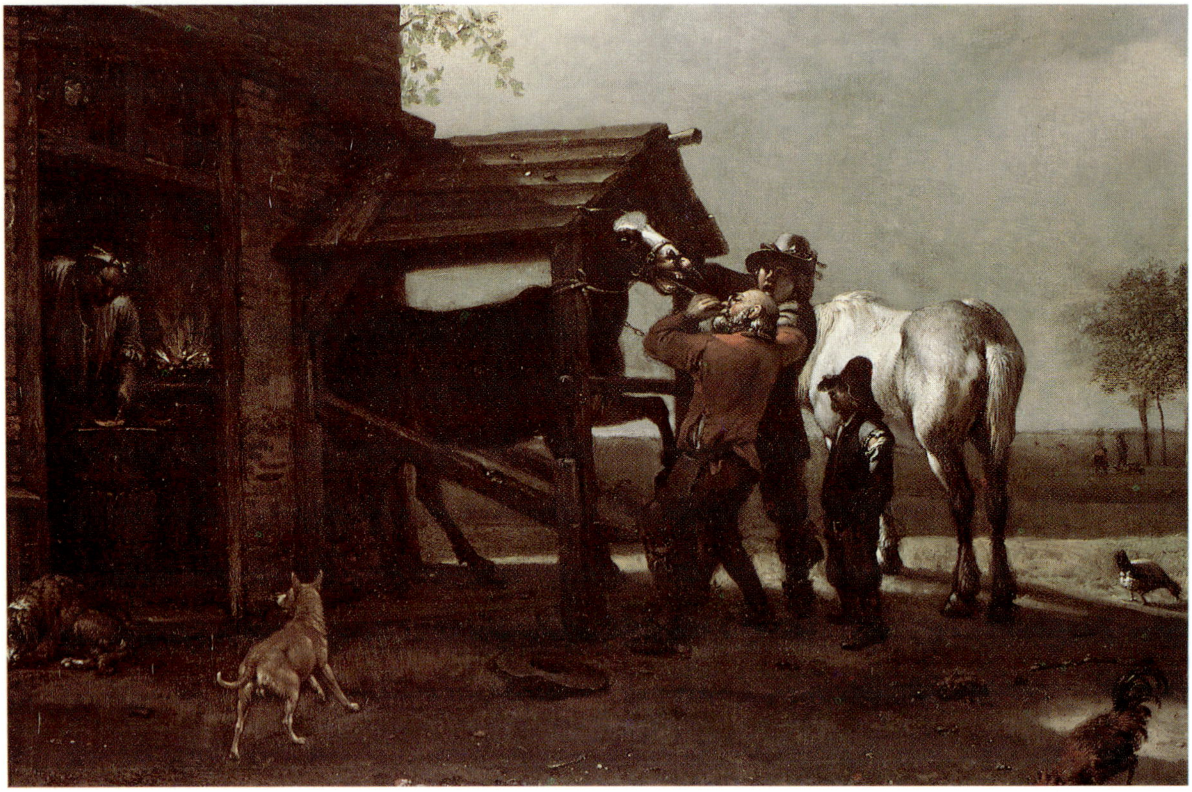

3 ***A Farrier's Shop*** **(a detail), Paul Potter (1625–1654). Widener Collection, National Gallery of Art, Washington, DC.**

4. Superstition played a varied role during the period of the masters of the horse. The blacksmiths were totally captivated by such beliefs, although the educated class and horse-healing books on the lines of Ruffus were influenced only to a minor degree and believed strongly in humoral pathology. Implanting of tooth roots through the face into the alveolus was called the *Wurzelstecken*. The site used was accessed through the masseter muscle, ventral to the facial crest. It was already practised in the 1st century, at the time of Pinicus, and continued its popularity in central Europe into the 20th century to combat the *wurm* (worm), which was any unknown disease, probably a sign of infection. The implanted root was even surrounded sometimes with the tip of an amputated tongue in the hope of increasing its effectiveness. The iatrogenic complications of the treatment included tetanus, sepsis, oedema of the masseter muscle and the inability of the animal to eat.

5. As horses were important and valuable items, procedures based on fraudulent motives were common. As young animals were not an attractive purchase due to their limited workload, the falsification of their age through early extraction of the primary teeth was sometimes performed to encourage the eruption of the permanent set. The practice of tampering with the appearance of horses to make them seem younger goes back to the Middle Ages. The oldest of the methods was to shorten the incisor teeth, but the best-known technique employed was termed 'bishoping' in England (see Glossary). Originally this involved burning a concavity in the dentine of the incisal tables with a hot iron to mimic the infundibula of the front teeth (**4**). The practice evolved over the centuries, so drills were used to deepen the defects, and to intensify the discoloration silver nitrate was applied. Numerous equine handbooks gave advice, even in the 20th century, on how such deceitful methods could be recognised. Another technique to make a horse appear younger involved inflation of the supra-orbital skin by blowing air subcutaneously with a quill, through a small incision. Horses that bit had their incisor teeth cut down or holes drilled in them in a belief that 'when the horse opens his mouth the wind blows down the teeth'.

6. Preventative treatment was rare, but there are

records of the anterior teeth of horses being smoothed with files at this period to prevent trauma to the soft tissues.

The period of enlightenment

The close of the period of the Masters of the Horse and the commencement of the period of enlightenment began in 1762 with the establishment of the first veterinary academy at Lyon, France by Claude Bourgelat (1712–1779). Veterinary surgery started to develop a scientific basis for understanding disease and the rationale for treatment.

As early as 1805 in the *Dictionary of the Veterinary Art* by Thomas Bordman it was acknowledged that the lampas resolved with time. By the middle of the 19th century a number of veterinary authors were strongly criticising burning the *lampas* as a 'barbaric and useless procedure'. They recognised it to be an 'imaginary disorder' and advocated a conservative approach to the treatment of the inflamed oral mucosa. In a book dated 1862 entitled *The Illustrated Horse Doctor*, Edward Mayhew (1813–1868), an English veterinarian, conveys an exceptionally deep and compassionate understanding of the extreme suffering dental disease and its thoughtless treatment inflicts on the horse. But as late as 1914 in Luis Merillat's book *Animal Dentistry and Diseases of the Mouth* there are still descriptions of burning the *lampas*, partially amputating the tongue and repelling the cheek teeth of horses without an anaesthetic.

The first dental operations on horses that used ether as an anaesthetic were performed in 1847, one year after its introduction by the Boston dentist W.T.G. Morton.

The visiting card of an established horse dentist from Portland, Connecticut, USA, emphasised the humane technique he used for the treatment of equine dental disorders (**5**).

By tradition, much of the routine dental work on horses over the centuries has been performed by farriers, stable employees and self-taught 'horse dentists'. After the end of the American Civil War, schools of equine dentistry sprang up in the United States for the training of non-professional personnel (**6**). Their heyday was between 1880 and 1895, but with the proliferation of private and state veterinary colleges their purpose became redundant. Nevertheless, even at the end of the 20th century some veterinary surgeons consider the routine maintenance of horses' teeth beneath them, an attitude that has probably contributed to the slow progress made in this field.

The first technique advocating an extra-oral, non-repulsive technique for the extraction of the upper cheek teeth was suggested about 1900, by

4

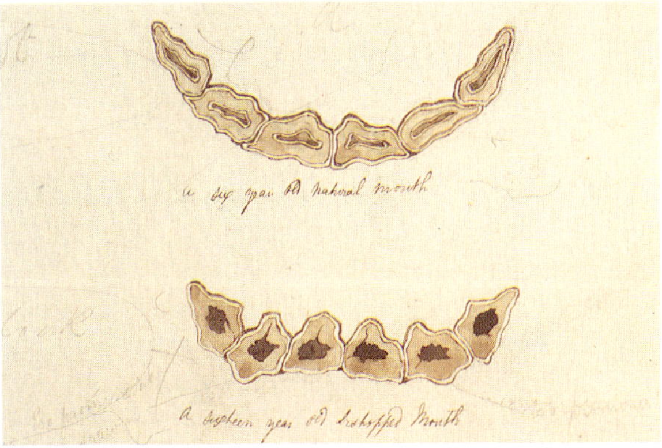

4 Original watercolour c.1850 by Edward Mayhew for his book *The Illustrated Horse Management*, which compares the appearance of natural infundibula with 'bishoped' incisors. (From the collection of the Royal College of Veterinary Surgeons' Wellcome Library, London.)

5

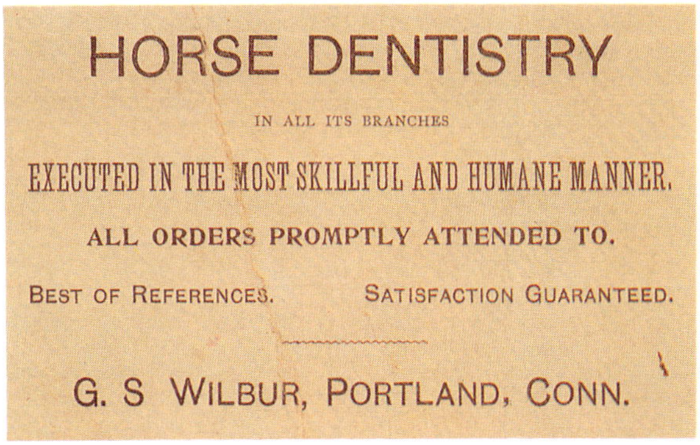

5 Late 19th century visting card of a horse dentist.

W.L. Williams, Professor of Surgery at the New York State Veterinary College. The procedure was called Williams' Operation. Although the basic idea was sound, the vertical incision advocated was contrary to the surgical anatomy of the region. The procedure did not gain popularity.

One of the most well-known European itinerant horse dentists in the early 20th century was Scottish-born Freddie Milne (1867–1942). He came from a horse racing family and spent most of his working life as a trainer in Hungary and Germany. When he retired from training in Vienna in 1924 he turned to equine dentistry and travelled the racecourses of Europe. Around 1933 he had caricature paintings of him exhibited at the Eiffel Tower, Paris as a curiosity. The cost of

6

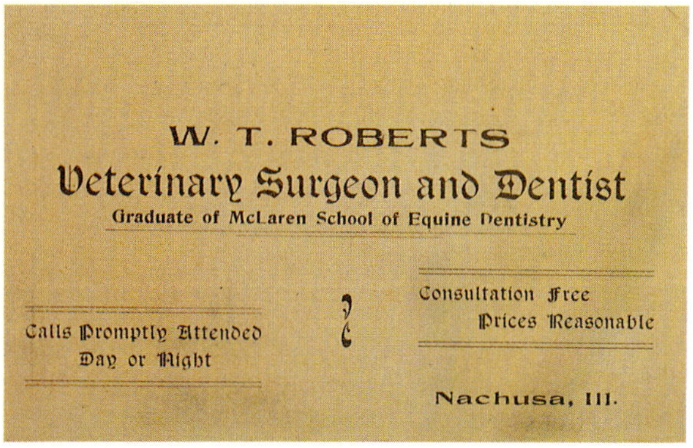

6 North American visiting card of a horse dentist from the late 19th century professing graduation from a 'School of Equine Dentistry'.

7

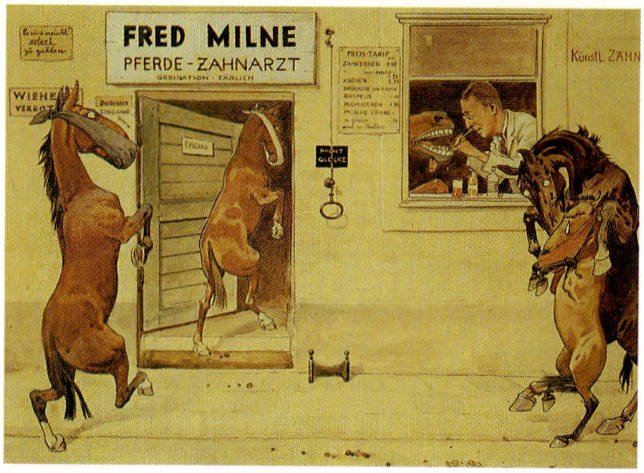

7 Painting of the equine dentist Freddie Milne that was exhibited in the Eiffel Tower, Paris.

8

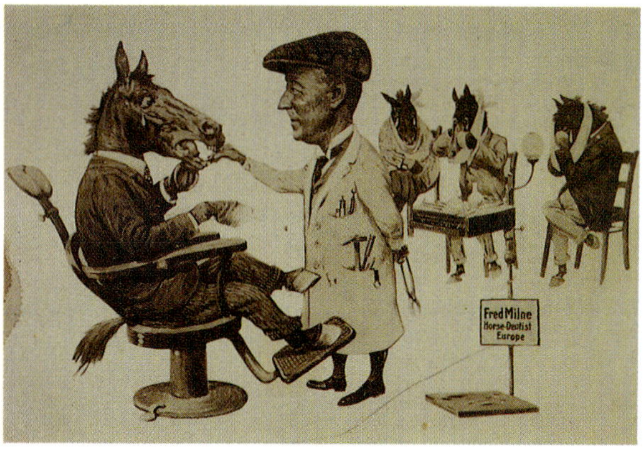

8 Caricatures of Freddie Milne also appeared on postcards.

9

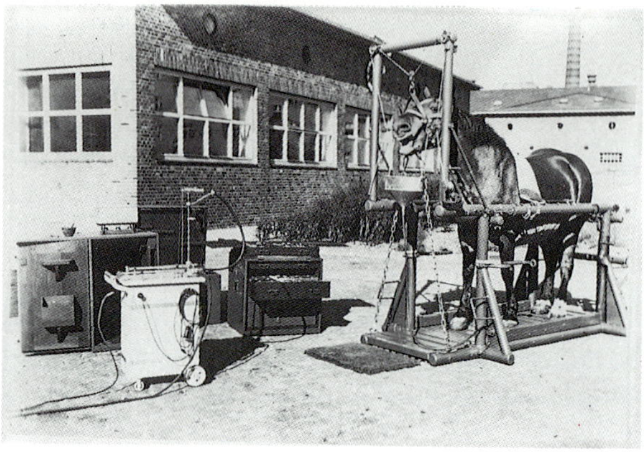

9 Military 'dental station' that was designed and used by Erwin Becker in the Second World War.

fillings, crowns and dentures are shown on the 'price list' (**7**). Humorous anthropomorphic depictions of horses and their dental treatment by him were also published on postcards (**8**).

In the 1930s a German veterinarian named Erwin Becker (1898–1978) revolutionised the treatment of enamel pointing by mechanising the floating of horses' teeth with an electrically operated, rotary, Carborundum disc. He treated over 50,000 military horses with his portable 'dental station' (**9**). His equipment was highly sophisticated in design, even incorporating continuous irrigation to cool the teeth being treated and a safety guard to protect the soft tissues. Commercial mechanical rasping units, which speed up and make the procedure less strenuous, have generally proved unpopular with operators.

In 1981 Evans, Tate and LaDow of the University of Pennsylvania introduced the 'lateral buccotomy' approach for the extraction of horses' upper cheek teeth. A modification of the Williams' Operation, the technique minimised the trauma, complications and prolonged aftercare the repulsion technique often creates to the maxillary sinuses.

Pigs

The examination of the mouth of pigs for the presence of cystic tapeworms, which can be traced back to the fifth century BC, is also discussed in Aristotle's *Historia Animalium*. In France it was necessary for pigs to be examined in the market by the *langueyeur* (a person specialised in the examination of the tongue of pigs for the presence of cysts); this practice, which originated before 1465, continued into the 20th century (**10**). The disarming of young pigs was also performed in the marketplace. The animals had their canines and incisor teeth broken off at gum level with pliers. Veterinary surgeons engaged in meat inspection still report large periapical abscesses occurring in animals having had such mutilations.

10

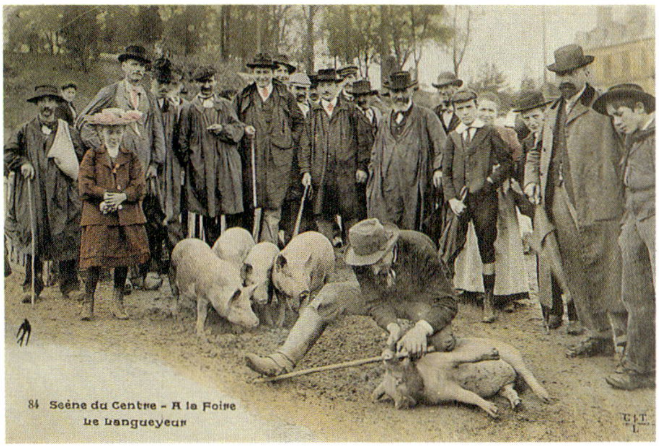

10 Pigs receiving dental attention in a French marketplace c. 1900.

Sheep

In 1980 a Scottish dentist named Adam Thompson introduced the Ewesplint, designed to overcome the 'broken mouth syndrome' of the anterior teeth of sheep (**11**). The device aimed to extend the breeding life of the animals feeding in a harsh environment by cementing a prefabricated steel splint over the mobile teeth. The initial enthusiasm for the system did not gain popularity due to the relatively high cost of the splints.

11

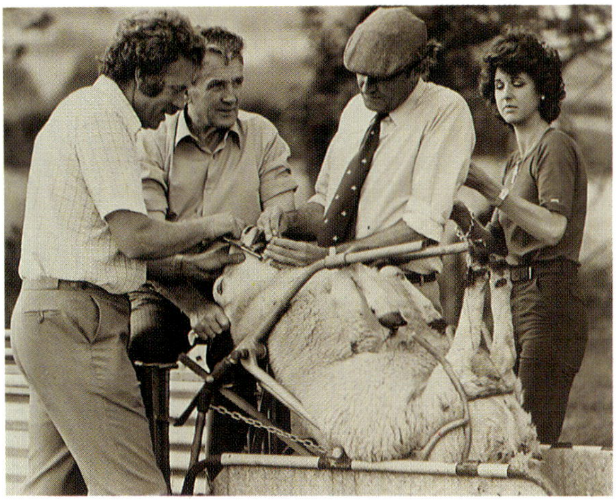

11 A Ewesplint being fitted.

Captive wild animals and comparative odontology

With the popularity of private menageries, and the development of zoological gardens in the early 19th century, the incidence and relevance of dental disease was soon recognised. One of the earliest cases reported was in the Exeter 'Change, Strand, London in 1826. An elephant bull named Chunie had to be destroyed by an infantry firing squad after becoming dangerously unmanageable due to the pain created by an infected fractured tusk. The skull of the animal was exhibited in the museum of the Royal College of Surgeons of England, until 1941, when it was destroyed during an air attack on London.

In 1832 in Britain the *Liverpool Advertiser* recorded the dental treatment of zoo animals

12

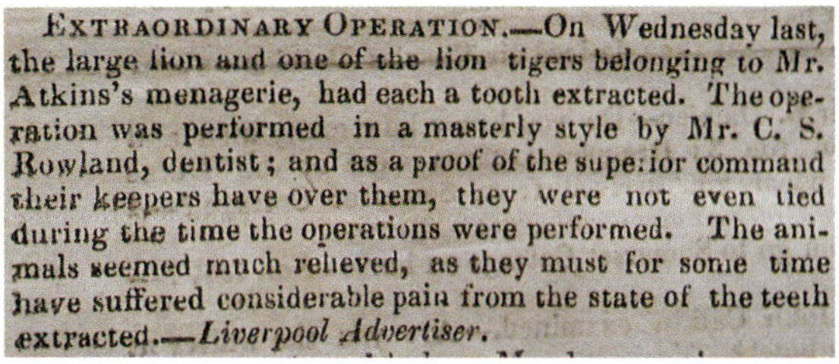

EXTRAORDINARY OPERATION.—On Wednesday last, the large lion and one of the lion tigers belonging to Mr. Atkins's menagerie, had each a tooth extracted. The operation was performed in a masterly style by Mr. C. S. Rowland, dentist; and as a proof of the superior command their keepers have over them, they were not even tied during the time the operations were performed. The animals seemed much relieved, as they must for some time have suffered considerable pain from the state of the teeth extracted.—*Liverpool Advertiser*.

12 One of the earliest reports on the dental treatment of zoo animals was published in Britain in 1832.

13 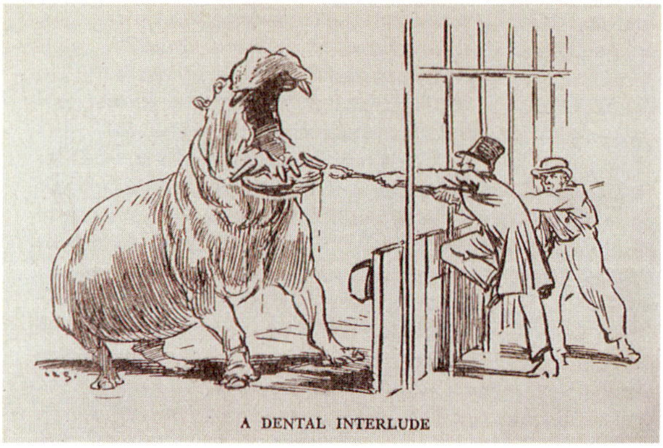

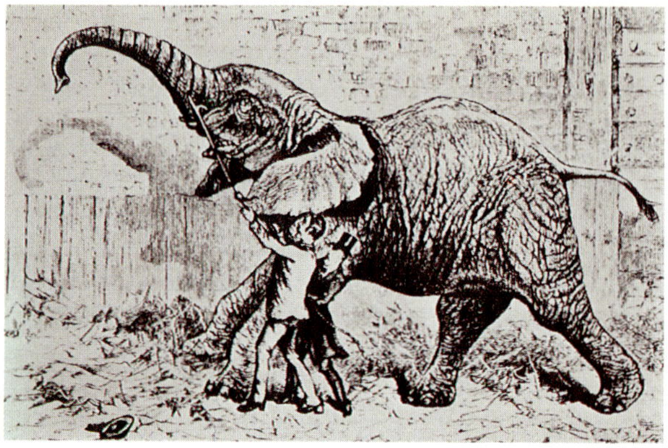 14

13 In 1873 at London Zoo A.D. Bartlett extracted a fractured incisor from a hippopotamus with custom-made dental forceps. Drawing by L.R. Brightwell c. 1920.

14 Jumbo, the famous London Zoo elephant having an abscess, caused by a fractured tusk, incised.

(**12**), while in 1845 Sir Richard Owen, the then Director of the Natural History Museum, published one of the first major works on comparative odontology, entitled *Odontographics.*

The variety of 'exotic' animals in zoological collections created a great interest in the subject of comparative general and dental anatomy. The Odontological Society of Great Britain was formed in 1859, with a membership that included dentists, physicians, surgeons and anatomists.

Also in 1859, Abraham Dee Bartlett (1812–1897), a taxidermist by profession, was appointed as the London Zoo's superintendent. The notes made by him reveal an early and exceptionally deep understanding of the significance of dental disease and the importance of a healthy mouth. He wrote on numerous topics, from continuously-growing teeth to kangaroo dentitions. On one occasion, when a hippopotamus fractured an incisor in 1873, he was responsible for its preventative extraction as he feared 'the consequences may be serious' in leaving the broken tooth (**13**).

The earliest illustration of zoo animal dental treatment dates back to to 1878 (**14**). Jumbo, the famous African bull elephant at London Zoo, fractured both of his tusks, apical to the tusk sheaths. The erupting tusks impacted into the soft tissues and formed abscesses below the eyes, which apparently caused great pain. Bartlett and Jumbo's keeper, Matthew Scott, incised these abscesses using a razor-sharp, hook-shaped instrument 18 inches in length. Apparently, no restraint was used. The animal's condition improved dramatically and it was reported that the tusks erupted at the point of incision rather than at their normal position under the upper lip. It is interesting to note that when the animal was killed in a train accident in Canada in 1885 post-mortem photographs indicated that the tusks were at a normal labial position and intra-oral examination revealed rotated and deformed molars, which some writers have blamed for his aggressive behaviour.

About 1881 the first dental operation was performed under general anaesthetic at the London Zoo. A private dental practitioner was invited to extract a decayed tooth from a baboon.

Sir John Bland-Sutton (1855–1936), a general surgeon with a lifelong interest in zoology, was keenly aware of the threat dental disease presented to the life of animals. In 1884, while still a lecturer in anatomy and comparative anatomy at the Middlesex Hospital, London, he wrote the first scientific paper on the dental diseases of non-domestic species, entitled 'Comparative oral pathology', which he presented to the Odontological Society of Great Britain. He became a Huntarian Professor of the Royal College of Surgeons of England in 1888–1889, and was appointed Vice-President of the Zoological Society of London in 1928.

In 1883 Professor W.H. Flower (1831–1899), Director of the Natural History Museum, London, defined new dental terminologies in the *Encyclopaedia Britannica.*

By the early 1920s the Zoological Society of London had regular dental consultants who assisted with the dental problems arising within the collection (**15**). One of the best known of these part-time 'zoo dentists' was Mr Sydney Kemp, who also worked with private menageries in other parts of Britain.

Sir Frank Colyer (1866–1954), an oral surgeon and Dean of the Royal Dental Hospital, London from 1904–1909, was appointed Honorary Curator of the Museum of the Odontological Society of Great Britain in 1900, a post that he held until his death. The collection, which is now housed in the Royal College of Surgeons in London, is the product of his dedication, and he made an invaluable contribution to the field of comparative dental pathology. The publication of his book *Variation and Diseases of the Teeth of Animals* was a milestone on the subject. Colyer mainly used specimens in the Odontological Museum as his reference material and followed the system set by Sir John Tomes in his book entitled *A System of Dental Surgery* and Bland-Sutton's paper of 1884.

With the growth of small animal dentistry in the 1980s, increasingly more cases of zoo animal dental procedures were reported in the literature. The extraction of an infected elephant tusk was a traumatic and time-consuming procedure until 1984, when Dr Boyd Welch of Florida introduced the 'internally collapsing' technique. A small group of dentists who developed an expertise in the dental treatment of non-domestic animals, and some veterinarians also interested in the field, wanted to share their knowledge and techniques. From this idea grew the first Exotic Animal Dentistry Conference, which was held in Milwaukee, Wisconsin, USA, in 1986.

15

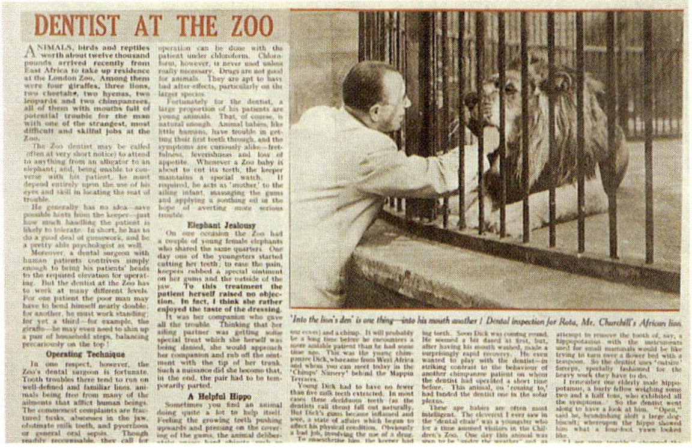

DENTIST AT THE ZOO

15 A 1920s magazine article on the variety of dental treatment being performed at the London Zoo.

Small domestic companion animals

From the first century there are accounts in *Historia Naturalis,* by the Roman writer Gaius Plinius Secundus (Pliny the Elder, AD 23–79) that the preventative treatment of rabies was often applied to the mouth. He perpetuated and rendered popular the Ancient Greek myth that the lyssa — fine, elastic, rod-like structure, situated in the ventrorostral border of the dog's tongue — was a worm responsible for rabies. Excision of the lyssa was often performed on puppies in a belief that it would prevent the disease. The practice is believed to have been continued by ignorant people into the late 19th century. Even veterinarians were often unaware of exactly what structure the lyssa was, frequently mistaking it for the lingual fraenum.

In 1859 Goubaux reported in the *Mémoires de la Société Vétérinaire* on the 'aberrations in the dentitions of domestic animals'.

By the late 19th century the excision of the lyssa was being frowned upon by veterinary surgeons as a useless and painful operation. A very early illustration of canine dentistry was in George Fleming's book, entitled *Rabies and Hydrophobia*, dated 1872 (**16**). He believed that cutting off the tips of dogs' canine and incisor teeth with pliers, and filing the rough edges, would prevent the spread of rabies.

16

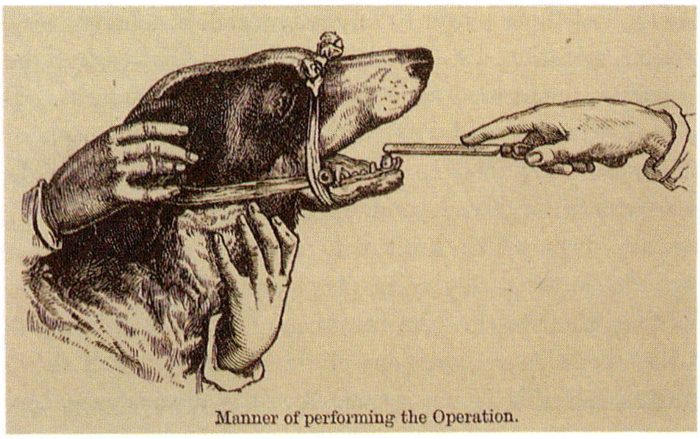

16 1872 illustration advocating the cutting down and smoothing of dogs' canines and incisors to prevent rabies.

Sir John Bland-Sutton in his 1884 paper stressed that indiscriminate breeders perpetuated hereditary occlusal abnormalities in dogs.

By the end of the 19th century clinical cases were being reported in the treatment of domestic pets. The first case of denture prosthodontics was published in the *Journal of Comparative Pathology and Therapeutics*, 1897. Not surprisingly, the treatment was not well received by the dogs and

17

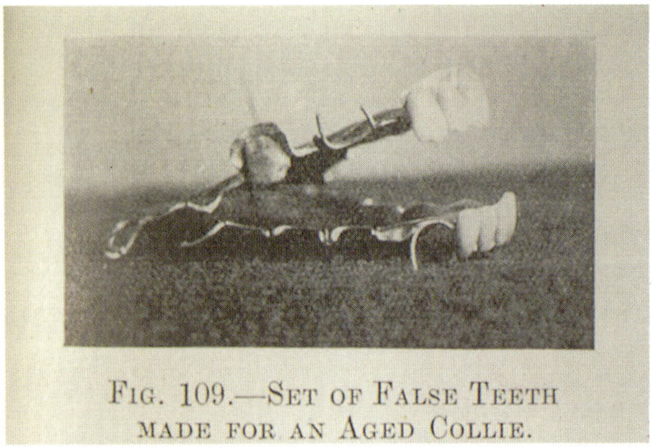

17 Dentures made for a dog in 1897.

18

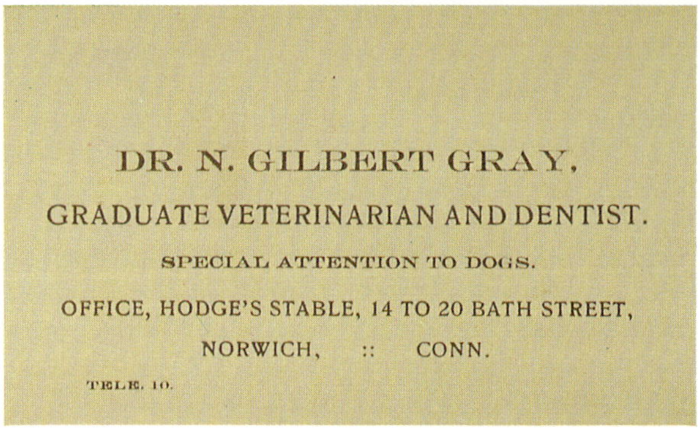

18 A visiting card of a veterinary surgeon and dentist, c. 1900, professing a speciality in dogs.

19

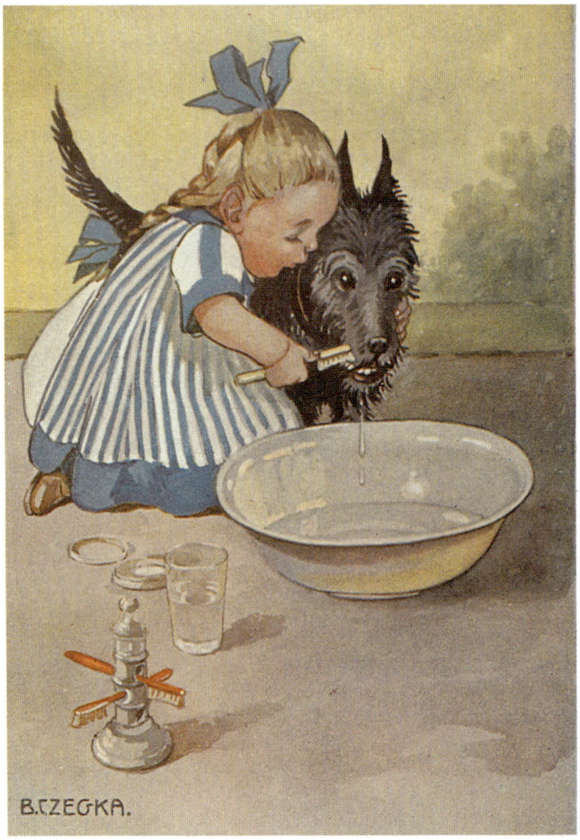

19 Preventative home dental care for dogs is depicted in this 1930s postcard.

20

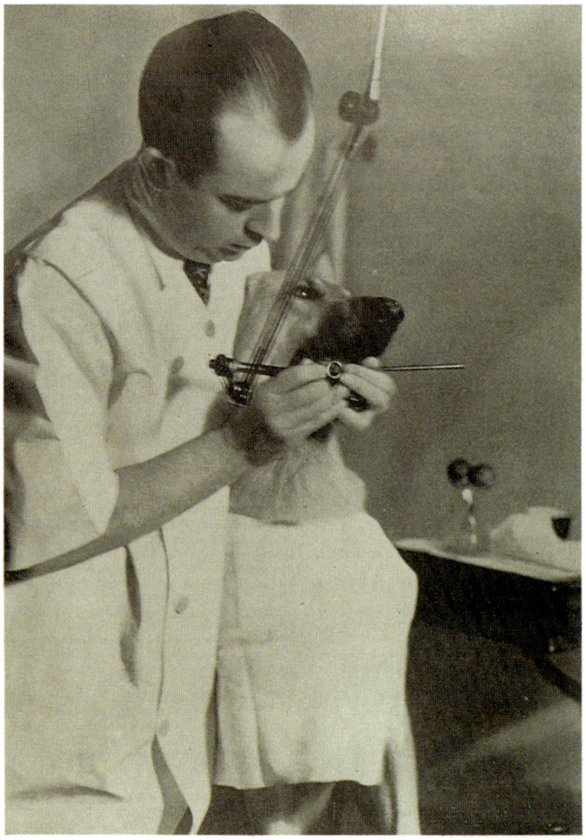

20 1930s book caption: 'A Good Patient — Canine dentistry is wellnigh as elaborate and efficient as the human variety. The above dog's teeth are receiving general attention.'

some were quickly lost by the patient. In 1928 the *Daily Mail* reported a reward for finding a denture belonging to a rat catcher Jack Russell terrier that had been lost within three days of fitting. Other pets were less fortunate and had dentures wired in for retention, although some successes were claimed in self-retained appliances (**17**). In Professor Frank Hobday's book, published in 1890, entitled *The Surgical Diseases of the Cat and Dog*, the aetiology and treatment of periodontal disease in dogs was already discussed, as well as the cause of malar abscesses and their association with occlusal trauma.

In 1914 Luis Merillat, Vice-President of the American Veterinary Medical Association, wrote on the filling of carious cavities in animals: 'The rarity of the indication will doubtless always prevent its introduction into the veterinary college curriculum'. In the early 1900s some individuals were advertising their small animal dentistry speciality (**18**). Some of the extraction techniques did not follow basic principles. In the 1941 edition of *Dollar's Veterinary Surgery* it is advocated that 'repulsion is the only method that will succeed in taking out sound permanent canine teeth in the dog'.

Preventative home dental care for dogs was already thought about and illustrated in this 1930s postcard (**19**), well before the introduction of DVM toothpaste for dogs, which was the first such product specially formulated and marketed in the United States for canine use in 1975. From the early 1920s animal dentistry was depicted in a comical way in magazines and postcards, which was a popular medium until about 1950. In some lay books, such as *Hutchinson's Dog Encyclopaedia*, *c*. 1934, the anthropomorphic and humorous attitude many people had towards the topic is reflected (**20**).

By 1939 the veterinary literature regularly published papers on the dental diseases and the dental treatment of companion animals. Endodontic treatment of dogs canine teeth was already illustrated in the German *Tierarztliche Operationslehre (Veterinary Operative Surgery)* by Berge and Westhues published in 1961.

During the 1970s a major change took place in veterinary dentistry. There was a great interest by a small group of enthusiasts who realised the prevalence of dental disease in the domestic pet population and recognised its clinical significance. It was understood that some special instrumentation was required for the different anatomy and dimensions of the veterinary environment and the dental trade was approached regarding the manufacture and supply of such items. It was this commercial sector who were the most far-sighted. They recognised the potential market 'small animal dentists' and their patients represented. The discipline was promoted partly on its economic significance. The American Veterinary Dental Society was formed in 1977.

Small animal dentistry was one of the greatest growth areas in veterinary surgery in the 1980s. There were countless seminars and practical sessions designed to introduce the subject to practitioners. By the end of the decade a number of veterinary and dental surgeons were concerned with the way the subject was evolving (*J. Veterinary Dentistry*, 1989, Vol. 6, No. 3, pp. 4–6) Some commented on the risk of iatrogenic diseases that may be created through 'reckless' or 'careless' treatment (*J. Veterinary Dentistry*, 1988, Vol. 5, No. 1, p. 3).

The future of veterinary dentistry

Without doubt the future of veterinary dentistry is assured. Its clinical significance is well documented, and its economic impact and importance on small animal practices proven. The only question is which direction it will take regarding treatment objectives and techniques. Certainly, as with any developing speciality, growing pains and a levelling out in understanding needs to take place. Judging by some of the trends advocated in the small animal field, it is debatable if a practical and ethical balance will be found. Many practitioners, enthusiastic with their newly found interest, attempt to apply the full range of human dental techniques to their small animal patients with apparently little understanding as regards the necessity or prognosis of the treatment. Some of the more bizarre canine cases reported include bleaching discoloured root-filled teeth, complex periodontal surgery, fixed bridgework to replace missing incisors and premolars, mandibular ostectomies and osteotomies to correct malocclusions, an artificial crown decorated with a diamond, intraosseous implant-supported crowns and bridgework, and extra-oral traction used in conjunction with orthodontics.

Equine dental surgery has slowly evolved over the last 150 years. The value of some of the animals has proved to be a strong incentive to improve on the rather primitive methods of the 19th century. Some progressive practitioners understand the limitations and risks involved with the old-fashioned techniques and are working to advance the conservative and surgical techniques in the field. We shall probably see a range of new instruments and equipment to help in these cases.

Wild animal medicine and anaesthetics have become highly specialised over the past two decades. Dental techniques on these animals have also become well documented, and specialised instruments are being designed and continually improved upon. The majority of zoo veterinarians and curators realise that animals in their collection are too rare and valuable to allow operators with questionable motives, objectives and limited experience to become involved in their treatment. Unfortunately, there is evidence that some of the unacceptable trends being introduced in the area of small animal dentistry are being practised in this field. On the other hand, there are still many establishments worldwide where active dental disease of the collections are left untreated, with fatal consequences, while others still use barbaric techniques more in line with the Middle Ages and have not kept up with the advances that have been made, or the assistance that is available, in this highly specialised subject. Worldwide there are only a few individuals who have made the necessary investment in time and equipment, and had the stamina to have remained in the field longer than a few years. Because of the paramount importance attached to wildlife conservation it is likely that in the next decade the dental treatment of captive wild animals will be looked upon as having made the greatest progress and constructive contribution to the field of clinical veterinary dental surgery.

Some veterinary colleges are incorporating dentistry in the undergraduate curriculum. This is a positive step, as there is a section of the veterinary profession who still do not understand the importance of a healthy oral environment or appreciate animals' silent response to dental pain. A realistic and caring approach to the subject must be presented to the new generation of veterinary practitioners.

In the Middle Ages the operators had no scientific background against which to judge their inhumane ideas and techniques. It can only be hoped that with the advances in academic and clinical knowledge and in philosophical analysis, practitioners are now in a position to find the right balance; otherwise, history may judge some of the present trends in veterinary dentistry as cruel overprescribing of treatment and the discipline may again be looked upon as the comic subject depicted in the 19th and early 20th century.

2 Nomenclature and Conventions

Anatomy

Crossing the species and specialisation barriers, confusion can be created by the different terminologies used for anatomical orientation by veterinarians, human physicians/surgeons and dentists. This results from the different body posture of quadrupeds and bipeds; for example, *ventral* and *dorsal* positions on animals' heads are termed *inferior* and *superior* when applied to humans.

Dental and oral anatomy

Difficulties are also created by the same or similar word having a different meaning in another discipline. In general anatomy, *proximal* and *distal* indicate positions and directions close to and away from the centre of the body (torso), or from the point of origin of an organ or limb. In dentistry, *approximal (proximal)* is a collective term that refers to surfaces of the teeth that face adjoining teeth of the same dental arch. The point of reference used for naming them precisely is where the median plane of the face bisects the jaws between the first incisor teeth. Following the natural curvature of the jaws, *mesial* and *distal* refer to surfaces of the teeth that face towards and away from this point, respectively. *Rostral* (towards the nose) and *caudal* (towards the tail) are standard veterinary terms and are used in this atlas to describe gross facial and oral positions (**21**); when describing dental anatomy, surfaces or relationships the more accurate *mesial* and *distal* terms are used (**22**).

Anterior teeth are the incisors and canines lying in the rostral aspect of the jaws, while posterior teeth are the premolars and molars positioned caudally.

Lateral and medial are inaccurate names for the outer and inner surfaces of the teeth in the

21

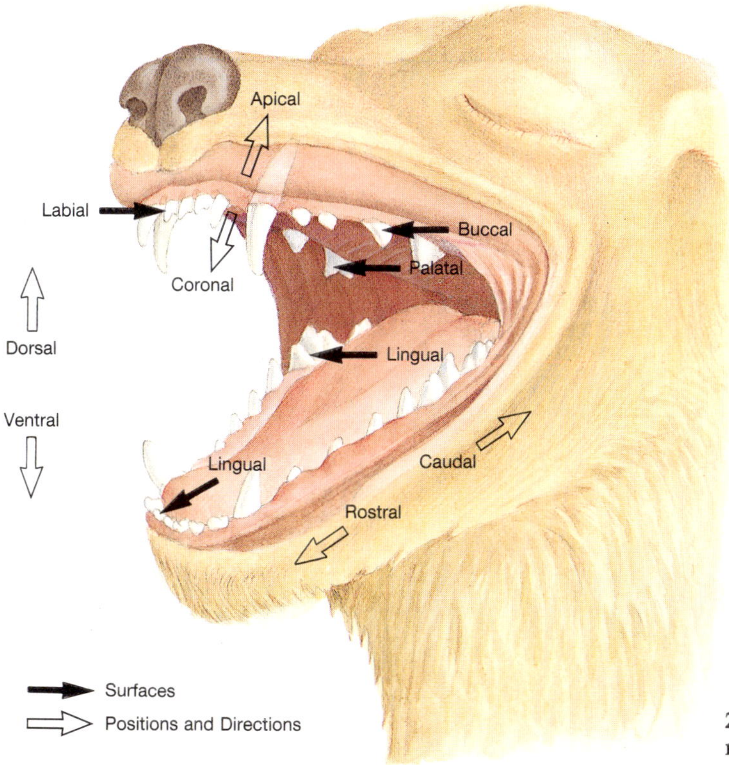

21 Illustration of general oral nomenclature.

22

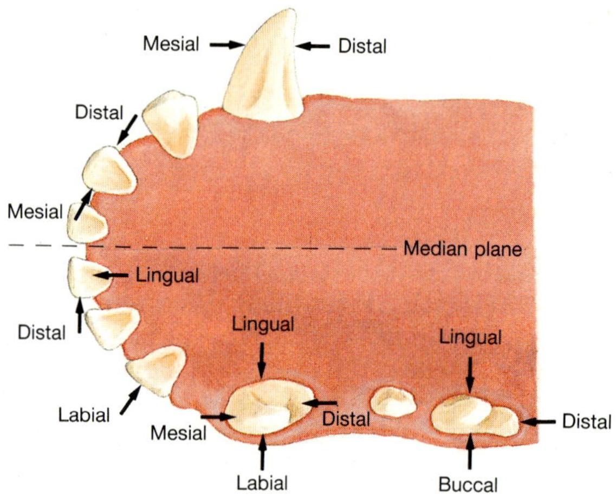

22 Illustration of dental surfaces.

curved or angular dental arches. *Labial* is the term used for the outer surface of the anterior teeth and associated tissues facing the labialis (lip) muscles, while *buccal* is the equivalent for the posterior teeth that face the plane of the buccinator (cheek) muscles. *Palatal* and *lingual* are surfaces of the teeth and associated tissues that face the roof of the mouth in the upper jaw and the tongue in the lower jaw, respectively.

Apical and *coronal* are terms for a direction towards or a relationship to the root extremities and crowns of the teeth, respectively. For such situations ventral and dorsal, or inferior and superior, are unsatisfactory expressions as teeth are reversed in their orientation in opposing dental arches.

The term *deciduous* is ambiguous; the more accurate term *primary* will be used when discussing the first set of teeth among the diphyodonts. In dentistry the first set of posterior teeth are regarded as *molars* because their root and occlusal morphology are more similar to that of permanent molars than premolars. The permanent premolars do not have precursors, and in this atlas the primary posterior teeth of all diphyodonts are termed *primary molars.*

The terms medial, central and lateral for incisors are not used in this atlas as it is confusing with species that have more than two incisors per quadrant. The terms first, second and third are used.

Some veterinarians name the major parts of the mandible the horizontal and vertical ramus. These are not accurate terms. The word *ramus* means part of an organ that branches from another part. The correct terms are the *body of the mandible* — the main component of the mandible which accommodates alveolar processes and the teeth — and the *ramus of the mandible* — the part that lies caudal to the alveolar processes where it dorsally forms the coronoid process and the condyle of the mandible.

The author has introduced some new terms in this atlas and has modified others that have been in general use since the 19th century but which he considers misleading or inaccurate. The rationale for these changes is discussed where the terms appear in the text. A list of these words is given in **Table 1.**

Table 1. Use of new terminology in this atlas

New	*Old*
Elodont	Continuously growing teeth
Anelodont	Teeth with a limited period of growth
Dental anatomy	
Constricted apex	Closed apex
Dilated apex	Open apex
Endodontics	
Partial coronal pulpectomy	Pulpotomy
Total coronal pulpectomy	Pulpotomy

Systems of dental notation

To date a universal dental notation system, one where individual teeth could be identified and recorded in clinical files, for any dentition, in a simple form of dental shorthand, has been lacking. The present systems have been developed with the dental formula of a single mammalian primate family, the *Hominidae* (man), in mind.

Palmer's dental notation

Palmer's dental notation, the oldest system of tooth designation, utilises grid symbols to indicate the dental quadrants of the maxilla and mandible. The quadrant symbols represent a view as if looking at the patient's mouth from the front. In this system

┼

indicates the four quadrants of the mouth. The vertical line of the symbol represents the midline of the dental arch, while the horizontal line depicts the occlusal plane. In the human dentition the permanent teeth are numbered from 1, which indicates each first incisor, to 8, the notation for the third molars in all quadrants, while the primary teeth have capital letter designations from A to E in each quadrant. In this system, for example

⌊6

indicates the upper left first permanent molar;

53⌉

is the notation for the permanent lower right canine and second premolar in the same quadrant.

International two-digit system

In 1971 the international two-digit system was adopted by the FDI (Fédération Dentaire Internationale), dispensing with the grid notation as with the increased use of computerisation quadrant symbols became impractical. In this system the first digit indicates a quadrant, from 1 to 4 in a clockwise sequence, starting at the patient's upper right for the permanent dentition:

1	2
4	3

The second digit indicates a specific tooth in the permanent dentition from 1 to 8, as in Palmer's notation. In an effort to keep the system strictly numeric, it is somewhat clumsy in the recording of the primary dentition. In this system, for example, 12 indicates the permanent upper right second incisor while 44 denotes the permanent lower right first premolar.

Universal dental notation system

The animal kingdom exhibits a great variety in the arrangement of its dentition and a two-digit system would be impractical when working with different types of animals. A combined alphanumeric system is ideal for universal veterinary use and can be easily utilised in a computerised environment. The author has taken the opportunity to devise and introduce in this atlas the following system of dental notation which is logical and simple to use with all species.

Quadrants

In this system the numeric designation of the quadrants, as in the two-digit system, is retained. A hyphen (-) is used to separate this symbol from the tooth notation and a solidus or forward slash (/) indicates a division between quadrants of the same mouth.

Tooth types

Because of the great variation in numbers and arrangement of the teeth of different animals, the tooth groups (incisors, canines, premolars and molars) need to be indicated (see also Chapter 4).

The different types of permanent teeth are indicated with upper case letters: I = incisors, C = canines, P = premolars and M = molars. The primary groups of teeth are written in lower case letters: i = incisors, c = canines, and m = molars.

Specific teeth

Within each tooth group, individual teeth are identified numerically, number 1 being the most mesial tooth in the series. In practice, the upper left permanent canine is indicated as 2-C. The upper left permanent first premolar and first and second molars, and the lower right first permanent premolar in the same mouth, are noted as: 2-P1, M1,2 / 4-P1.

Homodont dentitions

Within the homodont dentitions the quadrants are identified numerically as above, but of course no tooth type is noted. For example, upper right eight, 14 and 16 would be written as: 1-8, 14, 16.

Illustrations

The system adopted in this atlas to identify each picture is:
Figure number — Summary — Case number and letter to identify place in sequence — Species.
Example: **682 Intra-oral view of infection — Case 1b — Bennett's Wallaby.**

Summary

This is a brief summary of the condition or treatment.

Case numbers

Case numbers are only used where more than one illustration is used per animal. The position of each photograph in the sequence is denoted using a lower case letter after the case number. Case numbers start at No. 1 in each chapter, or section of animal family in Chapter 14.

Species

Photographs are of domestic dogs unless otherwise stated in brief caption, title of chapter (e.g. equine); sub-section of a chapter (e.g. feline periodontal disease); or sub-heading of family in Chapter 14. In a sequence where case numbers are used, the name of the species is only given for the first picture of the sequence.

Convention for radiographs

- Lateral radiographs — nose faces to the left of the page.
- Dorsoventral and ventrodorsal radiographs — nose faces towards top of page unless otherwise stated.

Clinical photographs associated with the radiographs are orientated in the same direction. All other photographs are reproduced facing the direction they were clinically.

Convention for tooth sections

Histological sections are positioned so apices are towards the bottom of the page.

3 Dental Anatomy

To describe the basic dental anatomy, the carnivore/omnivore dentition is used as a model. Throughout the book, variations in the dental anatomy of other types of teeth are described.

The anatomy of the tooth

In **23** the cross-section of a dog's canine tooth is shown. Enamel is the outer cover of the crown of the tooth. It is the hardest substance in the body and has approximately 2% organic content and no innervation. Dentine constitutes the bulk of the tooth. It has approximately 30% organic content and the dentinal tubules, which pass to the pulp cavity, have a form of innervation. The dental pulp occupies the cavity at the centre of the tooth. The hollow that is situated in the crown of the tooth is termed the pulp chamber, and the channel in the root portion, the root canal. The pulp itself consists of a collection of nerve fibres, blood vessels and connective tissue. Cementum, which is histologically very similar to bone, is bonded to the dentine surfaces of the roots. The teeth are supported by alveolar bone, which consists of cortical plates, a compact lining to the sockets termed the lamina dura, and trabeculated cancellous and bundle bone.

The teeth are attached to the alveolar bone of the sockets by the periodontal ligament, comprising collagenous and elastic fibres which act as a form of retention for the teeth. The cementum layer of the teeth and the lamina dura of the alveolus are penetrated by 'Sharpey's fibres' of the periodontal ligaments. The width of the periodontal space and the strength of attachment of the ligament is dependent on the functional aspect of the teeth. For example, the periodontal ligament of a carnivore is much tighter than that associated with an elephant's tusk or a rabbit's incisor.

It is often claimed that the periodontal ligament is the cushioning mechanism of the teeth. Strong evidence has been put forward that the plexus of vessels of the periodontal ligament

23

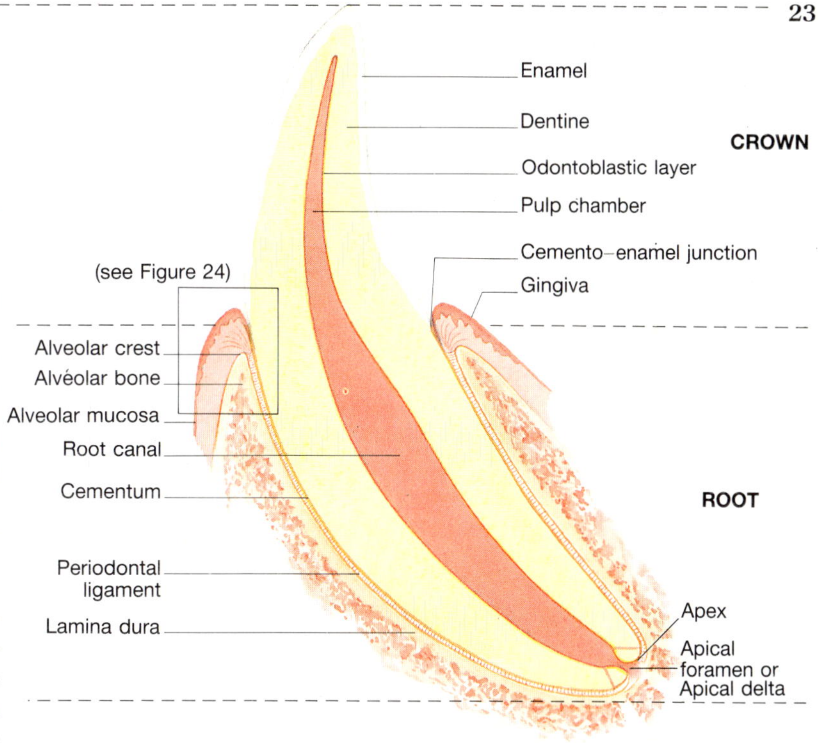

23 Cross-section of a dog's lower canine.

24

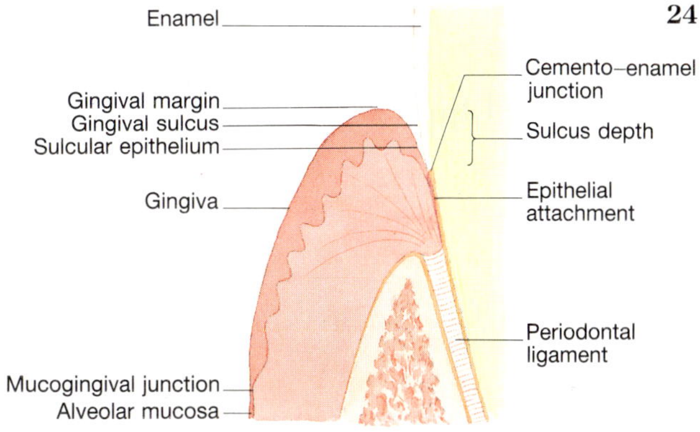

24 Detailed periodontal anatomy.

25

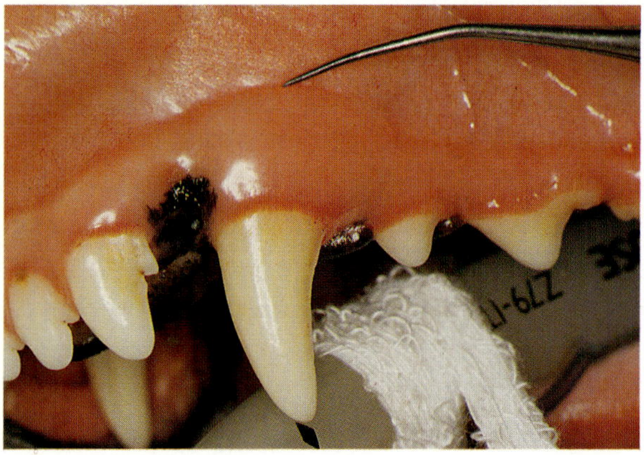

25 The mucogingival junction is a line of demarcation between the keratinised gingiva and the non-keratinised alveolar mucosa.

in conjunction with the vascular reservoir in the alveolar bone create a very important haemodynamic damping system, which acts as a hydraulic pressure loading and support mechanism against functional forces acting on the teeth.

Detailed gingival anatomy is shown in **24**. The alveolar bone is invested with a mucous membrane, which acts as a defensive barrier to the periodontal apparatus and the bone. The keratinised tissue, which is firmly bound to the extra-alveolar cementum of the teeth and the alveolar bone is termed the gingiva. The coronal border of the gingiva is not attached to the tooth but forms the wall to the gingival sulcus, its most coronal point being the gingival margin. The lining of the sulcus is called the sulcular epithelium and it is fused at its apical point to the tooth by the epithelial attachment. This interface between gingiva and tooth may be on enamel, cementum or both, depending on the level of gingival recession or tooth eruption.

Formerly the term 'free' gingiva was used to describe the unattached coronal aspect of the marginal gingiva, while the band of tissue apical to it was termed the 'attached' gingivae. The 1977 International Conference on Research in the Biology of Periodontal Disease recommended dispensing with the terms 'free' and 'attached' as in a healthy periodontal condition there is negligible sulcular depth.

A definite change is visible labially, buccally and lingually at the mucogingival junction **(25)**, where the gingiva stops and the non-keratinised, loosely attached alveolar mucosa commenses. The alveolar mucosa is well vascularised, while the gingiva derives its blood supply primarily through its periosteum. The mucosa of the hard palate resembles gingival tissue. It is keratinised and remains firmly bound to the maxilla to resist trauma from the passage of food.

The apical foramen is the aperture through which the vascular supply and innervation to the pulp enters the root canal. The different types of apical foramina are depicted in **26**. Root apices are often classified as 'open' or 'closed' because on radiographs the dilated foramina are self-evident as opposed to the constricted form of apical anatomy where the detail of the apertures cannot always be seen. These terms are anatomically incorrect as healthy teeth retain a vascular supply to their pulp tissues throughout life and the apical communication to the root canals does not become occluded. Elodont teeth grow throughout life and maintain a dilated apical foramen, while the apical foramina of anelodont teeth become constricted once the teeth are fully mature. Many anelodonts, especially the carnivores, do not have a single apical foramen per root but a complex delta formation at the root apex.

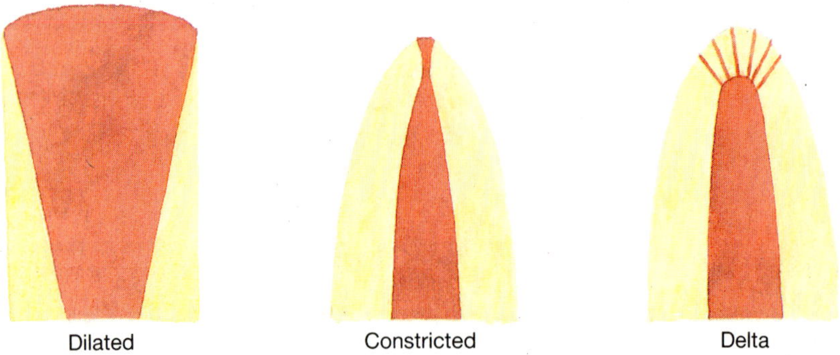

26 Types of apical foramina: dilated, constricted and delta.

Development of a brachyodont dentition

The layer of cells surrounding the outer surface of the dental pulp inside the pulp cavity are termed odontoblasts; they fulfil the pulp's primary function, which is the development of the tooth. The secondary role of the pulp is protective, through the deposition of secondary dentine if it receives chronic, low-grade external stimuli, as in the cases of attrition and abrasion.

The development of the permanent dentition is well illustrated by radiographs of dogs' hemimandibles. At the age of three months **(27)**, the unerupted tooth buds are seen in their crypts. The teeth rapidly develop in the following three months. By the age of six months **(28)**, the roots are developed to their full lengths, although the walls of the crowns and, especially, the roots are very thin. The volume of the pulp chambers and root canals are large and the apical foramen of the lower canine is still dilated. By the age of two years **(29)**, secondary dentine has been deposited to the extent that only relatively narrow root canals remain, the size of the pulp chambers has been reduced and the apical foramina are constricted or a delta formation is present.

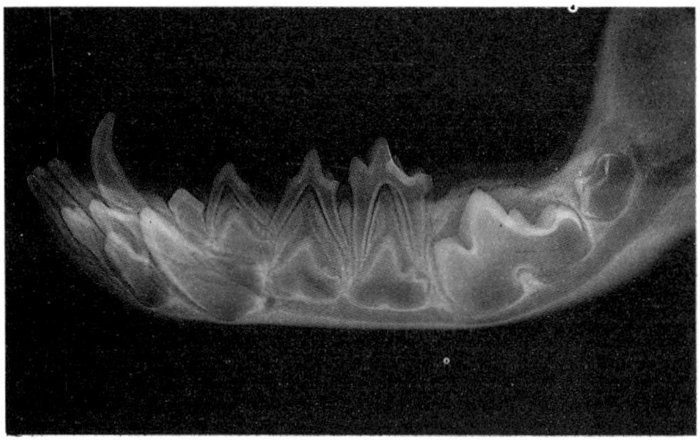

27

27 Radiograph (× *0.8*) **of a three-month-old dog's hemimandible with primary teeth present and permanent tooth buds developing in their crypts.**

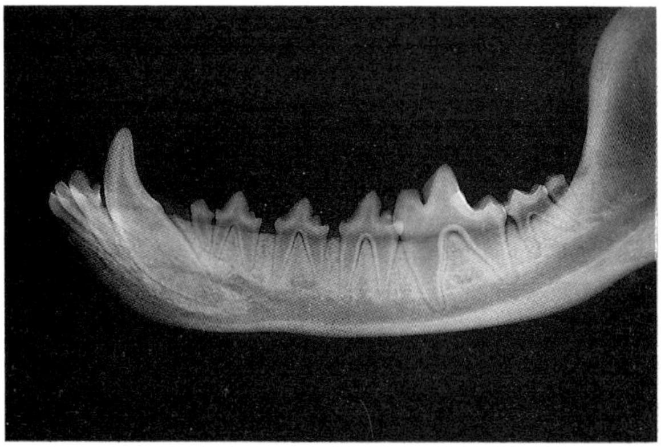

28

28 Radiograph (× *0.7*) **of a six-month-old dog's hemimandible illustrating the relatively large pulp chambers and root canals that are present in these immature permanent teeth.**

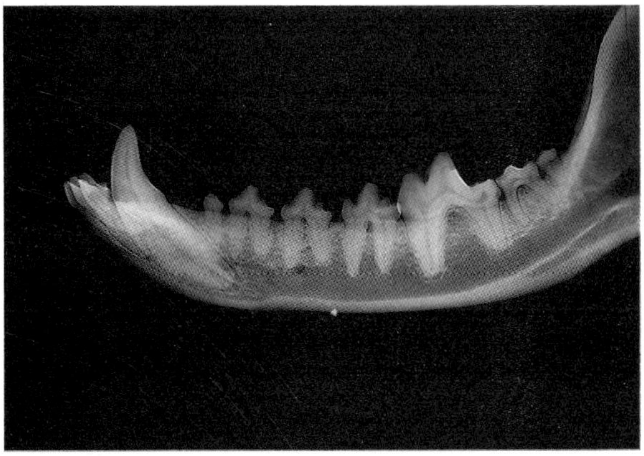

29

29 Radiograph (× *0.7*) **of a two-year-old dog's hemimandible shows how the volume of the pulp cavities has been reduced through the deposition of secondary dentine.**

4 Comparative Odontology

The term 'teeth' is applied to calcified structures that contain dentine. They are usually found in or at the mouth. The survival of a species can often be attributed to the adaptation of its dentition to the environment. In nature, animals with a damaged mouth or dentition are at a serious disadvantage, and are likely to succumb to premature death.

The function of the dental apparatus is varied throughout the animal kingdom. By and large the primary functions of the teeth are prehension and preparation of food for digestion. In some instances incision has replaced the function of prehension, as in the case of primates.

The next stage is the division of food, followed by mastication and insalivation, where the combined action of the dentition and oral musculature mixes the food with saliva, helping with digestion.

One of the most important secondary functions of the teeth is that of defence; in carnivores, teeth are also used as a killing apparatus. They can also serve in sexual dimorphism and mate selection. In some cases, as with tusks, which are modified incisors or canines, teeth are used as secondary prehensile instruments, or as tools of excavation. The canines of the walrus are also used as an aid in locomotion.

The incisor teeth of many animals are used for grooming. In the case of the lemur, comb-shaped lower incisors in conjunction with a specially modified tongue projection have been adapted for this purpose. The beaver's incisors are used as instruments of construction, while the 'fangs' of some snakes are used to inject venom.

In man, the anterior teeth play an important part in the action of phonation as well as having an important role in aesthetics and sexual attraction.

There are numerous possible dental classifications — the systems have varied according to classical taxonomy, mode of jaw movement, tooth anatomy, cusp morphology or mode of attachment to the jaws. Whatever classification is used it will inevitably be one of convenience or compromise.

The primary objective of this chapter is to describe and classify the different types of teeth. In the second half of this chapter the contrasting characteristics of the different dentitions are outlined following a unique practical approach, primarily on the basis of tooth physiology, function and anatomy. This format is relevant to dental development, eruption patterns and dental diseases, their consequences and possible treatment. When teeth from different classifications are present in the mouth of an animal, they are discussed under both groups of dentitions.

These classifications are not attempts to redefine the taxonomy tables but a practical and applied guide to the variety of dentitions encountered in the treatment of animals.

Nomenclature

The author believes it is vital, in a book that deals with the dental anatomy, diseases and treatment of a wide range of animals, to review critically the traditional terms and update them where desirable, for the benefit of the subject and its students. This is also necessary to ensure that veterinary and dental surgeons have a common ground from which the animal patients' dental care can begin.

The terminologies currently in use derive largely from Ancient Greek, incorporating some Latin. The inherent ambiguity of some of the original terms has contributed to the misuse and confusion that has occurred in understanding the different types of teeth.

Hypsodont and brachyodont were the two main classifications introduced by W.H. Flower in 1883 in the *Encyclopaedia Britannica*. As recently as 1990, these terms were being vaguely defined in an important dental text as 'high crowned' and 'short crowned' teeth.

The definition of continuously growing teeth has also created confusion. As late as 1952, references are made in textbooks to 'teeth with perpetual pulps', erroneously implying that all other types of mammalian teeth lose their pulp tissue with age. Other important modern works demonstrate a lack of understanding of the subject by using the term 'hypsodont' for both continuously growing teeth and teeth of a limited period of growth. One author uses 'continuously growing' and 'continuously erupting' to describe the same teeth.

Further disarray was created when attempts were made to introduce a concise name, such as *hypselodont,* for the continuously growing teeth. Additional difficulties were created as the etymological synonyms hypselodont and hypsodont were often confused.

Classification of teeth

When examining the variety of teeth present in the animal kingdom, it is clear that the logical division — on the grounds of anatomy and physiology — is between *continuously growing teeth* and *teeth that have a limited period of growth.* As indicated above, the nomenclature in this respect has been rather confused. In this atlas the author has taken the opportunity to introduce new scientific names which he has devised in order to replace clumsy and ambiguous phrases with concise and rational terms. The neologisms are compound words of Greek and Latin derivation.

Elodont teeth

New term. [from *elo-* (prefix) to increase in length (abbreviated from Latin: *elongare*) + *-odont* (suffix) type of tooth (from Greek: *odon, odous* tooth)]

An *elodont* is a type of tooth that grows throughout life on its pulpal axis (height or length) and never develops anatomical roots. The apical foramina of these teeth remain dilated throughout life (**30**). Their lengths increase at their apices, but the position of the apices remains stationary in the alveolus. As these teeth increase in length, the occlusal/incisal surfaces extrude intra-orally, but their total length is maintained constant through masticatory attrition at those surfaces. Extra-orally positioned teeth, such as the tusks of elephants, the canines of wild boar and hippopotami, are exceptions and any wear is through abrasion on non-dental structures. The exposure of the pulp through continuous coronal wear is prevented by the deposition of secondary dentine at the coronal extremity of the pulp chambers. The unique characteristic of elodont teeth is the parallel or divergent walls of the pulp cavities and the lifelong dilated apical foramina; by comparison, in anelodont teeth (see below) the root canals progressively narrow and the apical foramina become constricted with age. The shape of the elodont pulp cavities facilitates a rich blood supply to the pulp tissue, and a high activity within the odontoblastic layer sustains continuous apical growth and often allows for repair to take place on exposure of the pulp chambers. At the same time, any damage to the integrity of the dental arches can rapidly become life-threatening, as the intra-oral teeth in the group rely on continuous wear through accurate articulation and constant attrition against their opposite numbers: otherwise, rapid overgrowth occurs. The sharp, chisel-shaped incisor edges are maintained through a slower rate of wear labially. This occurs either by enamel being only present labially, or being thicker on that surface.

30

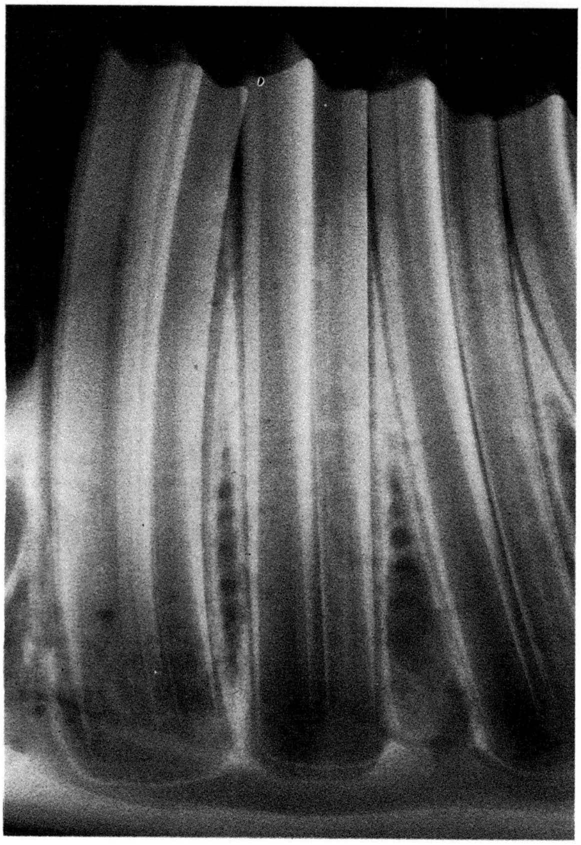

30 Radiograph (*×6.3*) of an elodont premolar illustrates the permanently dilated apical foramina.

Anelodont teeth

New term. [from Greek: *an-* (prefix) not + *elo-* (prefix) to increase in length (abbreviated from Latin: *elongare*) + *-odont* (suffix) type of tooth (from Greek: *odon, odous* tooth)]

31

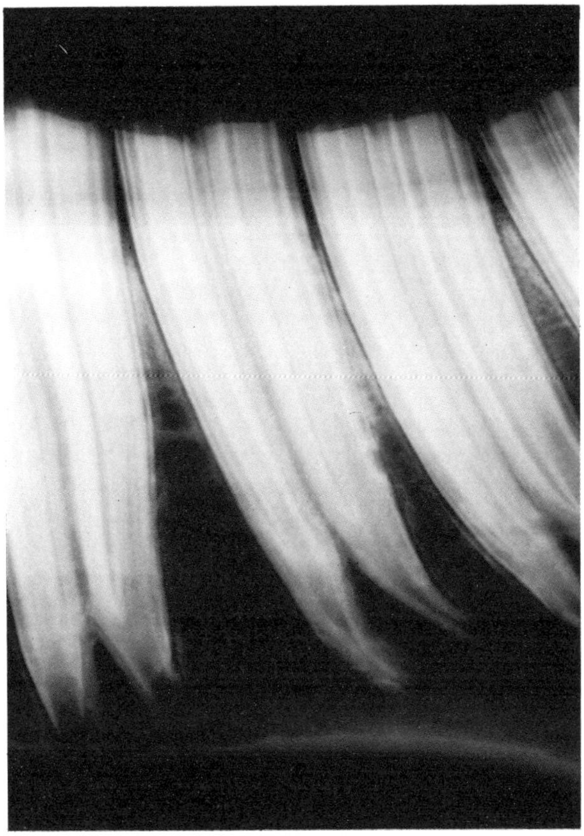

32

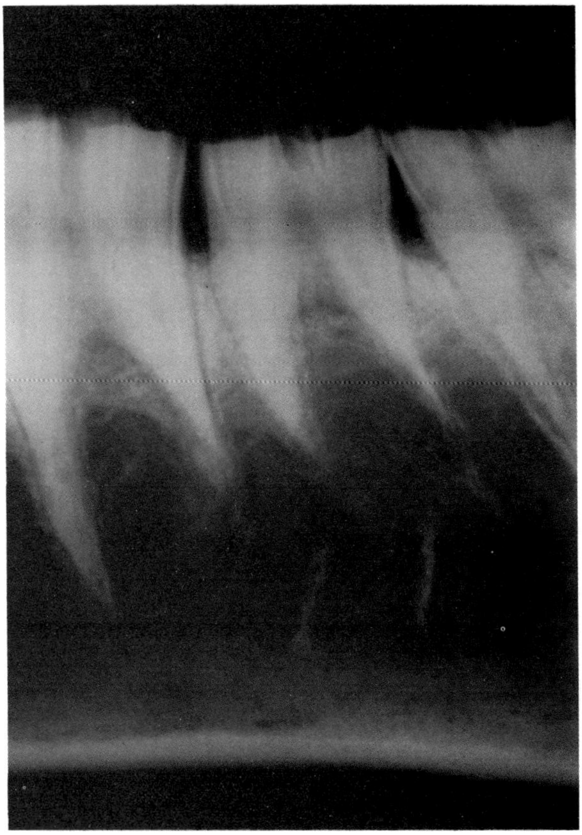

31 Radiograph *(× 1.2)* **of a hypsodont molar at a moderate stage of apical development and minimal coronal wear.** Note the constricted apical pattern and also the long reserve crown in comparison to the short roots.

32 Radiograph *(× 1.2)* **of a hypsodont molar of an old animal where coronal wear, normal for such an age, has resulted in a short anatomical crown that is similar in length to that of the roots.**

An *anelodont* is a type of tooth that has a limited period of growth. A definite demarcation exists between the anatomical crowns and roots of such teeth. The apical foramina of the root canals become constricted once the teeth have completed their longitudinal development.

The group can be subdivided into the hypsodont and brachyodont teeth, terms that imply long and short teeth, respectively, but it is the crown/root ratio that is the most important and relevant feature, not the physical size of the crowns.

Hypsodont teeth

A hypsodont tooth has a long anatomical crown when fully mature which has been subjected to minimal occlusal attrition. Much of this crown is held in reserve subgingivally in the alveolar bone. In comparison with the length of the crown, the root is relatively short. Depending on the tooth in question, the root apices complete their development at different stages of life. Some of the 'cheek teeth' continue apical development and progressive constriction of the apical foramina into early middle age. Once fully formed, no further longitudinal growth takes place at the root apices. These teeth erupt throughout the life of the animal as occlusal wear takes place; so, in youth, there is a considerable length of reserve anatomical crown in the alveolar bone (**31**).

It is important to note that the hypsodont teeth are quite different from the continuously growing elodont teeth. As occlusal wear takes place, eruption of the teeth into persistent occlusion and function causes the reserve crown length in the alveolar bone to decrease. The clinical crown height of the cheek teeth, the part of the tooth which is visible in the mouth, and the anatomical root length remain the same from the time of tooth maturity, but the position of the root apex migrates coronally as the height of the anatomical, i.e. reserve, crown decreases. By having a length of reserve crown in the alveolar bone that erupts continuously until the crown's length is exhausted hypsodonts are able to maintain a functional dental apparatus well into old age (**32**).

Because of the dependence on accurate articulation of the teeth, which is responsible for even wear, any disturbance to the integrity of the dental arches as a result of trauma, malocclusion or tooth loss can have serious repercussions in the form of tooth drifting, food packing, irregular tooth wear or pathological overeruption. The threat to life, however, is usually not as acute as it would be among the continuously growing elodont teeth. It is important to note that the apical foramina of these teeth are constricted once fully mature, not dilated as they would be in the elodont teeth. Therefore they do not possess the healing potential of the pulp that those teeth exhibit.

Brachyodont teeth

Brachyodont teeth are defined as those where, at tooth maturity, the lengths of the roots are longer than the anatomical crowns (canid (**33**)). The teeth remain relatively stationary in the alveolus, the root apices usually reach maturity at a earlier age than the hypsodonts and the apical foramina of the root canals become constricted at that time.

33

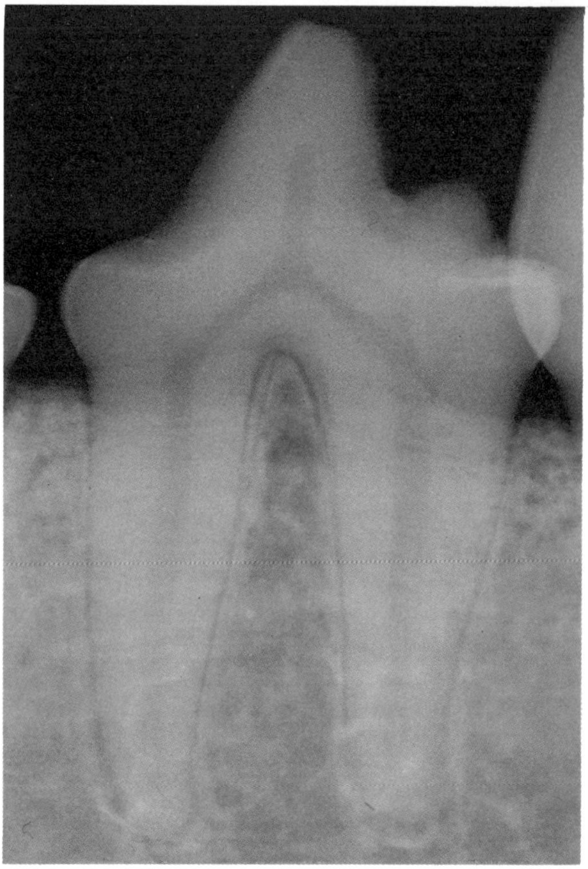

33 Radiograph *(×5.5)* **of a typical brachyodont posterior tooth demonstrating the root lengths, which are longer than the crown height dimension.**

Classification of dentitions

The major division of the dentitions is between the homodonts and the heteredonts (**Scheme 1**). The homodonts have the most primitive type of teeth. They are uniform in shape throughout the mouth, whereas the heterodonts contain teeth of different forms and function. All homodonts are anelodonts.

Homodonts

The homodont group can be further divided into subgroups:

- Monophyodonts. These have a single set of teeth, and include the toothed cetaceans (Odontoceti — dolphins and killer whales). The crowns of the teeth are covered with enamel and have a pulp chamber that becomes filled with secondary dentine with age.
- Polyphyodonts. These have an endless succession of teeth. Their lifestyle is usually so violent that tooth loss is common. Polyphyodont teeth are usually classified according to type and position of attachment (pleurodont, acrodont and thecodont — for definitions see the Glossary). For clinical purposes the group may be further subdivided into:

  (a) Those where teeth are replaced vertically, through the sockets of the lost teeth (e.g. in *Crocodilia* (**34**), the developing teeth are visible on the radiograph in the pulp chambers of the teeth in function). The thecodont teeth are attached through gomphosis; that is, held in the alveolus by a root and socket formation.

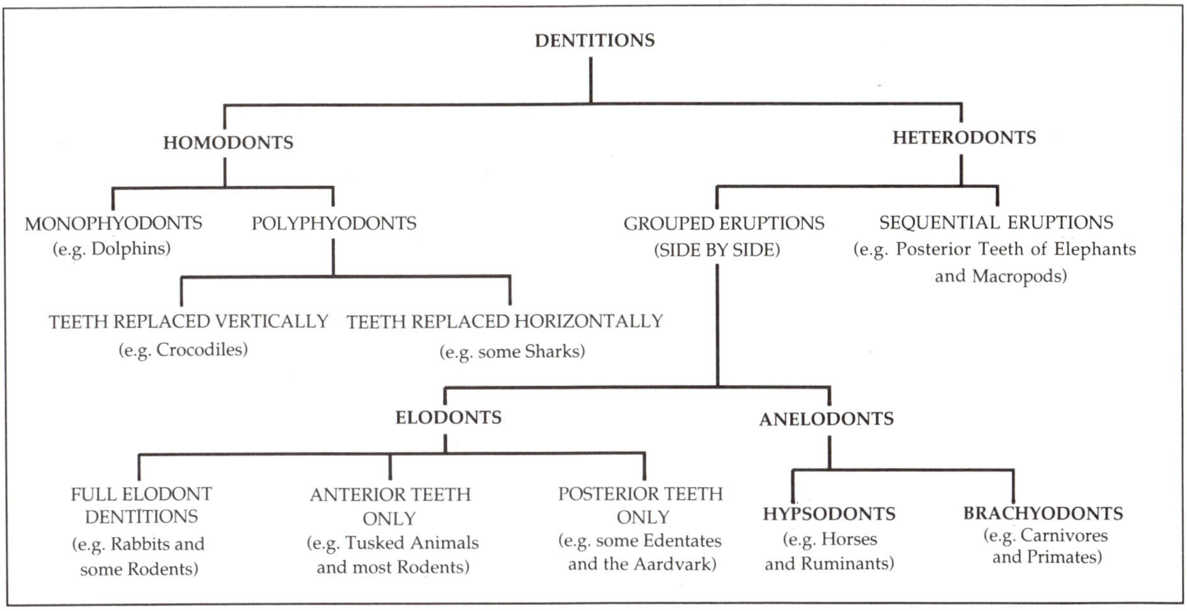

Scheme 1

34

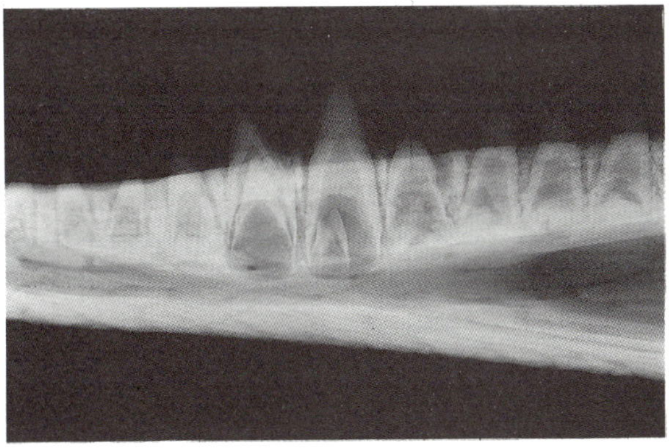

35

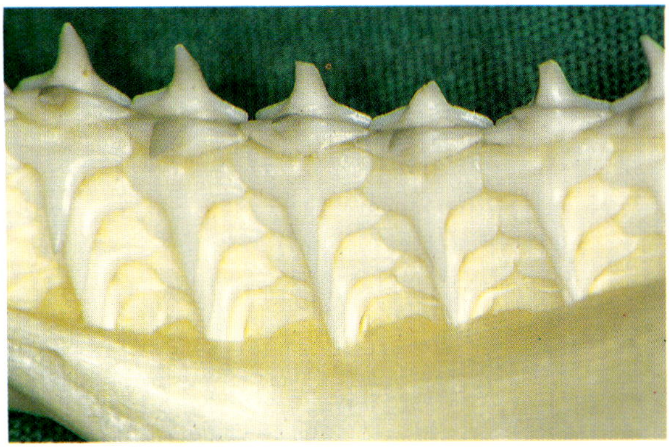

34 Radiograph (*×1*) of a crocodile's hemimandible showing the next set of teeth developing in the pulp cavities of these polyphyodont teeth.

35 In polyphyodont sharks, teeth are replaced horizontally from a caudal direction (*×1.5*).

(b) Those where lost teeth are replaced horizontally, from a caudal direction (e.g. in the predatory sharks (**35**) — the teeth are attached through a fibrous attachment directly to the mucous membrane that covers the surface of the cartilaginous jaws), while in pleurodont *reptilia* (e.g. lizards) the teeth are anchylosed to the jaws.

Heterodonts

Heterodonts can be classified into two main groups according to the way the posterior teeth erupt:

- Dentitions where the posterior teeth erupt in a grouped (side by side), vertical direction.
- Dentitions where the posterior teeth erupt in a sequential, horizontal direction.

Dentitions erupting in a grouped, vertical direction

Dentitions in this group may be divided into:

- Elodonts — some or all of the teeth are continuously growing.
- Anelodonts — none of the teeth grow continuously.

36

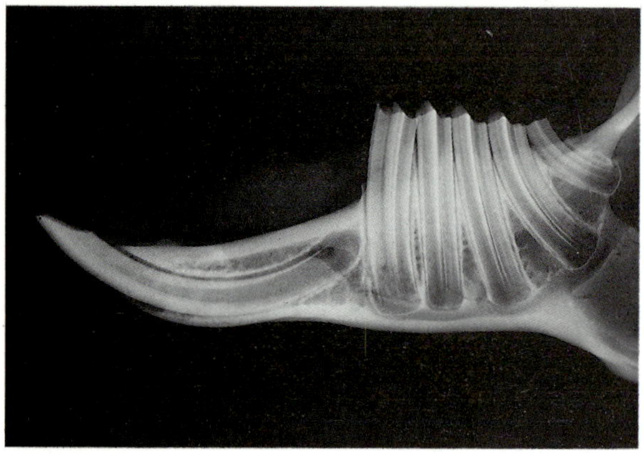

36 Radiograph *(× 1.5)* **of a lagomorph's hemi-mandible reveals dilated apical foramina of both the elodont incisor and cheek teeth.**

37

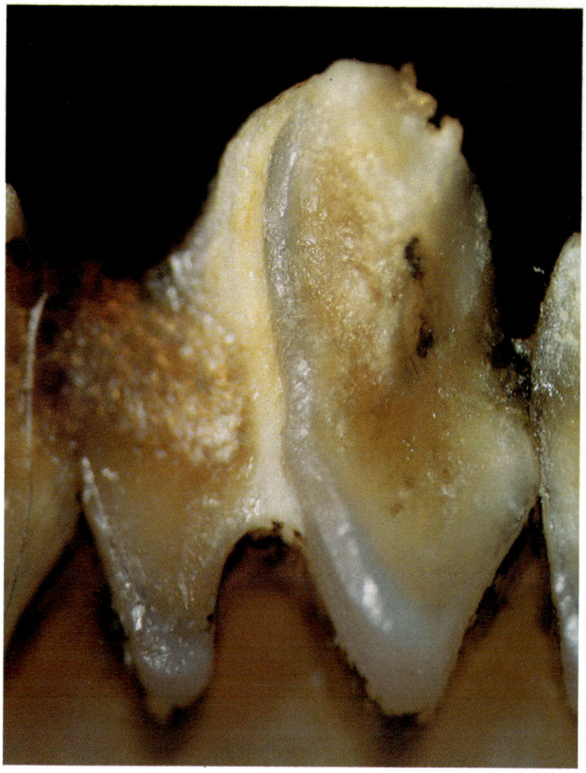

37 The enamel pattern *(× 24)* **on the occlusal surface of a lagomorph's molar is suited to continuous wear.**

Elodonts

Dentitions that contain elodont teeth are mono- or diphyodonts. For practical purposes the group may be subdivided according to the location of these teeth in the mouth.

(a) *Anterior and posterior teeth continue to grow throughout the life of the animal.* To this group belong the lagomorphs (e.g. hares, rabbits (**36**)) ; some rodents (e.g. guinea pig and chinchilla); and the wombat, which is the sole representative of marsupials in this group. The occlusal surfaces are not fully covered with enamel, an efficient grinding surface to the cheek teeth throughout life being maintained by vertical layers of enamel and dentine, which have different rates of wear, e.g. rabbit (**37**).

(b) *Only the anterior teeth are continuously growing.* This group includes most rodents that are omnivorous in their diet, e.g. rats (**38**), mice and squirrels; the tusks of elephants; hogs; the canines and incisors of the hippopotamus; and the upper incisors of the hyrax family. The posterior teeth are often brachyodonts. It is often stated that the vicuña's incisors are rodent-like and permanently growing. The author believes this to be incorrect. The vicuña has enamel only on the labial surfaces of its incisors, which encourages a chisel-shaped incisor edge to be created. These teeth have an exaggerated time of root development and the apical foramina are dilated until an advanced age. This way, lost tooth substance through incisal abrasion in a harsh dietary environment is compensated for through apical growth. There is histological evidence that the apical foramina become constricted, as in other hypsodont teeth, but at an even later stage in life. At that stage, amelo- and dentinogenesis ceases and eruption continues to compensate for coronal abrasion. Eventually, the teeth may exfoliate through lack of root support.

(c) *Only the posterior teeth are continuously growing.* To this group belong some of the edentates and the aardvark (**39**), which is the sole member of the order *Tubulidentata*. The aardvark was removed from the *Edentata* when that order was revised. Although the word 'edentate' implies no teeth, the *Edentata* contains not only species with no teeth but ones with a highly reduced dentition. One early criterion for inclusion, the absence of incisors in the premaxillary bone, was changed to the acceptance that no incisors or canines in both arches qualified an animal for the order. The order was re-classified into three families: the armadillos, the sloths; and the truly edentulous American anteaters.

Aardvarks are diphyodonts, although the primary dentition is rudimentary. The order *Tubulidentata* is so termed because of the structure of the teeth. The pulp chambers are narrow channels (**40**) at the centres of vertical prisms of osteodentine, which makes up most of

38

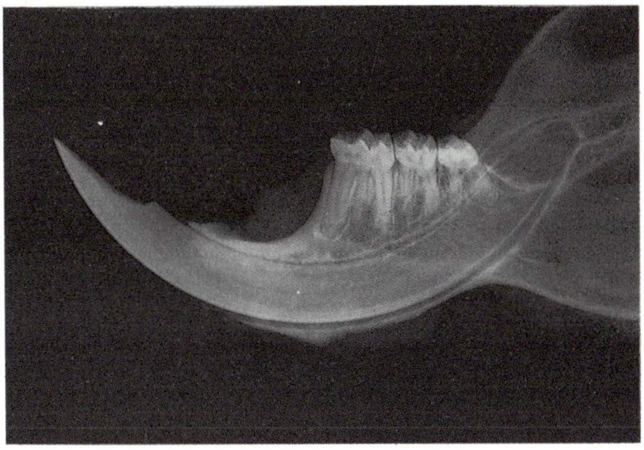

38 **Radiograph** *(×2.7)* **of a rat's hemimandible illustrates the elodont incisor and the brachyodont cheek teeth.**

39

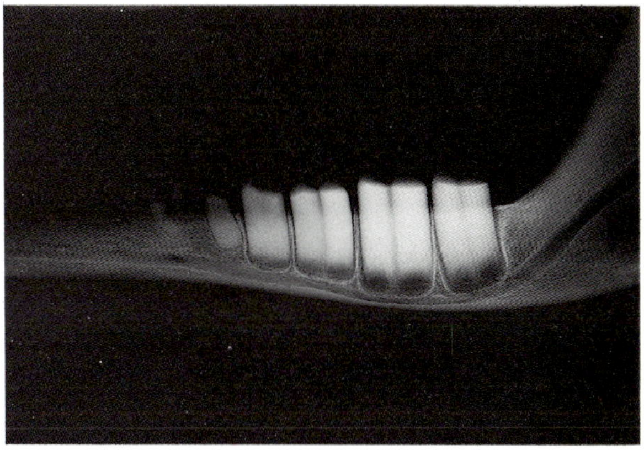

39 **Radiograph** *(×0.8)* **of an aardvark's hemimandible shows the elodont cheek teeth.**

the tooth structure (enamel being absent). The dental formula for this animal is unclear, but up to seven posterior teeth may exist per quadrant of the permanent dentition. The teeth are simple, columnar, structures, but their sizes vary in the dental arches. There is a groove at the mid-point of the buccal and lingual surfaces of the molars (**41**), forming a bicolumnar structure, hence the classification as a heterodont.

Anelodonts

The anelodont group is subdivided into hypsodonts and brachyodonts. They are both diphyodonts, having a primary and a permanent set of teeth.

Hypsodonts are usually grazing/browsing ungulates whose anatomical crowns shorten through occlusal attrition with age. The crown/root ratio varies according to family. The *Equidae* have long reserve crowns when young which shorten with age through attrition (horse — seven years old (**42**), 15 years old (**43**) and 22 years old (**44**)), while the *Bovidae* and *Camelidae* (Bactrian camel — five years old (**45**)) have relatively shorter crowns in relation to their root lengths.

The occlusal surfaces are rough, for breaking up the vegetable diet, and are not completely covered with enamel. The desired surface is achieved either by having a convoluted occlusal pattern or ridges of enamel, cementum and dentine, which wear at different rates and maintain the surface texture (lower molar of a horse (**46**)), or by having infundibuli in the occlusal anatomy (upper molar of a horse (**47**)) and/or multi-lobed selenodont molars of the

40

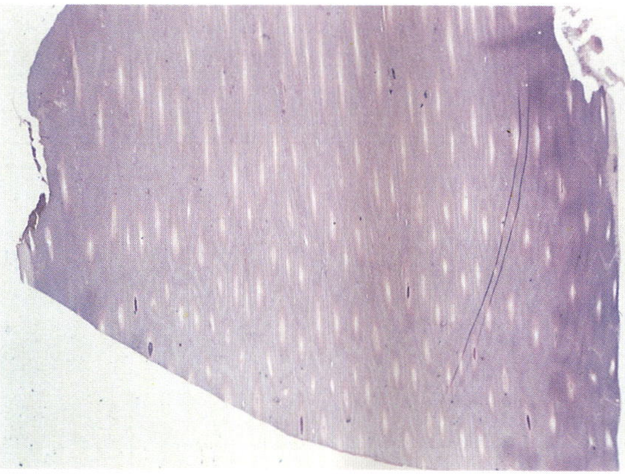

40 **Oblique longitudinal section of an aardvark's molar reveals the multiple pulpal tubuli** *(×8)*.

41

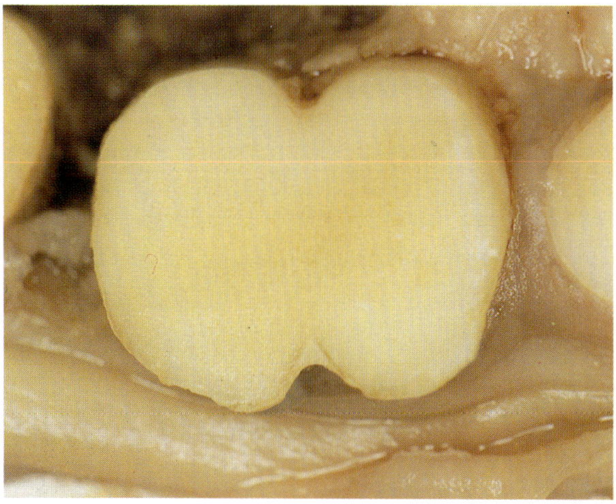

41 **The occlusal view** *(×3.9)* **of an aardvark's molar demonstrates its bicolumnar morphology.**

42

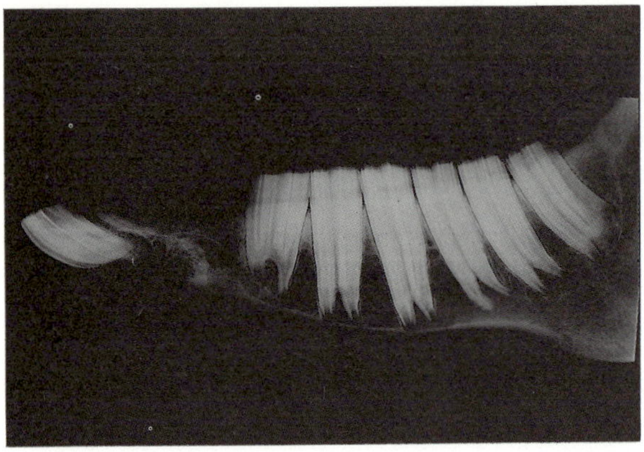

42 Radiograph ***(× 0.24)*** **of a seven-year-old horse's hemimandible illustrates the long reserve crowns of the hypsodont teeth and the proximity of the root apices to the ventral border of the mandible.**

43

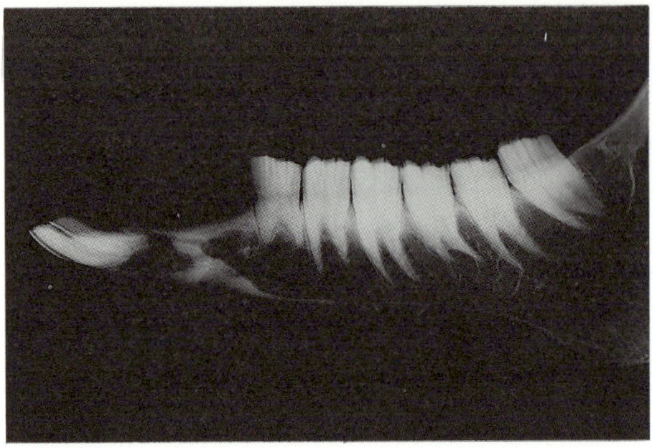

43 At 15 years of age, root maturity has been completed in the horse ***(× 0.25)*****.** Reduction of the reserve crown height has taken place and tooth eruption has compensated for the wear.

44

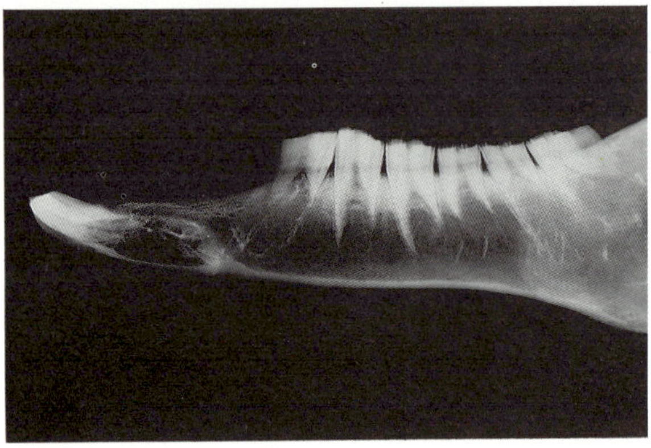

44 Radiograph ***(× 0.25)*** **of a 22-year-old horse's hemimandible illustrates the lack of reserve crown remaining in the alveolar bone due to the level of attrition present at this age.**

45

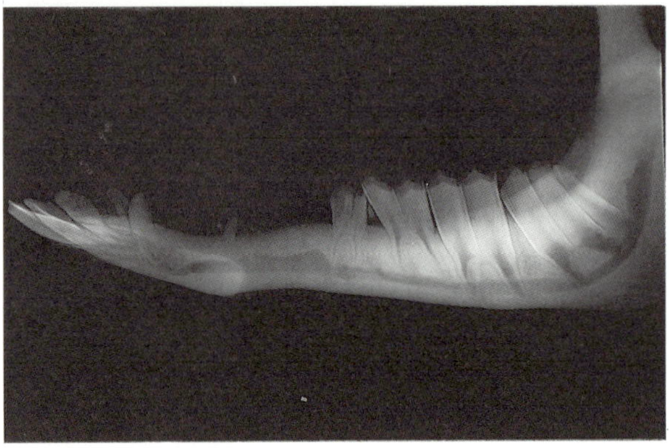

45 Radiograph ***(× 0.2)*** **of a five-year-old Bactrian camel's hemimandible demonstrates the less columnar shape of these hypsodont cheek teeth.**

46

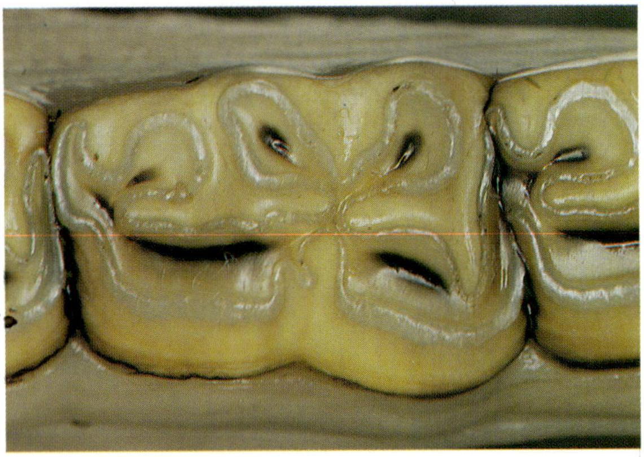

46 Occlusal view ***(× 2.2)*** **of a horse's lower molar.** A layer of cementum surrounds the convoluted ring of enamel that travels vertically through the crown of the tooth. The bulk of the tooth at the centre of the enamel ring is composed of dentine. Although some staining is present, the tooth lacks an infundibulum.

47 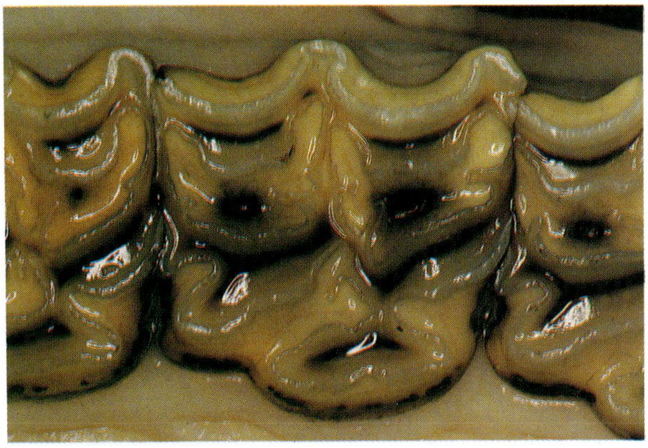

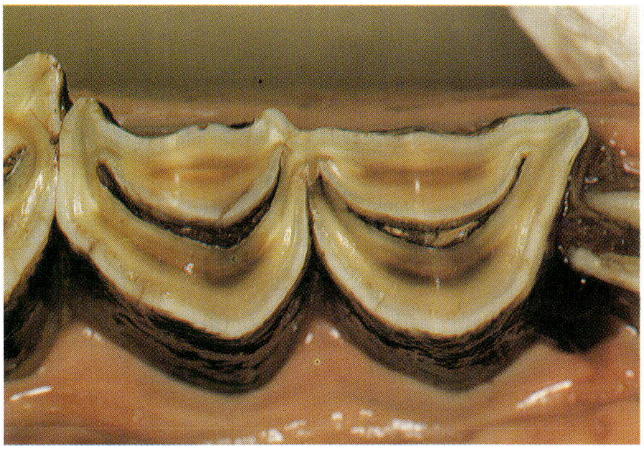 48

47 Occlusal view *(× 1.9)* **of a horse's upper molar.** These teeth differ from the lower cheek teeth as rings of enamel at the centre of the upper teeth produce two 'cement lakes', which are the infundibula lined with cementum. A developmental channel is present at the centre of each infundibulum.

48 Occlusal view *(× 1.3)* **of a multi-lobed selenodont molar of a camelid, with crescent-shaped infundibula.**

Camelidae, where the well-differentiated crescent-shaped cuspal pattern closely follows the well-differentiated root morphology (**48**).

Brachyodonts are usually omnivores, carnivores or non-grazing herbivores. The *Felidae*, *Canidae*, *Ursidae* and Primates are included in this group. The crowns of these teeth are fully covered with enamel. The dentition may be non-specialised, and have a flatter occlusal surface of the posterior teeth in some omnivores (bear (**49**); human (**50**, **51**); rat (**52**)) or have become progressively more specialised, as in true carnivores (cat (**53**, **54**)), which have sharp, blade-like secodont carnassial posterior teeth, for cutting up meat, and long well-retained roots in the alveolus. Compared with teeth of the other groups, brachyodont teeth suffer relatively little wear of their occlusal surfaces, although in omnivores the enamel cover is often lost through dietary attrition with age.

It is interesting to note that the more specialised the dentition becomes in respect of killing and processing the carcass, the less drifting and pathological over-eruption takes place if the integrity of the arch is violated. In omnivores a moderate degree of tooth displacement may occur, while in carnivores little or no change in the position of the remaining teeth takes place if the integrity of the dental arches is disrupted.

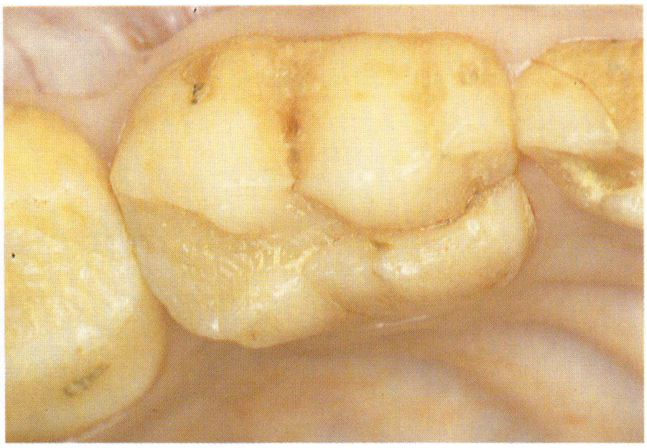 49

49 The molar of a bear has blunt, cone-shaped bunodont cusps on its occlusal surface *(× 1.6)*.

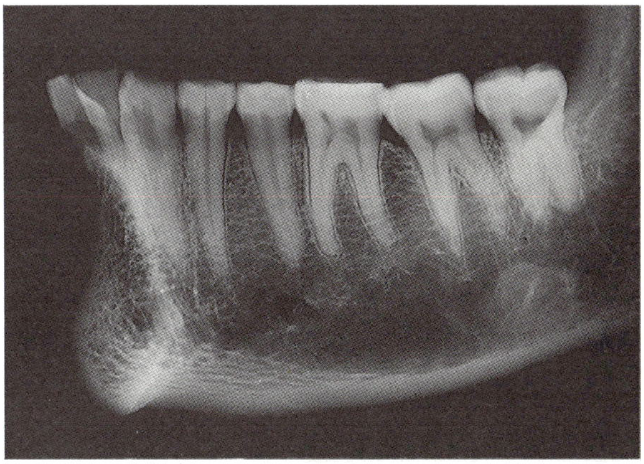 50

50 Radiograph *(× 1.1)* **of a human hemimandible illustrates the brachyodont pattern seen in omnivores' posterior teeth.**

51 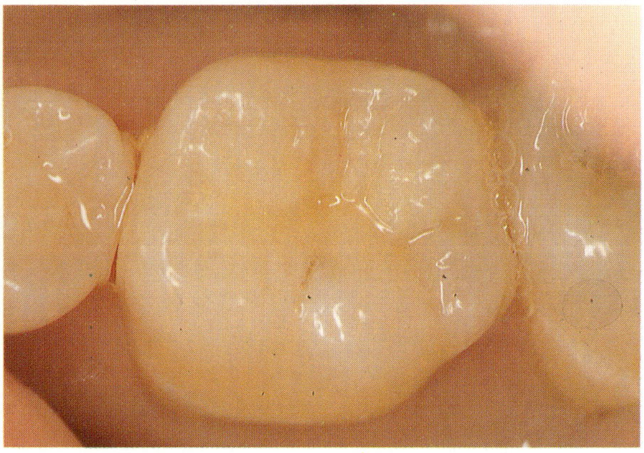

52 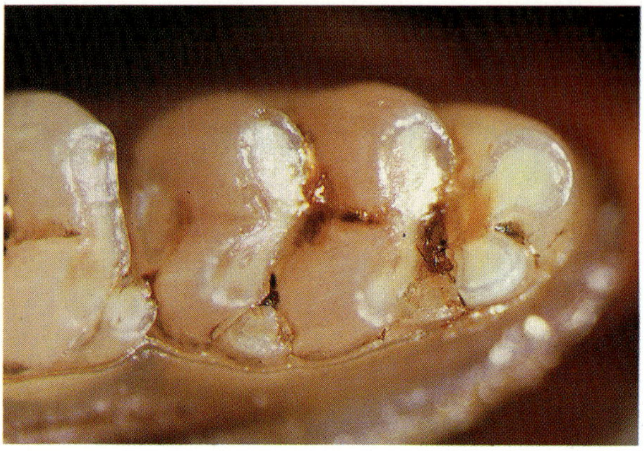

51 The occlusal surface of the human molar also demonstrates the relatively blunt cusps seen in omnivores (×*4.4*).

52 The occlusal view (× *26*) of a rat's brachyodont molar reveals lophodont ridges of its enamel-covered crown, which are showing signs of attrition.

53 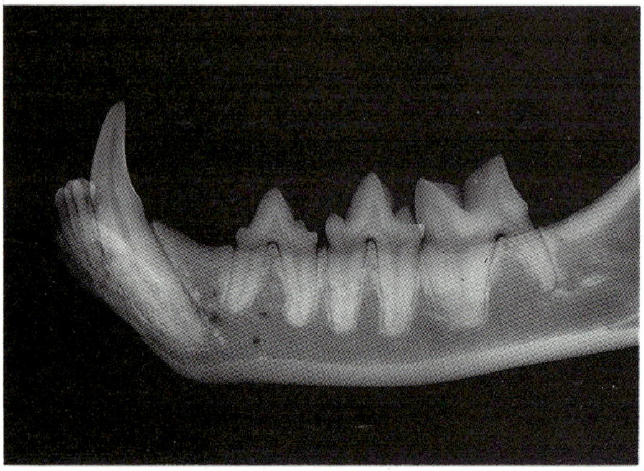

54 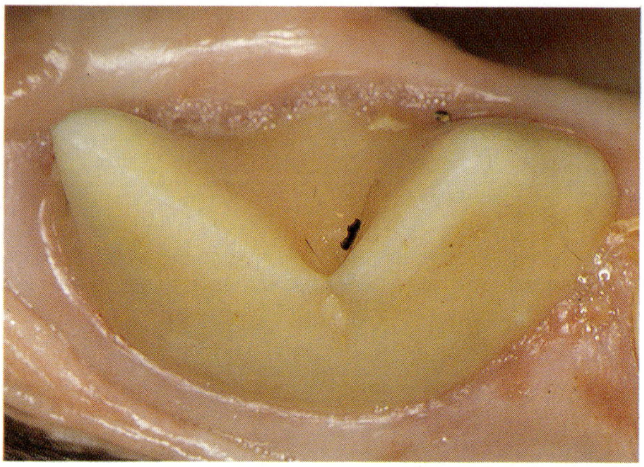

53 Radiograph (× *2*) of a cat's hemimandible demonstrates the relatively long and often divergent root formation of these brachyodont teeth.

54 Occlusal view (× *8.4*) of the cat's molar shows the sharp blade-like secondont crown formation perfectly suited to cutting and slicing meat.

Dentitions erupting in a sequential, horizontal direction

The cheek teeth of elephants, macropods (e.g. wallabies, kangaroos) and the manatee can be classified in this category, as they erupt sequentially in a horizontal, rostral direction rather than a grouped, vertical, side-by-side manner, as in other members of the heterodont group.

Elephants

Elephants have six molars per quadrant, which are progressively larger in all dimensions, the first three being sometimes considered as primary teeth as they are present in the juvenile. At any one time either a single complete, or one partially worn and one partially erupted molar are present per quadrant (**55**). As the mesially lying molar wears occlusally, mesial root resorption also takes place; at this area, parts of the unsupported tooth are broken off and exfoliated. A single molar is evident on the left side of the animal's jaw immediately after the loss of the rostral tooth (**56**).

The next tooth is formed in the caudal aspect of the jaws from individual plates containing longitudinal layers of enamel and dentine. These plates become fused together with cementum (**57**). The molars are hypsodonts and the multiple roots of the teeth are at different stages of development along the length of the tooth when it is in a fully functional position. There have been suggestions that the roots are continuously remodelled throughout the drifting process in

55

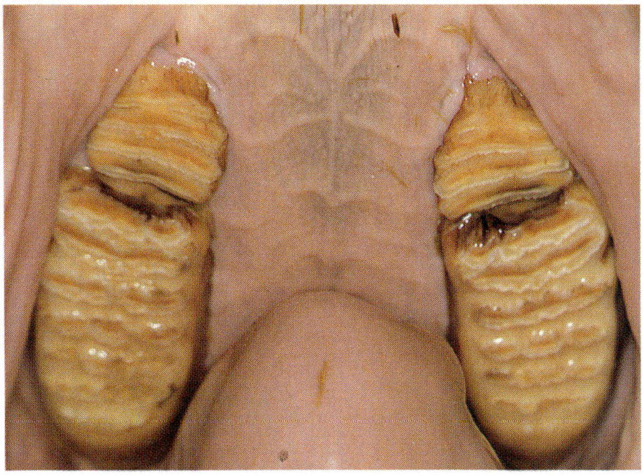

56

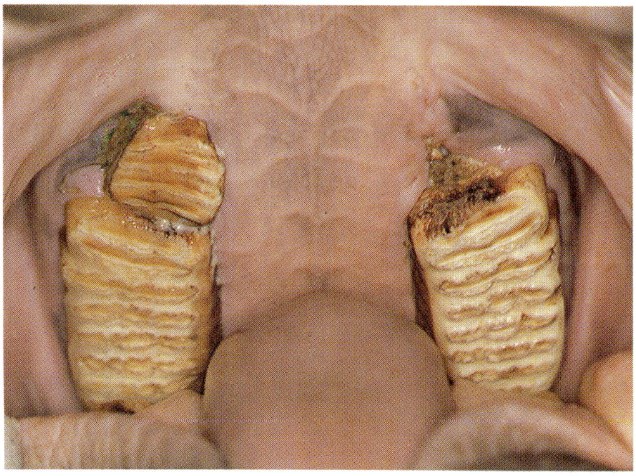

55 Occlusal view of a five-year-old Asian elephant showing well-worn second molars.

56 The same animal as in 55 six months later, immediately after the loss of the upper left second molar. Increased occlusal lengths of the third molars are also evident.

57

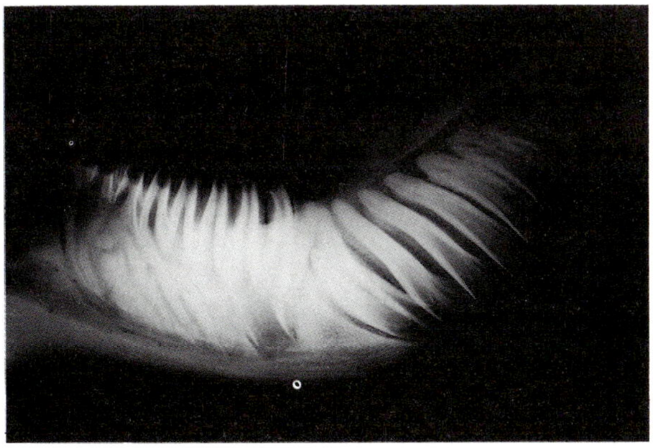

57 On this radiograph ***(× 0.25)*** **of a six-year-old African elephant the fourth molar can be seen developing in its crypt distal to the third molar that was in full occlusion.**

58

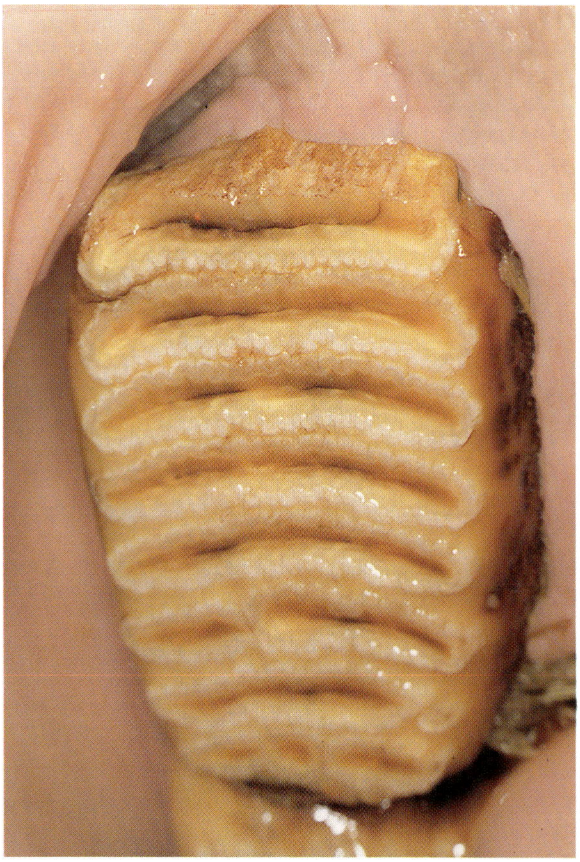

58 Occlusal view ***(× 0.7)*** **of an Asian elephant's molar illustrates the lophodont pattern, formed through ridges of enamel, dentine and cementum, that facilitates an efficient grinding mechanism.**

the mandible: the mesial roots are fully formed with constricted apical foramina, while the distal roots are dilated and continue longitudinal growth as the tooth drifts rostrally and occlusal attrition takes place. Once the root reaches the most mesial position in the socket, its apical foramina become more constricted before root resorption and partial coronal exfoliation occurs. Although teeth are prone to infections from occlusal perforation, they possess strong powers of secondary dentine deposition to wall off the mesial laminae before exfoliation occurs, which prevents exposure of the pulp chamber.

The occlusal morphology of enamel, cementum and dentine forms the lophodont pattern. The transverse ridges of different materials wear at different rates, producing a

59

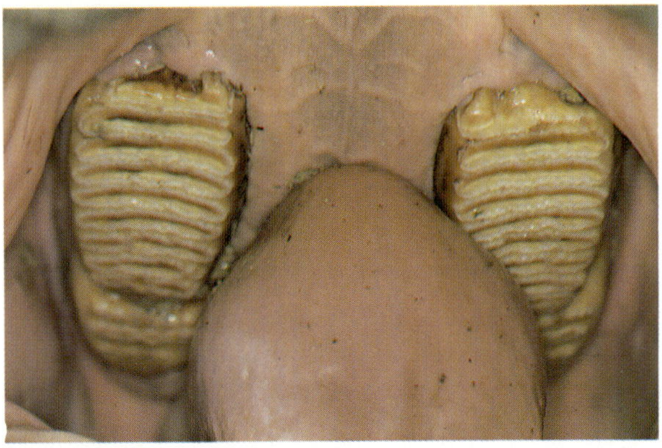

59 **Occlusal view of the same animal shown in 55 and 56 at 10 years of age showing the third molars fully functional, while the fourth molars are erupting distal to them.**

60

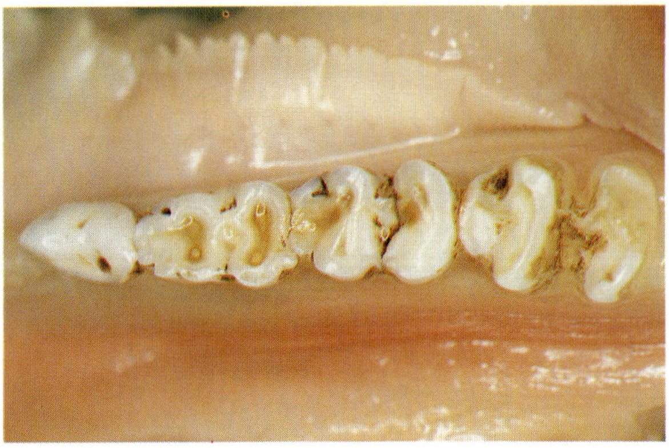

60 **Occlusal view *(×2.8)* of a one-year-old wallaby demonstrates the different stages of attrition between the primary teeth and the first permanent molar.**

61

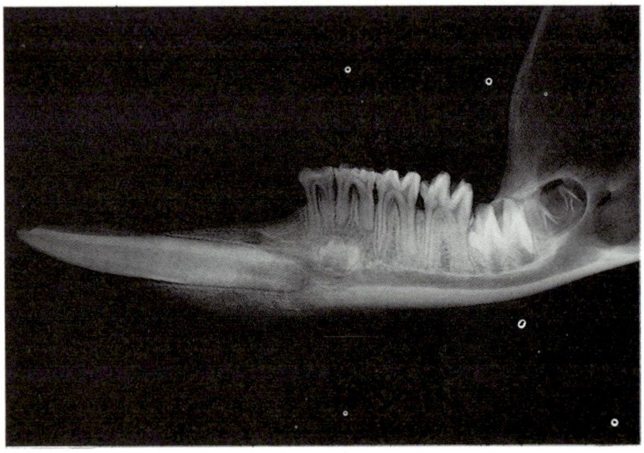

61 **Radiograph *(× 0.8)* of the specimen shown in 60 illustrates the developing second permanent premolar apical to the primary molars and the permanent molars developing in their crypts that will drift rostrally as the primary molars are lost.**

continuously rough surface that acts as an efficient grinding mechanism (**58**). The succeeding tooth lies immediately distal to its predecessor and drifts progressively into position once that one is reduced in length (**59**).

Macropods

The eruption of the permanent dentition of the macropods varies considerably. The cheek teeth may be hypsodonts or brachyodonts and drift in a rostral direction. The most rostrally lying primary molar is exfoliated because of occlusal wear and root resorption. The next tooth in the quadrant is present at the caudal aspect of the quadrant and erupts into the mouth in a horizontally drifting mode. In some species the exception is the third permanent premolar, which replaces the primary third molar in a vertically erupting fashion, as seen in the wallaby (**60, 61**).

The occlusal surfaces of the molars have marked lophodont ridges before they suffer from attrition. The lower incisors have often been classified as permanently growing, but this is contrary to critical assessment. There is a definite anatomical demarcation between the enamel-covered crown and the root, which is covered with cementum. Histological examination suggests that at middle age the apical foramina of the incisors are still not fully constricted, and irregular secondary dentine and cementum has contributed to the length of the root after eruption. There is no evidence of continuous amelogenesis, but it is believed that the root apex has an extended period of longitudinal development, as in some other herbivore teeth.

The dental formula

In the discussion of mammalian dentitions it is important to be able to convey the information in a precise and concise form.

To illustrate the dentitions an alphanumeric notation is utilised, where the number of teeth in each tooth category present and their arrangement in a maxillary quadrant are noted above a horizontal line, with the corresponding formula for the opposing mandibular quadrant underneath. As stated in Chapter 2, permanent incisors, canines, premolars and molars are abbreviated as I, C, P and M.

For example, the dental formula for the cat is:

$$I\frac{3}{3}:C\frac{1}{1}:P:\frac{3}{2}:M\frac{1}{1} = 15 \times 2 = 30$$

which is the total number of teeth present in the four quadrants. Simplified, this formula can be written:

$$\frac{3}{3}:\frac{1}{1}:\frac{3}{2}:\frac{1}{1} = 30$$

Common variations in the number of teeth in a tooth category and the dentition as a whole are indicated as 2–5 or 20–26. If teeth in adjacent tooth categories are morphologically the same, a variation in the total number of teeth present in the combined group is indicated as 7——9.

Dental formulae for permanent dentitions

The totals shown in the formulae are the normal variants and not necessarily the minimum and maximum totals as indicated by the dental formulae.

Order Marsupialia

Didelphidae (opossum)

$$\frac{5}{4}:\frac{1}{1}:\frac{3}{3}:\frac{4}{4} = 50$$

Vombatidae (wombat)

$$\frac{1}{1}:\frac{0}{0}:\frac{1}{1}:\frac{4}{4} = 24$$

Macropodidae (wallabies and kangaroos)

$$\frac{3}{1}:\frac{0-1}{0}:\frac{2}{2}:\frac{4}{4} = 32 - 34$$

Order Edentata

Myrmecophagidae (American anteaters)

$$\frac{0}{0}:\frac{0}{0}:\frac{0}{0}:\frac{0}{0} = 0$$

Bradypodidae (sloths)

$$\frac{0}{0}:\frac{0}{0}:\frac{1}{1}:\frac{4}{3} = 18$$

Dasypodidae (armadillos)

Nine-banded armadillo

$$\frac{0}{0}:\frac{7\text{——}9}{7\text{——}9} = 28 - 36$$

Giant armadillo

$$\frac{0}{0}:\frac{20\text{——}25}{20\text{——}25} = 80 - 100$$

Order Tubulidentata

Orycteropodidae (aardvark)

$$\frac{0}{0}:\frac{0}{0}:\frac{2-4}{2-4}:\frac{3}{3}=20-28$$

Order Insectivora

Talpidae (moles)
Erinaceidae (hedgehog)

$$\frac{1-3}{2-3}:\frac{1}{0-1}:\frac{3-4}{2-4}:\frac{3-4}{3}=30-46$$

Order Primates

Pongidae (great apes and gibbons)
Cercopithecidae (Old World monkeys)

$$\frac{2}{2}:\frac{1}{1}:\frac{2}{2}:\frac{3}{3}=32$$

Cebidae (New World monkeys)

$$\frac{2}{2}:\frac{1}{1}:\frac{3}{3}:\frac{3}{3}=36$$

Lorisidae (lorises)

$$\frac{1-2}{2}:\frac{1}{1}:\frac{3}{3}:\frac{3}{3}=34-36$$

Lemuridae (lemurs)

$$\frac{0-2}{2}:\frac{1}{1}:\frac{3}{3}:\frac{3}{3}=32-36$$

Order Carnivora

Canidae (dog types, foxes)

$$\frac{3}{3}:\frac{1}{1}:\frac{4}{4}:\frac{2}{3}=42$$

Ursidae (bears)

$$\frac{3}{3}:\frac{1}{1}:\frac{4}{4}:\frac{2}{3}=42$$

Ailuropodidae (pandas)

$$\frac{3}{3}:\frac{1}{1}:\frac{2-3}{3}:\frac{3}{3}=38-40$$

Procyonidae (racoons)

$$\frac{3}{3}:\frac{1}{1}:\frac{3-4}{3-4}:\frac{2}{2}=36-40$$

Mustelidae (weasles, skunks, otters)

$$\frac{3}{3}:\frac{1}{1}:\frac{3-4}{3-4}:\frac{1}{1-2}=32-38$$

Viverridae (civets)

$$\frac{3}{3}:\frac{1}{1}:\frac{3-4}{3-4}:\frac{1-2}{1-2}=32-40$$

Hyaenidae (hyenas)

$$\frac{3}{3}:\frac{1}{1}:\frac{4}{3}:\frac{1}{1}=34$$

Felidae (cats)

$$\frac{3}{3}:\frac{1}{1}:\frac{3}{2}:\frac{1}{1}=30$$

Order Pinnipedia

Otariidae (sea lions)

$$\frac{3}{2}:\frac{1}{1}:\frac{4}{4}:\frac{2}{1} = 36$$

Odobenidae (walrus)

$$\frac{2}{0}:\frac{1}{1}:\frac{3-4}{3-4}:\frac{0}{0} = 20-24$$

Phocidae (seals)

$$\frac{2-3}{2}:\frac{1}{1}:\frac{4}{4}:\frac{1}{1} = 32-34$$

Order Sirenia

Trichechidae (manatees)

$$\frac{0}{0}:\frac{0}{0}:\frac{0}{0}:\frac{6}{6} = {}^{*}$$

*Usually six molars are present per quadrant at any one time. Up to 40 molars per quadrant may be formed throughout the life of the animal.

Order Cetacea

Delphinidae (dolphin types)
12–50 teeth per quadrant, depending on the genus.

Order Proboscidea

Elephantidae (elephants)

$$\frac{1}{0}:\frac{0}{0}:\frac{0}{0}:\frac{6^{*}}{6^{*}} = 26$$

*The first three molars in each quadrant are sometimes referred to as primary molars.

Order Hyracoidea

Procaviidae (hyraxes)

$$\frac{1}{2}:\frac{0}{0}:\frac{4}{3-4}:\frac{3}{3} = 32-34$$

Order Perissodactyla

Equidae (horses)

$$\frac{3}{3}:\frac{0-1}{0-1}:\frac{3-4}{3}:\frac{3}{3} = 36-42$$

Tapiridae (tapirs)

$$\frac{3}{3}:\frac{1}{1}:\frac{4}{4}:\frac{3}{3} = 44$$

Rhinocerotidae (rhinoceroses)

$$\frac{1-2}{0-2}:\frac{0}{0}:\frac{3-4}{3-4}:\frac{3}{3} = 28-34$$

Order Artiodactyla

Suidae (pigs)

$$\frac{3}{3}:\frac{1}{1}:\frac{4}{4}:\frac{3}{3} = 44$$

Tayassuidae (peccaries)

$$\frac{2}{3}:\frac{1}{1}:\frac{3}{3}:\frac{3}{3} = 38$$

Hippopotamidae (hippopotami)

$$\frac{2}{2}:\frac{1}{1}:\frac{4}{4}:\frac{3}{3} = 40$$

Camelidae (camels and their South American counterparts)

$$\frac{1}{3}:\frac{0-1}{0-1}:\frac{2-3}{2}:\frac{3}{3} = 28-34$$

Cervidae (deer)

$$\frac{0}{3}:\frac{0-1}{1}:\frac{3}{3}:\frac{3}{3} = 32-34$$

Bovidae (bovids, cattle, sheep, goats, antelopes, etc.)
Giraffidae (giraffes and okapi)

$$\frac{0}{3}:\frac{0}{1}:\frac{3}{3}:\frac{3}{3} = 32$$

Order Rodentia

Caviidae (guinea-pigs)
Chinchillidae (chinchilla)
Hydrochoeridae (capybara)
Castoridae (beaver)

$$\frac{1}{1}:\frac{0}{0}:\frac{1-2}{1}:\frac{3}{3} = 20-22$$

Muridae (Old World rats and mice)

$$\frac{1}{1}:\frac{0}{0}:\frac{0}{0}:\frac{3}{3} = 16$$

Sciuridae (squirrels)

$$\frac{1}{1}:\frac{0}{0}:\frac{1}{1}:\frac{3}{3} = 20$$

Order Lagomorpha

Leporidae (rabbits and hares)

$$\frac{2}{1}:\frac{0}{0}:\frac{3}{2}:\frac{3}{3} = 28$$

5 Dental Development and Abnormalities

In the great majority of animals the development of the dentition, eruption times and the position of the teeth have little or no variation. Abnormalities that do occur may be due to external, developmental and/or genetic factors. The dog is used in this chapter as the model to illustrate the principles: because of the different size and shape of breeds and intensive and sometimes indiscriminate inbreeding, the dog probably suffers from more hereditary dental abnormalities than any other animal.

Normal dental development

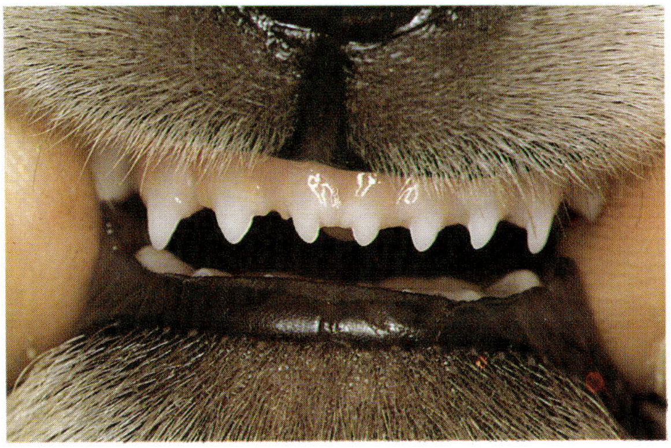

62

62 Primary dentition — Case 1a. The primary teeth are lighter in colour than the permanent successors. They are also smaller and have a finer root formation so they may be accommodated in the developing jaws.

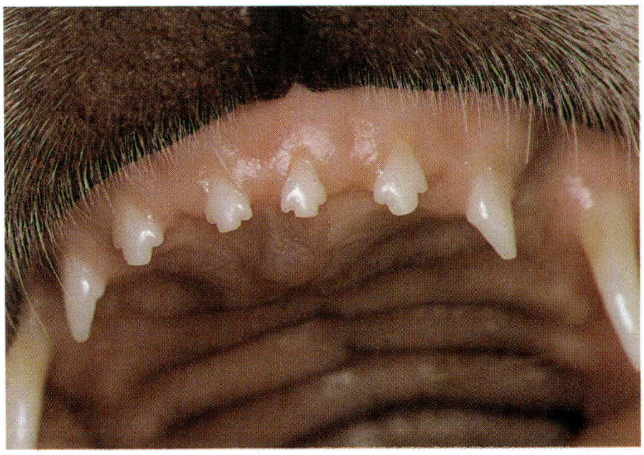

63

63 Primary anteriors spreading — Case 1b. As the individual grows, the spaces between the incisors increase, with the jaw needing to accommodate the larger teeth of the permanent dentition.

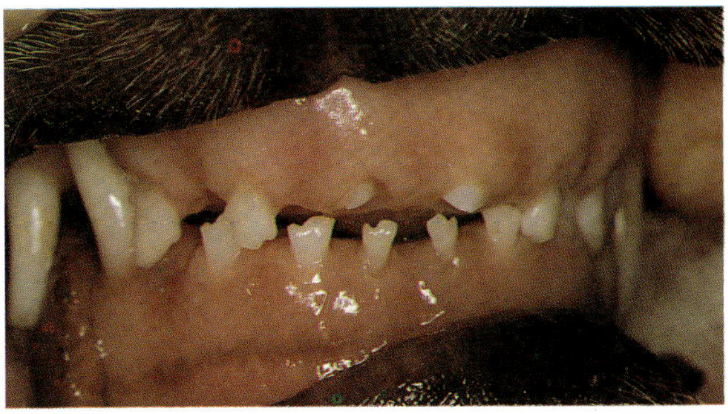

64

64 Primaries still in place — permanent teeth showing — Case 1c. Normally, the primary teeth are lost just before or as the permanent ones erupt. The pressure from the erupting second set usually encourages root resorption.

65 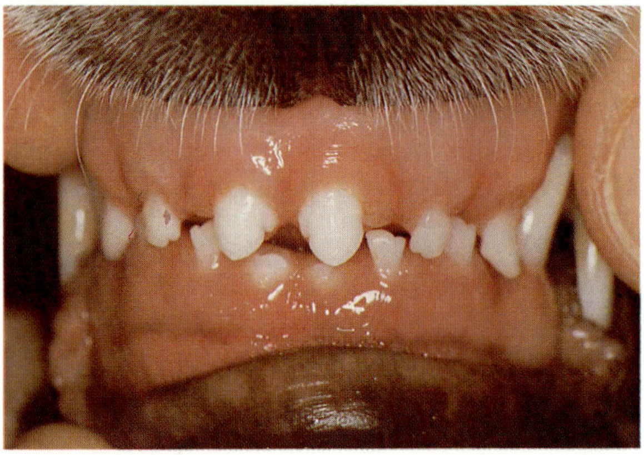

65 Four days later — Case 1d. The permanent incisors erupt very rapidly once the process commences. Any delay in the loss of the primary teeth may guide the permanent ones into an abnormal position.

66 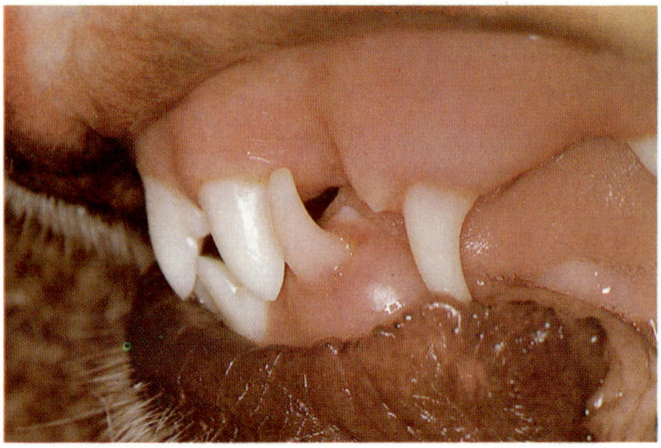

66 Permanent canines erupting — primaries still retained — Case 1e. A critical stage is reached where the shedding of the primary teeth allows for normal occlusion of the canine teeth.

67 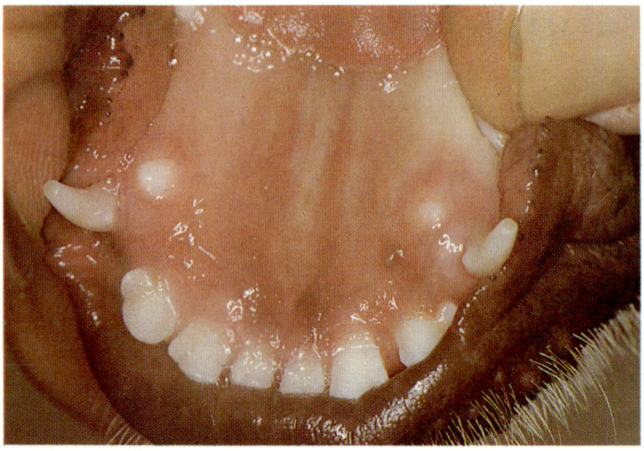

67 Occlusal view of erupting lower canines — Case 1f. The lingual position of the lower permanent canines can be clearly seen, but their coronal tips point labially.

68 Shed primary teeth — Case 1g. Fully formed primary roots are extremely long (*see* **358**). These teeth were lost naturally; the resorption is confirmed by the 'moth-eaten' appearance and thin walls of the residual root substance.

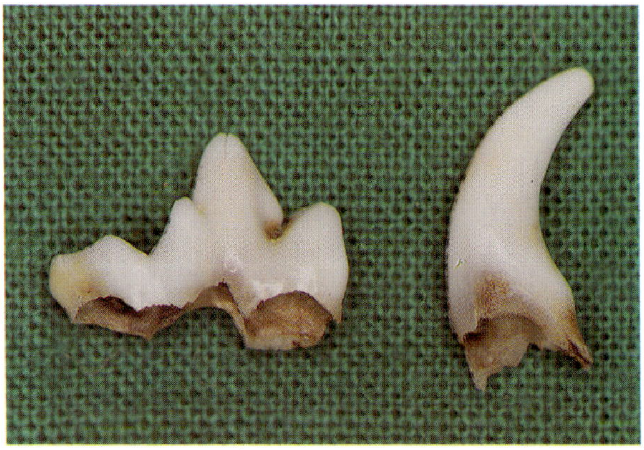

68

69 Labial view of erupting permanent canines — Case 1h.

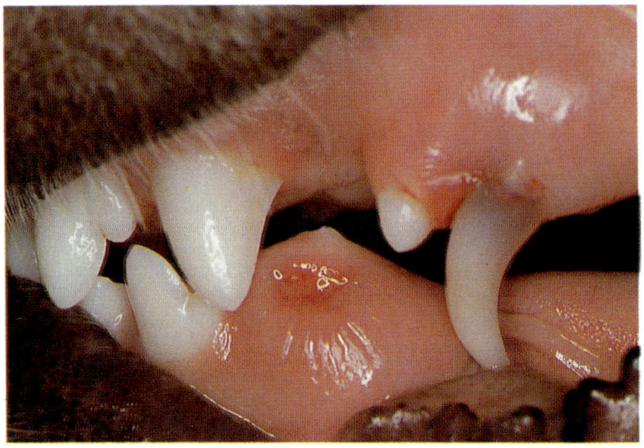

69

70 Primary canines lost and permanent canines erupting — Case 1i. Once the primary canines have been lost, the labial drift and eruption of the lower permanent canines is rapid.

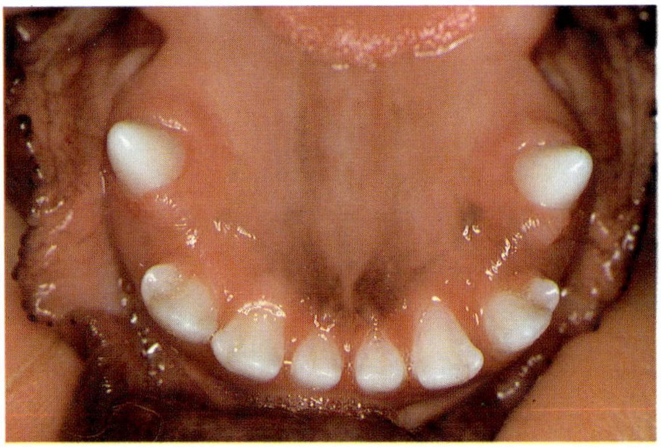

70

71

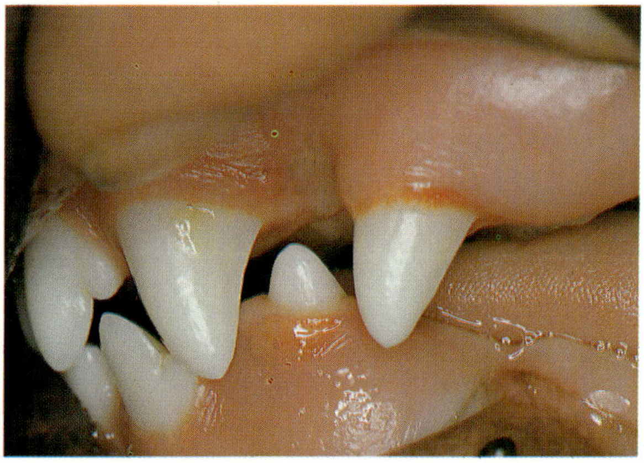

71 Labial view of erupting lower canines — Case 1j. After the loss of the upper primary canines the permanent successors can drift distally unimpeded. Thereby, an adequate diastema exists between the upper canine and third incisor so the eruption path of the lower canine is not obstructed.

72

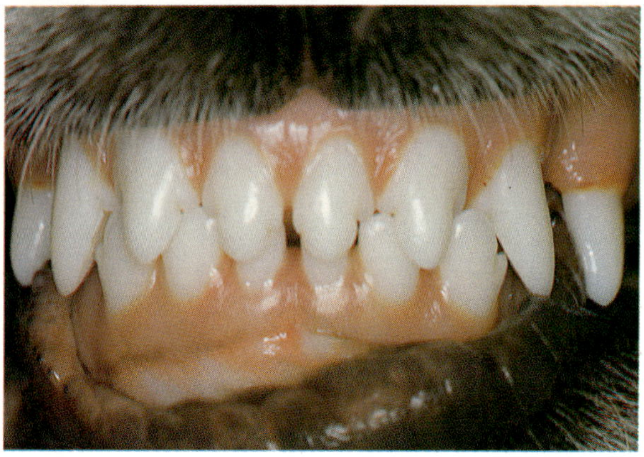

72 Incisor relationship — Case 1k. A good incisor relationship exists that is normal for the breed.

73

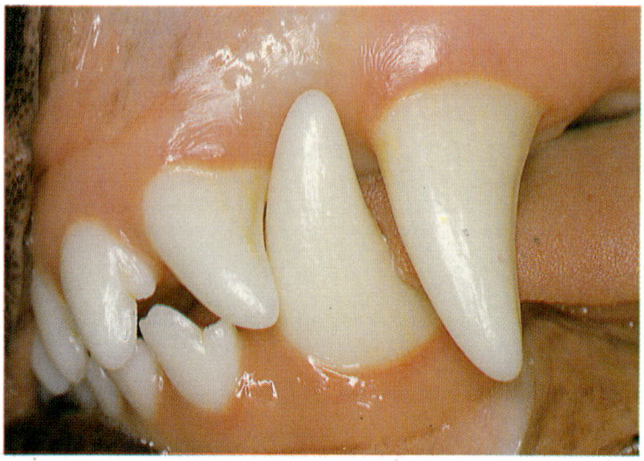

73 Canine relationship — Case 1l. The final mandibular canine relationship to the maxillary canine and third incisor indicates a normal bite. This is a more practical indicator to the jaw relationship of the dog than variations in the cuspal interdigitation of the posterior teeth.

Developmental disorders of the teeth

74 Delayed eruption — 18 months of age. On rare occasions, the eruption of the permanent dentition is delayed. Radiography of the jaws may be advisable as unerupted supernumerary teeth and dentigerous cysts can interfere with eruption. In this case there was no clinical reason.

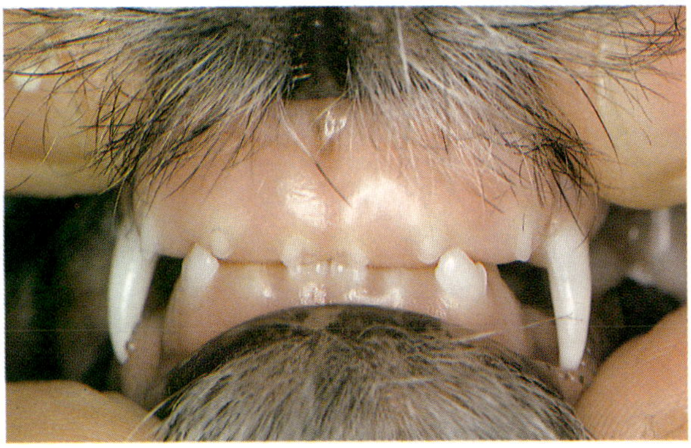

74

75 Incomplete dichotomy — partially divided tooth. The permanent incisor gave the impression of a longitudinal split of the enamel. The condition is the partial division of a single tooth bud. The aetiology may be hereditary or it may be through physical trauma to the primary predecessor having been transmitted to the underlying permanent tooth bud during development.

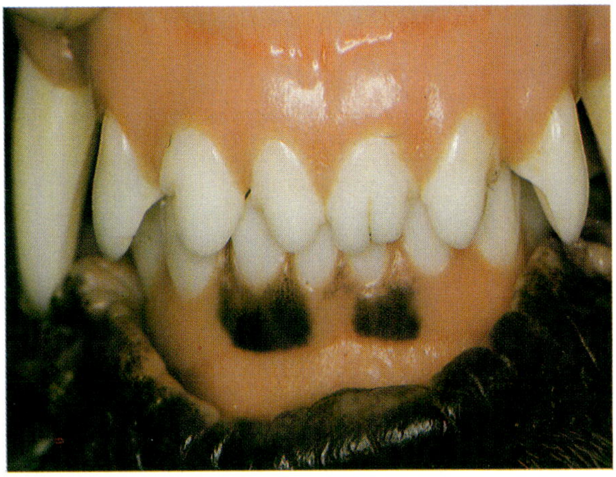

75

76 Incomplete dichotomy — a more severe example. An upper first permanent premolar gives the impression that it is two separate teeth. 'Show people' often confuse incomplete dichotomy with supernumerary teeth or partial anadontia. As these conditions may be hereditary, it is important for breeders that the correct diagnosis is made.

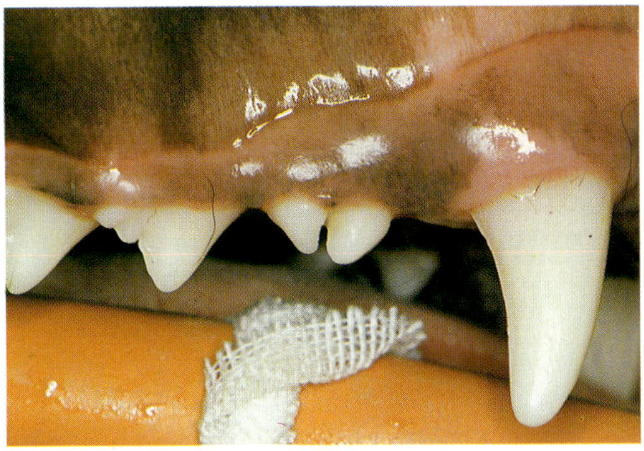

76

77

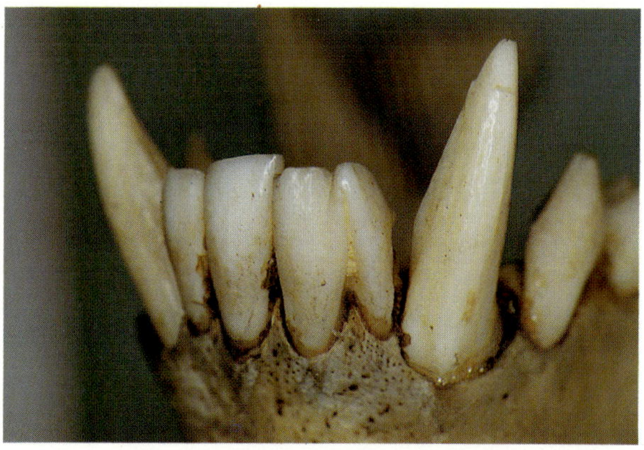

77 True gemination — Tantalus monkey (Royal College of Surgeons of England, Odontological Museum, London: Museum No. G13.4). The fusion of two separate tooth buds, gemination, is a rare condition and can give a similar appearance to incomplete dichotomy.

78

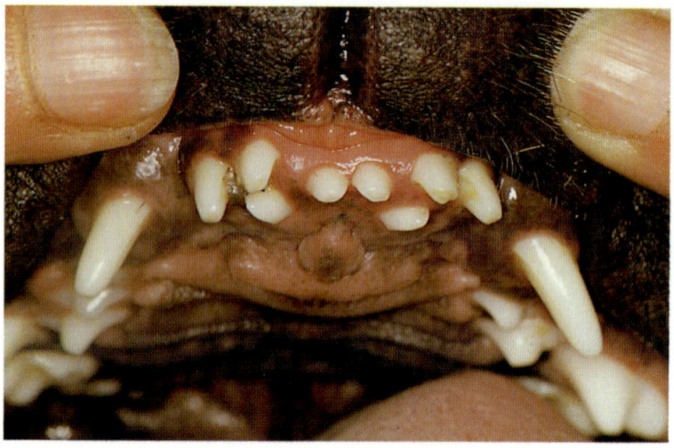

78 Polyodontia. Two extra teeth are present in the incisor region of the dental arch.

79

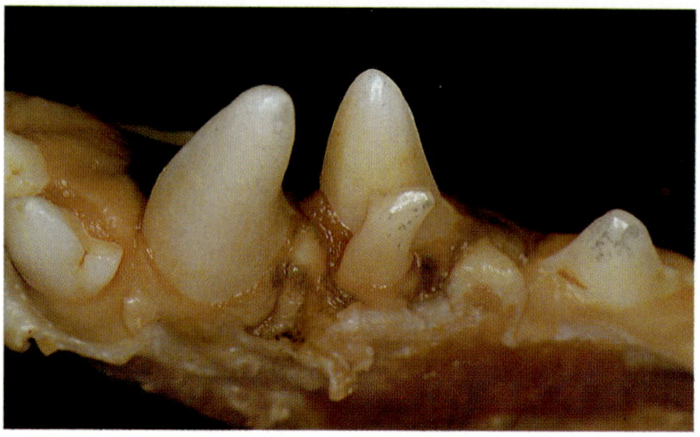

79 Supplemental canine (postmortem). An additional (supplemental) permanent canine tooth is present in the mandible; the primary canine was also retained.

80 Enamel hypoplasia. Amelogenesis imperfecta — disturbance in enamel formation — may result from defects in the formation of the enamel matrix or from hypocalcification of the enamel during the period of enamel formation. Dogs' teeth with such defects are usually termed 'distemper teeth'. The aetiology of the defects are not necessarily connected with the disease. It is often connected with periods of systemic illnesses, pyrexia or disturbance of the metabolism through gastroenteritis.

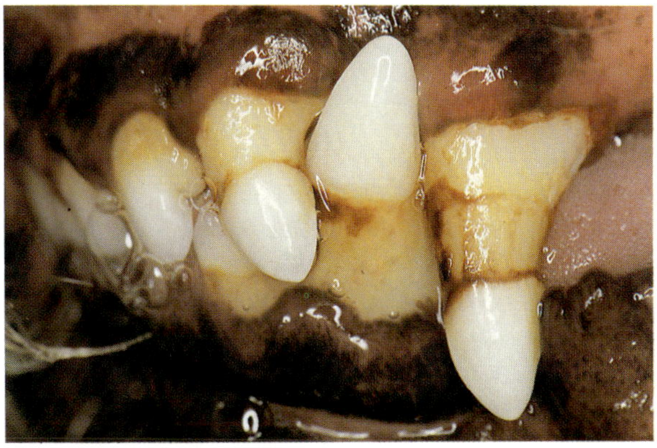

80

81 Enamel hypoplasia — domestic cat. Amelogenesis imperfecta is evident on the crowns of the primary canines and third incisors, while the permanent incisors are erupting with normal enamel, chronological proof that the disturbance in amelogenesis took place prenatally. Note the difference of the condition from that seen in the dog (**80**). The surface of the enamel does not have the irregular pitted texture, only discoloration.

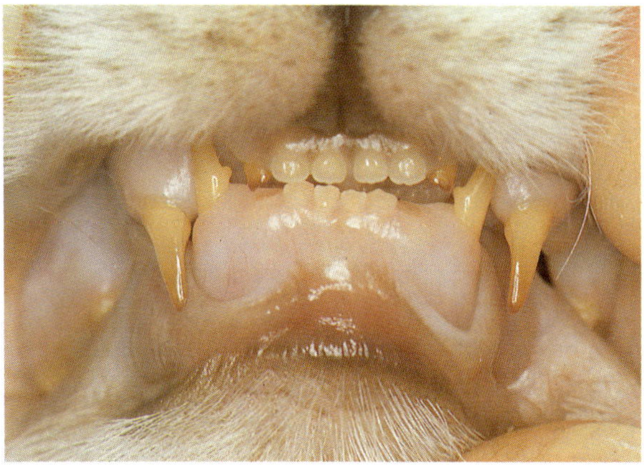

81

82 Tetracycline pigmentation. Tetracycline is absorbed by calcified tissues and causes permanent discoloration. In the dentition this only occurs during the period of development of the teeth at the time of tetracycline treatment. The pigmentation may be deposited in the dentine and enamel as bands. The more prolonged the treatment, the broader the areas effected. Occasionally, the crowns may be totally discoloured. The colours may vary from yellow to grey and green. As tetracyline effects a number of teeth developing concurrently it is not difficult to differentiate between this condition and isolated teeth discoloured through pulpal necrosis caused by trauma (see **232**).

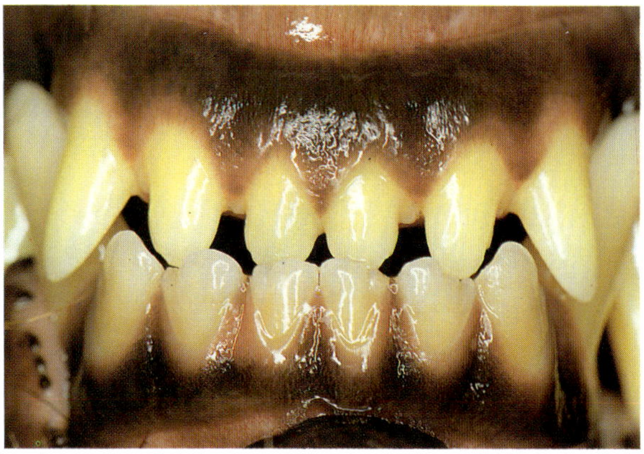

82

Malocclusion

The position of the teeth are often determined by the skeletal relationship of the mandible and the maxilla. Most of the discrepancies are of hereditary origin, although in some cases environmental factors can also play a role. Most malocclusions are minor and are not clinically significant, but to show breeders they are a primary concern. It is important that an accurate diagnosis is made and the owner is given the appropriate advice regarding prognosis, treatment and breeding repercussions.

Eruptive malocclusion

83 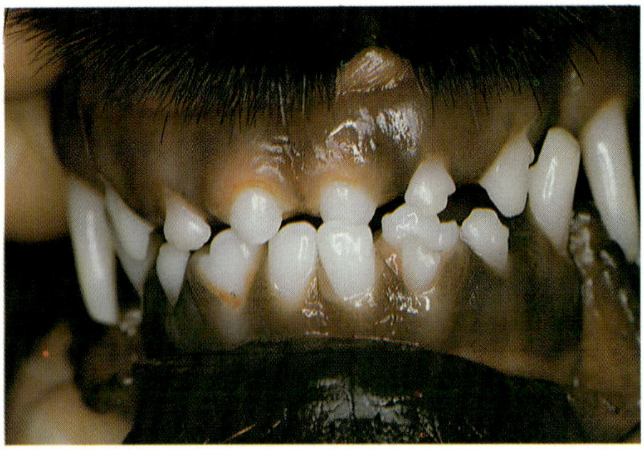

83 Mixed dentition — no crowding. The permanent lower first incisors were guided into their present labial positions due to primary incisors having been retained too long. No crowding of the anterior arch is apparent and the skeletal relationship appears normal.

84 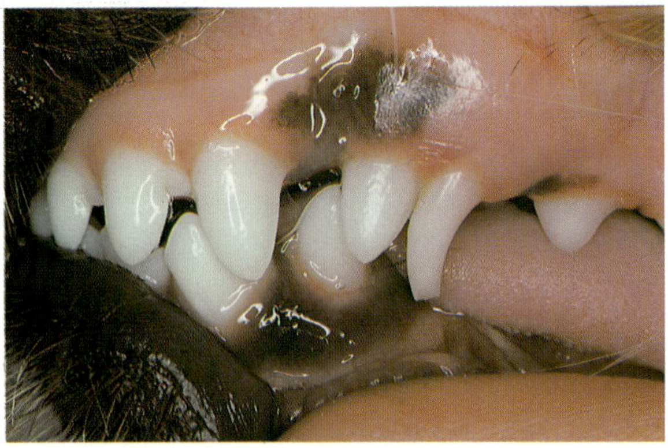

84 Lower permanent canine biting into palate. Upper primary canines have been retained distal to their permanent successors, which are crowding the incisor — canine diastema. This lack of space did not allow the lower permanent canine to erupt normally and it was guided into a palatal occlusion. With further eruption the canine will traumatise the palatal mucosa.

Traumatogenic malocclusion

This form of malocclusion is caused by trauma to the maxilla and/or mandible or to the teeth themselves at an early stage of development. Malocclusion caused by vigorous games with rubber rings or sticks must be included in this group, as these activities can force the position of the erupting teeth into an abnormal relationship.

85 The anterior view of the dentition exhibiting a 'wry mouth' — unilateral deformity in the malocclusion — Case 2a. The aetiology is not apparent from this aspect, although scar tissue is visible between the upper left third incisors and the canine.

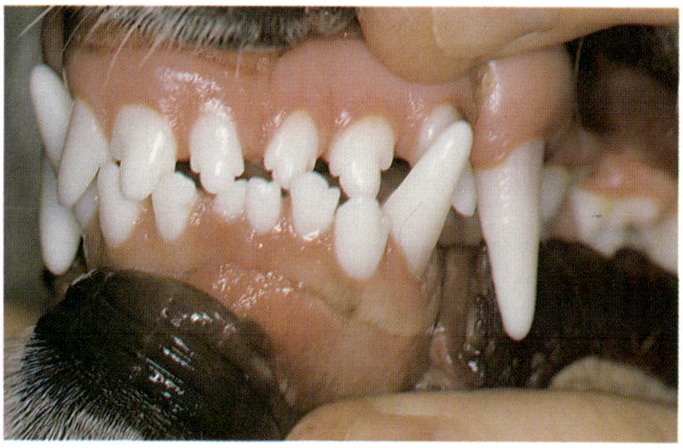

85

86 Lateral view — Case 2b. The lateral view of the malocclusion indicates that the premaxilla is deviated to the left. The gingival scar suggests a past injury.

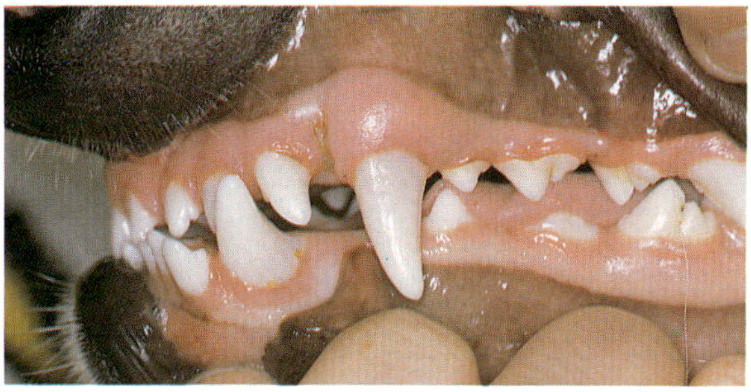

86

87 Dorsal view — Case 2c. The deviation of the nose and the mid-line of the fur on its dorsal surface indicates a distortion of the skeletal base. Trauma from a bite to the maxilla is the most likely cause of the deformity, which probably occurred at a very early age.

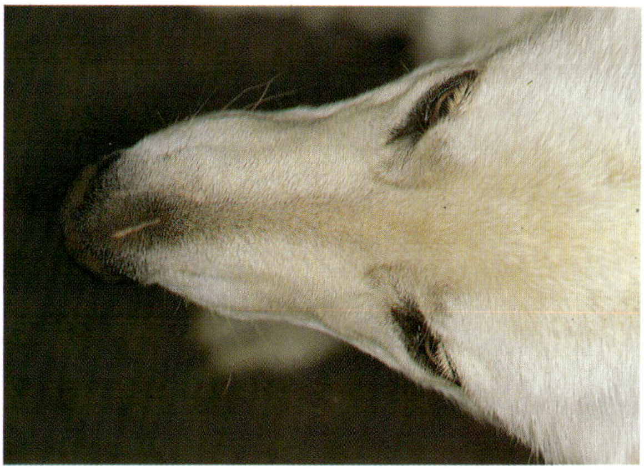

87

88
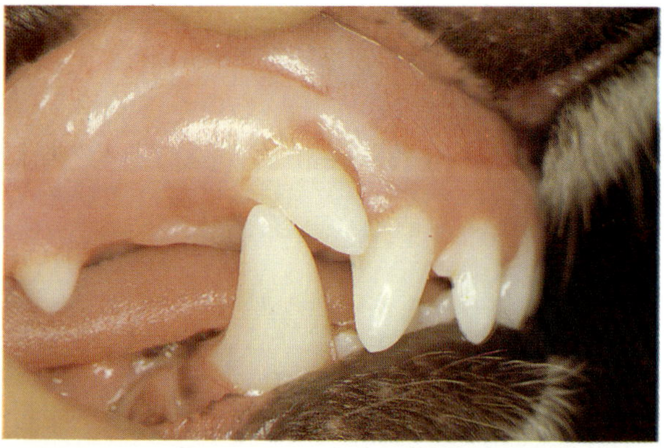

88 Impacted upper canine. This permanent maxillary canine lies horizontally, unable to erupt normally as its coronal tip is lying mesial to the lower canine. Impacted upper canine may be considered to be eruptive in origin, but certain breeds like shelties often demonstrate this condition, hence its classification as a hereditary malocclusion.

89
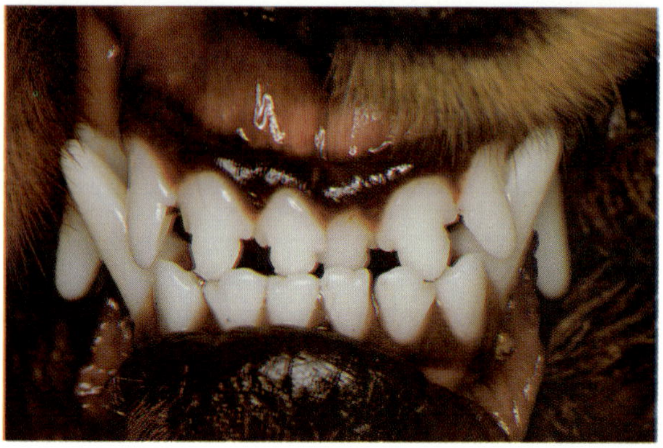

89 Crowded incisors. The incisor relationship is abnormal as a result of crowding of the teeth. Even though the discrepancy is minimal, orthodontic treatment is ruled out due to the lack of interdental space.

When there is a discrepancy in the classical scissor bite relationship of the upper incisors the condition is colloquially termed as 'overshot' or 'undershot'. These malocclusions are usually a result of a discrepancy within the skeletal bases.

Retrognathism is a clinical term for an 'overshot' bite, where the mandible lies in an excessively caudal position in relation to the upper jaw. The condition is most common among the dolichocephalic breeds, where the condition is usually caused by a brachygnathism. Retrognathism is usually evident through the mandibular incisors being excessively lingual to their maxillary counterparts and often the mandibular canines lie distal to the maxillary canines instead of being positioned in the maxillary third incisor/canine diastema.

90
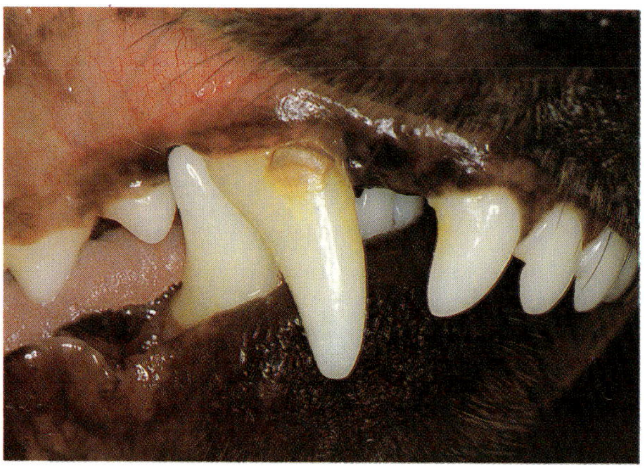

90 Canine relationship reversed in a retrognathic malocclusion.

Prognathism is the clinical term for an 'undershot' bite where the mandible lies in a protrusive position in relation to the upper jaw. The condition is often present as normal in the brachycephalic breeds, although it can occasionally be caused by an abnormally long mandible. Prognathism is usually evident in the labial position of the mandibular incisors in relation to their maxillary counterparts and often the mandibular canines also lie mesial to the maxillary third incisors **(91)**.

91
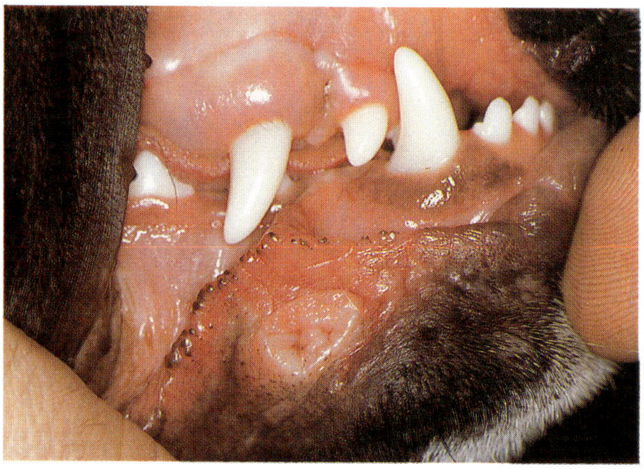

91 Prognathic occlusion that causes trauma to the lower lips from misaligned upper canine.

92

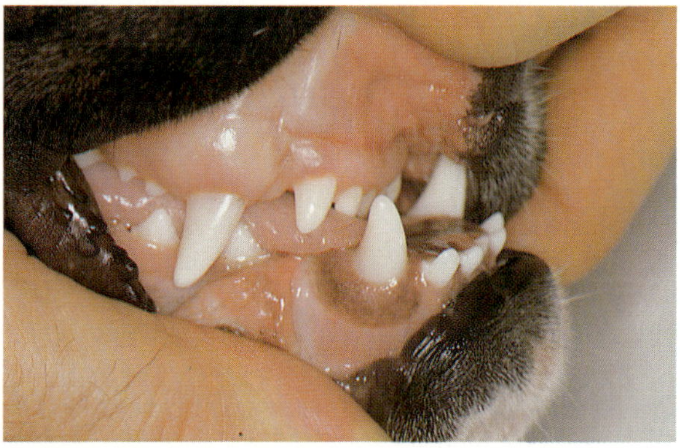

92 Severe prognathic malocclusion.

93

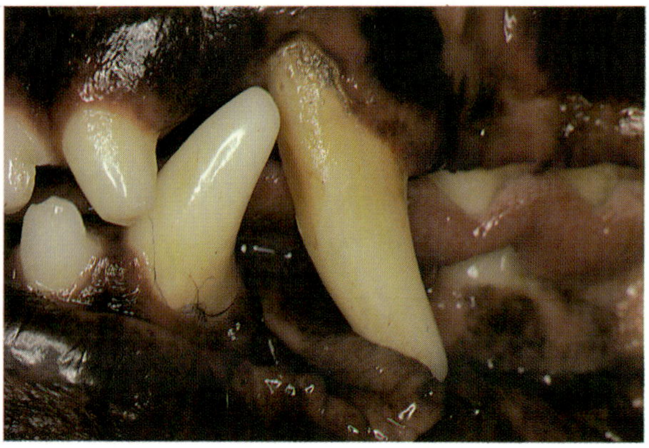

93 Wear pattern to upper canines. Although the lower canine is lying in the upper third incisor/canine diastema the prognathic malocclusion has forced it into a distal inclination. This has resulted in attrition to the mesial surface of the upper canine and the mesial gingiva has also been torn away from the root.

94

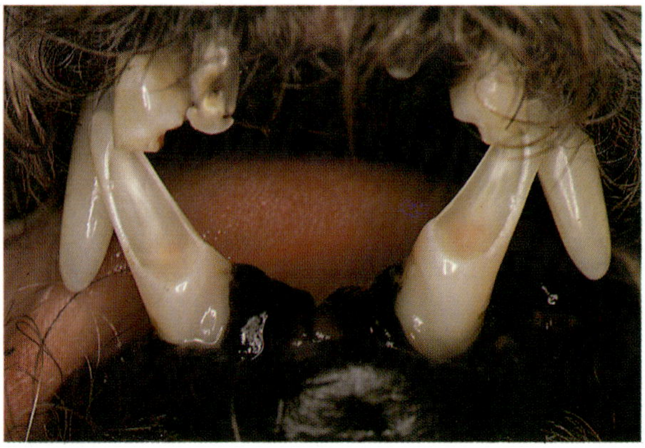

94 Wear pattern. Malocclusion has resulted in excessive wear to the tips of the lower canines.

95 **Prognathism, with crowding of the incisors.**

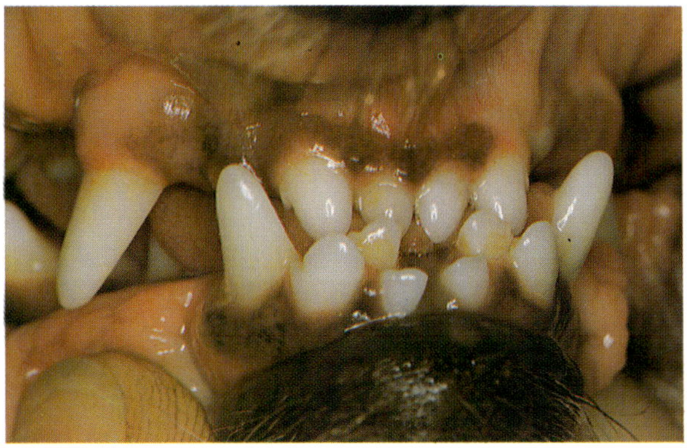
95

No attempts should be made to correct the malocclusions illustrated above either with appliance therapy or surgical measures for aesthetic reasons. If the malocclusions are responsible for a level of oral trauma, amputating the crowns of the teeth in conjunction with endodontic treatment or extractions should be considered.

Orthodontics

Ethical guidelines

Animal orthodontics, which generally means the correction of malocclusions in dogs, bears little resemblance to its human counterpart. Impressions, bonding of brackets and many of the professional adjustments we take for granted in human practice require general anaesthetics in a veterinary environment. Rarely can one justify multiple general anaesthetics for orthodontic reasons when considering the malocclusions of animals.

If malocclusions are indiscriminately corrected for show purposes the breeds will suffer hereditary abnormalities that could be easily prevented. Canine orthodontics, which requires broad diagnostic skills and experience to differentiate among eruptive, traumatic or genetic malocclusions, also requires strength of character and professionalism from the operator to resist the pressures from owners who obsessively want their animals' bite corrected for aesthetic and show purposes.

The basic principles of canine orthodontics should be:

- Not to correct occlusal discrepancies for aesthetic reasons.
- To consider active orthodontics only if the malocclusion is causing tissue damage, pain or infection, or is likely to give rise to it in the future.
- To treat a condition that is considered to be hereditary, but where active orthodontics is advisable to relieve pain and suffering, but also neutering the animal to prevent the condition being passed on further.

The principles of orthodontics

Orthodontics is the active correction of abnormal dental relationships. Orthodontic movements when analysed at their most basic level are only pushing and pulling forces. Rotating, torquing, tipping as well as body movements are all more sophisticated forms of the basic movements. The forces encourage osseous remodelling to take place in the form of osteoclastic and osteoblastic activity, which allows the teeth under traction to slowly move through the alveolar bone. Excessive forces can create undesirable movements, contribute to root resorption, devitalisation of the tooth being moved and premature tooth loss.

For satisfactory orthodontic movements to take place certain criteria must be fulfilled:

- Sufficient space must exist — not only interdental space but occlusal clearance as well — for the required tooth/teeth to move into. Many orthodontic movements are doomed to failure at the outset of treatment as this fundamental criterion is ignored.
- Sufficient force must be applied at the correct point of application.
- To each force there is an equal and opposite force. Sufficient anchorage must be utilised so that teeth other than the ones being treated are restricted in their movement during the application of orthodontic forces.
- The force must be maintained for a sufficient length of time for the movement to take place.
- At the completion of treatment, sufficient time must be allowed for a retention period, or relapse of the condition may occur. Occasionally the incisal relationship will be naturally retentive.

96

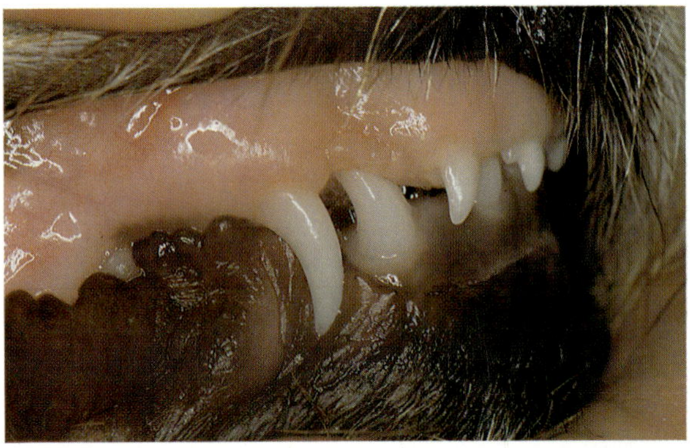

96 Primary canines biting into palate — Case 3a. The palatal traumatic occlusion of primary canines is an indication that the permanent successors will follow a similar eruptive pattern. The skeletal relationship may be normal.

97

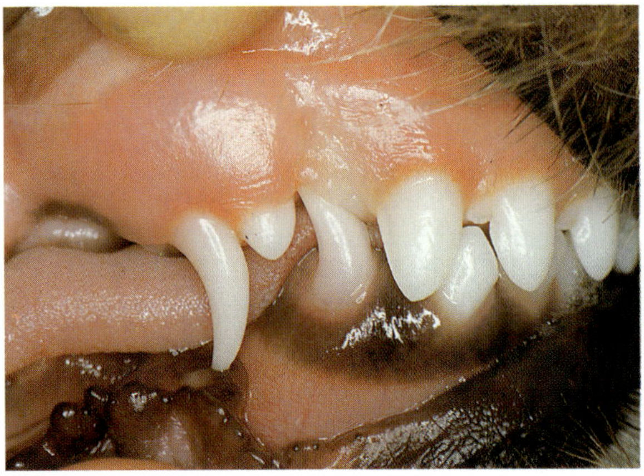

97 Upper canine erupting — Case 3b. This upper permanent canine is forced to erupt in an abnormally mesial position because the primary tooth has not been shed.

98 Lower canine erupting — upper primary still retained — Case 3c. The mesial position of the upper permanent canine has reduced the natural diastema between the upper third incisor and canine. This crowding has guided the lower canine into a lingual position, whereby it is erupting into a traumatic palatal occlusion. The extraction of the upper primary canines in these cases of malocclusion at an early stage can allow the necessary drifting of the upper permanent canines, so that the lower canines are able to erupt in a non-traumatic position (for surgical treatment of this case see **352–360**).

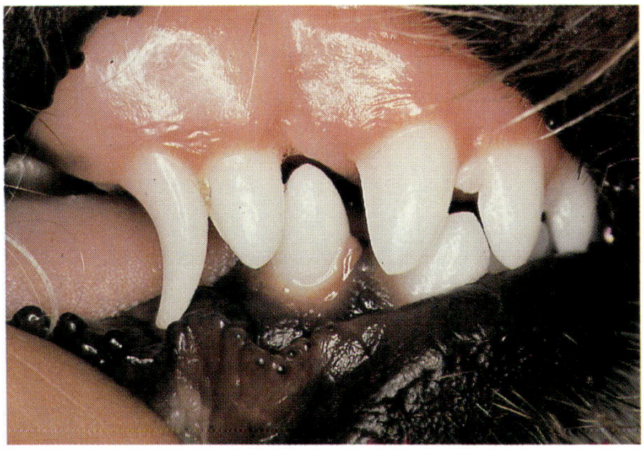

98

99 Older animal with traumatic bite — labial view — Case 4a. This case illustrates how a palatal malocclusion can present once the lower canine has fully erupted in a middle-aged animal.

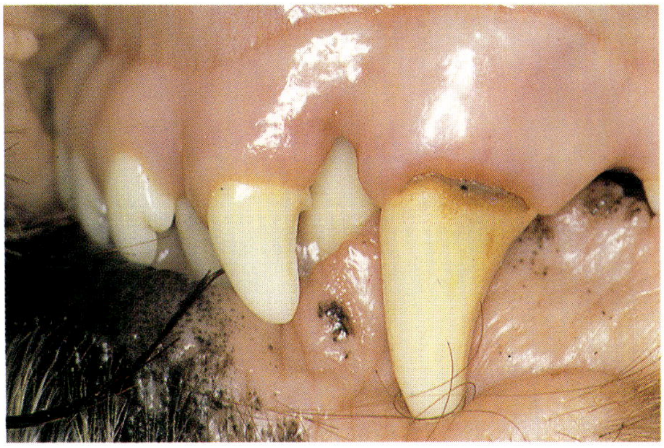

99

100 Occlusal view — Case 4b. A palatal view of the same animal shows how the gingiva is inflamed; it has been torn away from the third incisor root. The animal exhibited discomfort. At such an advanced state two treatment options are available: extraction, a surgically traumatic alternative, or reduction in the height of the tooth, a preferable alternative but one in which the pulp chamber will be exposed. This must be treated by endodontic therapy, otherwise acute pain, pulp necrosis and periapical infection will result.

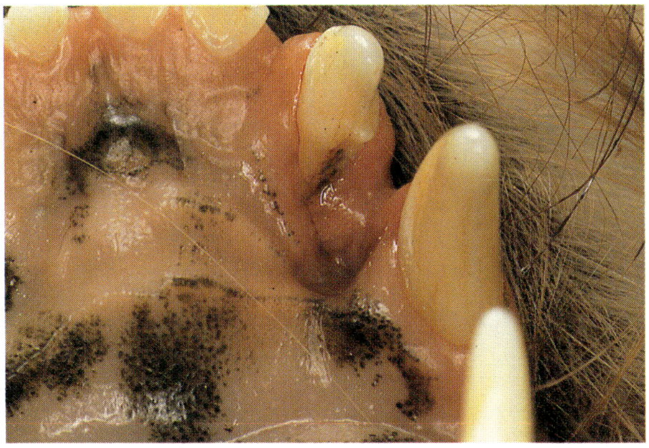

100

101

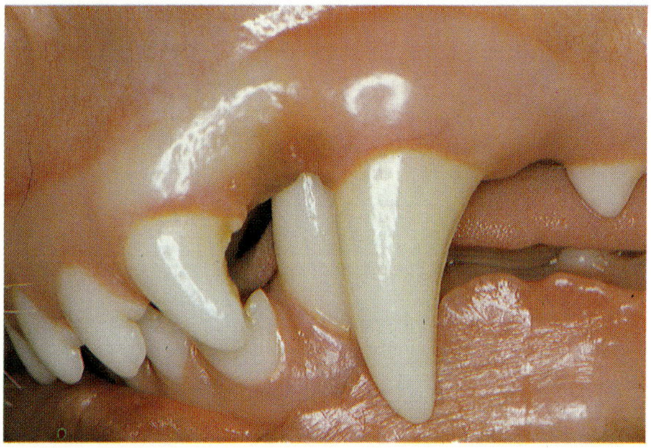

101 Early canine malocclusion — Case 5a. Young dog aged 10 months with traumatic palatal malocclusion of the lower left canine. The upper permanent canine is lying too mesial due to late loss of its primary predecessor. The crowding has reduced the incisor–canine diastema and forced the lower canine into a lingual malocclusion.

102

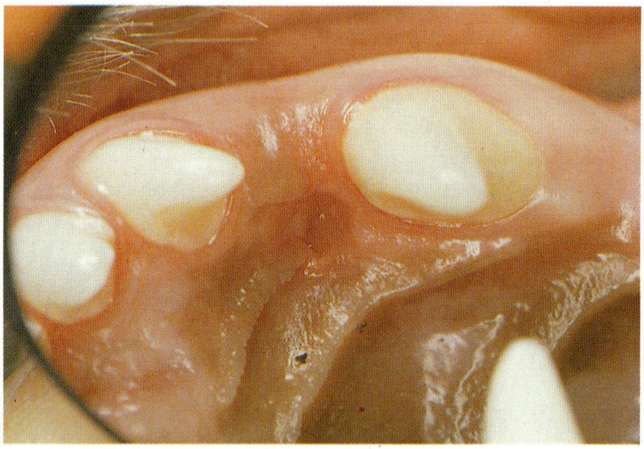

102 Occlusal view — Case 5b. Occlusal view already illustrates the potential trauma that can result.

Appliance therapy

The correction of malocclusion in the dental treatment of animals must be looked upon as the exception rather than the norm. Even if it is justifiable, before it is embarked upon the owners of the animals must fully understand the commitment they have to make for the treatment to succeed.

Traumatic palatal malocclusion

It is important that the correct initial diagnosis of the aetiology is made as a narrow-based mandible can give rise to malocclusions where orthodontic treatment is ruled out. It must be remembered that mandibular symphysis in the dog is a synarthrosis, and expansion forces applied to the lower canines can result in opening the symphysis, which will give rise to a false impression of tooth movement and a relapse to the original malocclusion at the completion of treatment.

103

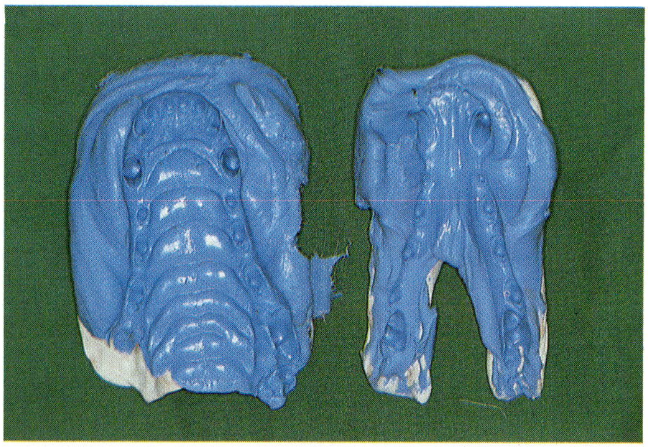

103 Silicone impressions — Case 5c. Thermoplastic resin impression trays are prepared before the general anaesthetic on a similar-sized model/skull. The trays can be checked for fit once the animal is anaesthetised and can be easily adjusted if necessary. For technique on handling tray material see Chapter 9. Irrespective of how placid an animal may be, meaningful impressions cannot be made without a general anaesthetic or deep sedation. Silicone, the material of choice for permanent impressions, allows the option of casting multiple plaster models. Although the cost of silicone is higher than alginate, this cannot be compared with the inconvenience of further impressions and anaesthetics if the models or the non-silicone impressions are damaged in the laboratory, or further appliances need to be made if the original one is destroyed, or lost.

104 Etching enamel — Case 5d. Once satisfactory impressions have been obtained, the teeth are prepared for bonded brackets during the same session as impressions are taken. Dogs' enamel needs to be etched for a longer period than human enamel.

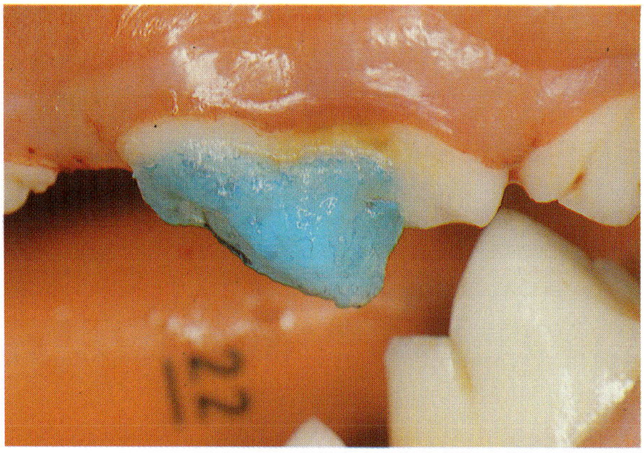
104

105 Close-up of etched enamel — Case 5e. If the typical matt appearance is not obtained, the enamel should be re-etched and then thoroughly re-rinsed with water.

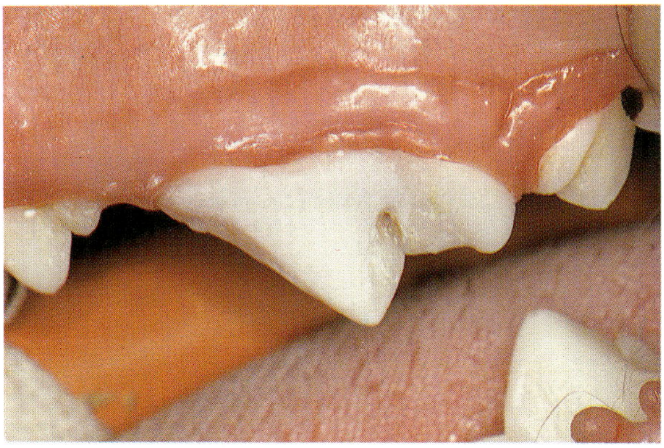
105

106 Bracket bonded — Case 5f. A 'two part' composite orthodontic resin is used to bond the bracket to the etched enamel. Light-cured materials or glass ionomer cements are definitely contraindicated. Each tooth and bracket is treated individually to completion. The material is painted onto the enamel and bracket in a creamy consistency. The bracket is then applied to the material on the tooth and allowed to set for a number of hours before elastics are applied.

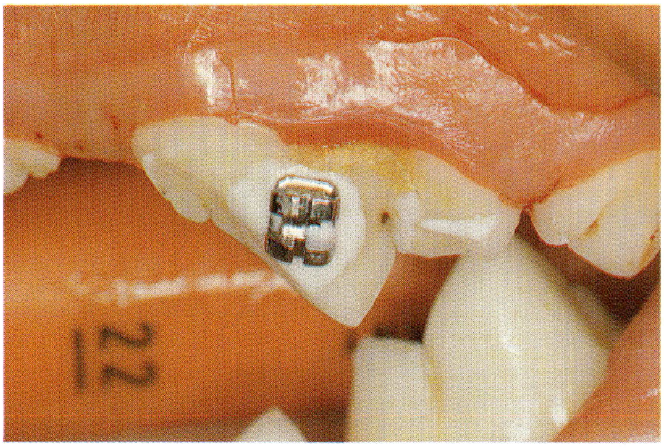
106

107

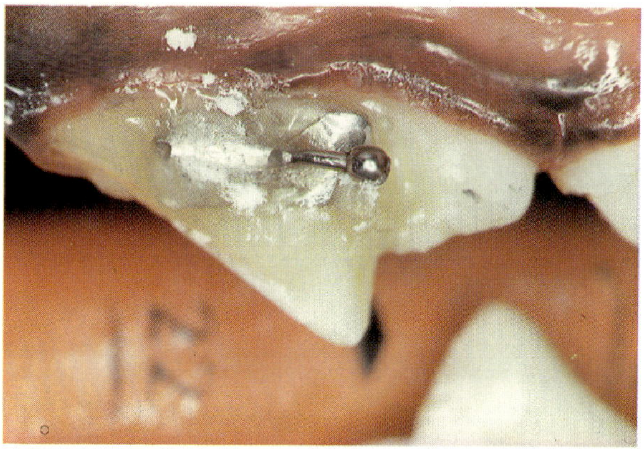

107 Custom-made bracket. A custom-made bracket with a large surface area and a hook is helpful when using heavier elastics.

108

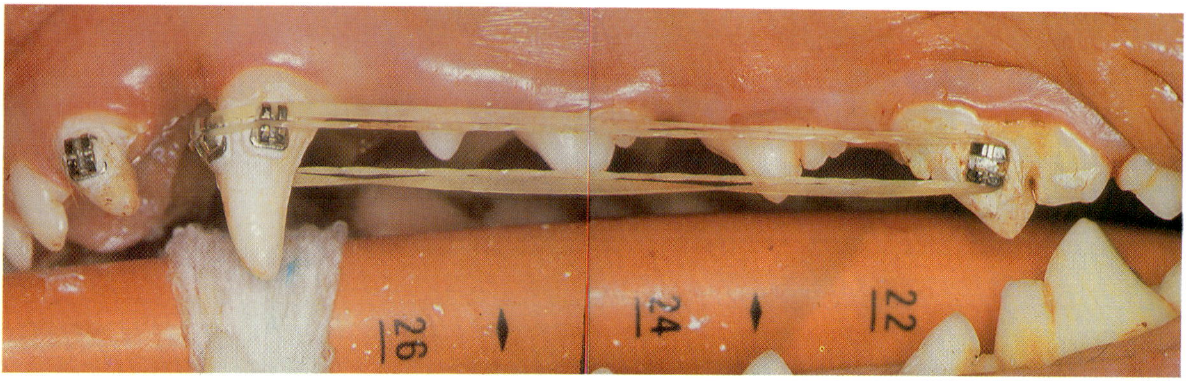

108 Retracting with elastic bands — Case 5g. The canine is retracted with latex orthodontic bands from the upper fourth premolar. The size and strength of the band need to be chosen carefully for the correct force to be applied. The owners have to change the bands on a daily basis.

109

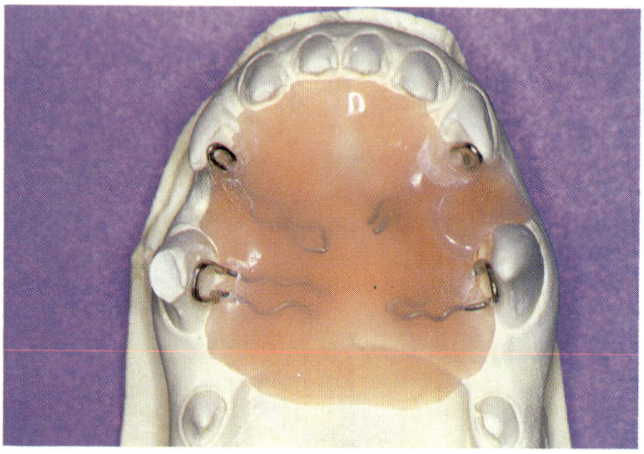

109 Removable appliance on model — Case 5h. The dental laboratory makes an acrylic appliance on the model obtained from the silicone impression.

110 Appliance held in place with small elastic bands — Case 5i. Once an adequate diastema has been created through the retraction of the upper canine, the removable inclined plane appliance can be inserted. The plate is held in place with small elastic ligatures and can be removed, cleaned and reinserted by the owner on a daily basis. Removable upper appliances are desirable for the movement of a single, lower canine tooth. They can be cleaned regularly and therefore cause minimal irritation to the palatal mucosa. The inclined plane's action is to push the lower canine labially as the teeth occlude. Another advantage of a removable appliance is that the progress of the correction can be checked without undoing ligature wires, as would be necessary in the case of a fixed plate, which may also require a general anaesthetic. Note the different brackets, as the ones bonded with composite resin were displaced within a few weeks. In the author's experience the bonding of the orthodontic brackets on dogs' teeth has proved to be more successful with ultra-fine grained methyl methacrylate than with composite resin.

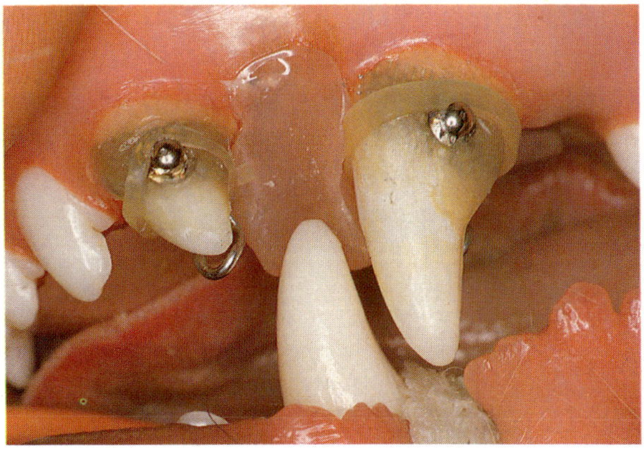

110

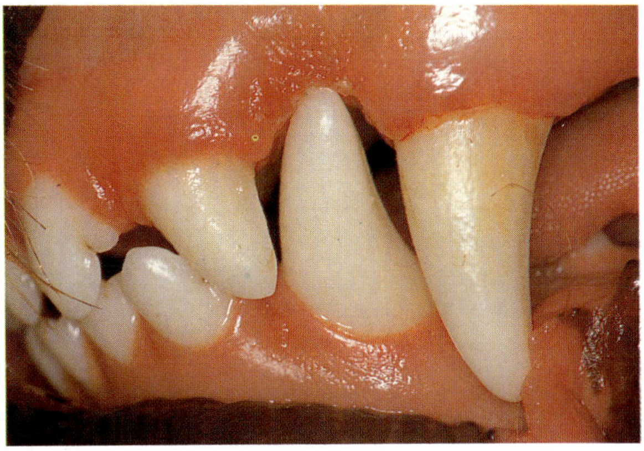

111

111 End result — Case 5j. Final occlusion after the brackets have been removed. The bonding technique does not damage the enamel. The lower canine had been out of appliance therapy for approximately four weeks prior to this photograph. Although some physiological rebound occurs once treatment is stopped, the tooth is still in a non-traumatic position and will remain so.

Expansion screw technique

112 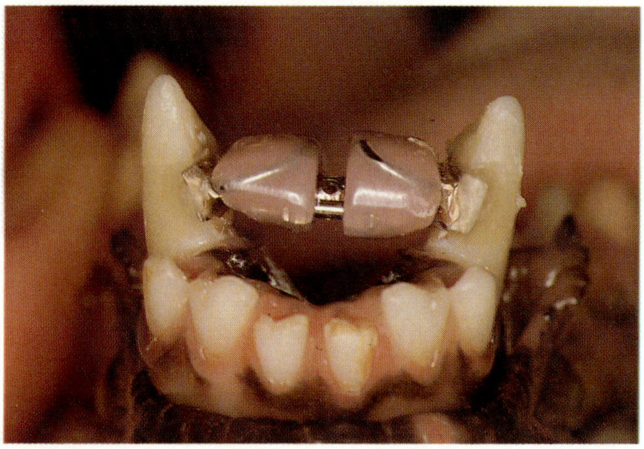

112 Commencement of treatment — Case 6a. If both the lower canines are in a lingual position, instead of an inclined plane, a specially modified expansion screw can be bonded onto the lingual surfaces of the teeth. By adjusting the screw on a regular basis, the tips of the lower canines are pushed labially.

113 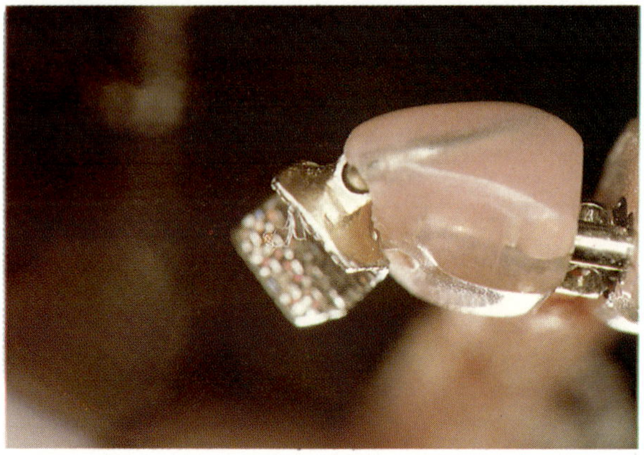

113 Hinge joint — Case 6b. As the teeth become labially inclined, so the angulation of the brackets needs to change in relation to the expansion screw; otherwise, the bond to the enamel will break. The appliance shown was custom-made and incorporates hinge joints at the brackets so that they follow the angulation of the teeth throughout the treatment.

114 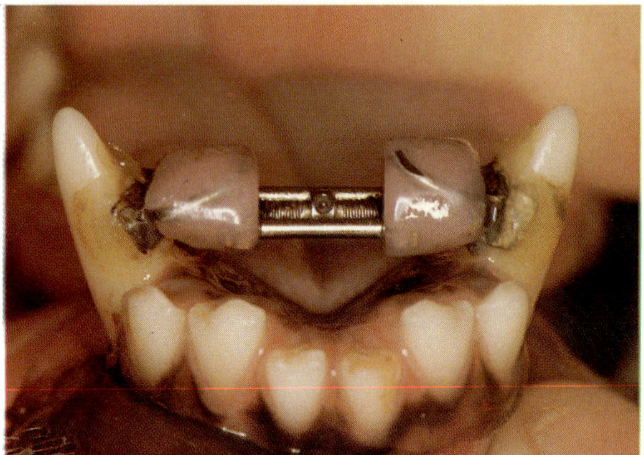

114 Expansion screw *in situ* at end of treatment — Case 6c. The position of the teeth was retained for two months for the alveolar bone to stabilise before the appliance was removed.

Complications of treatment

As previously emphasised, orthodontics in animals should be discouraged at all times unless the animal is suffering pain through its malocclusion or there is gross interference with function. Elective treatment for aesthetic reasons is cruel and unethical. As the photographs below illustrate, even the simplest orthodontic treatment can create unnecessary trauma and pain.

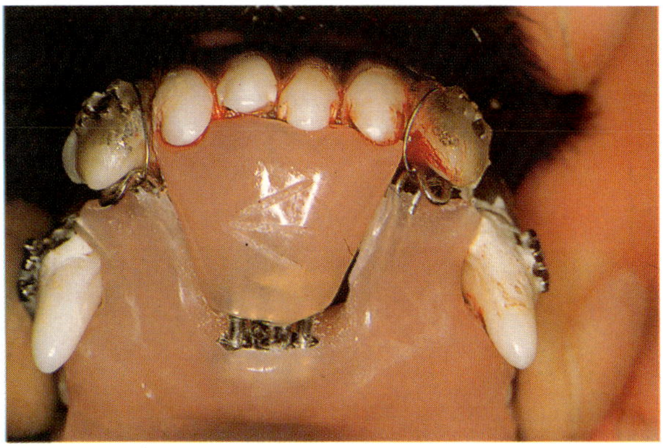

115

115 Fixed appliance — Case 7a. This appliance was wired to the bonded brackets of the teeth, the screw incorporated in the plate being designed to push the incisors over the bite.

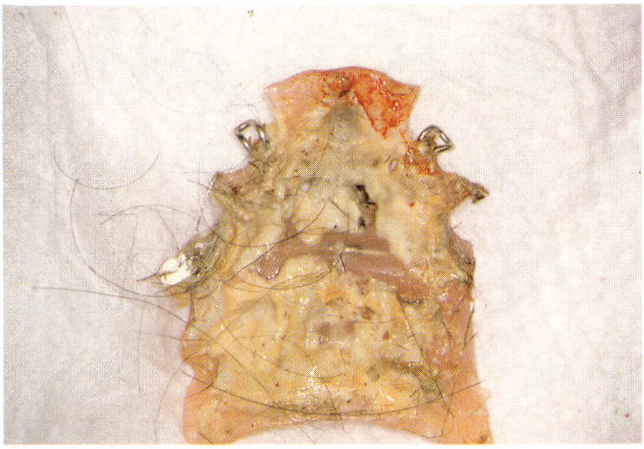

116

116 Food stagnation on plate — Case 7b. As the plate had been wired in the mouth for six weeks, and therefore could not be removed for cleaning, necrotic debris had collected under the appliance.

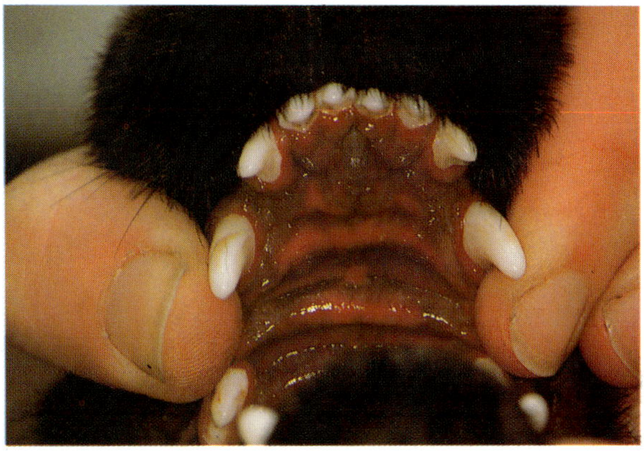

117

117 Inflamed palatal mucosa — Case 7c. The resultant palatal mucosa was extremely inflamed and bled spontaneously.

118

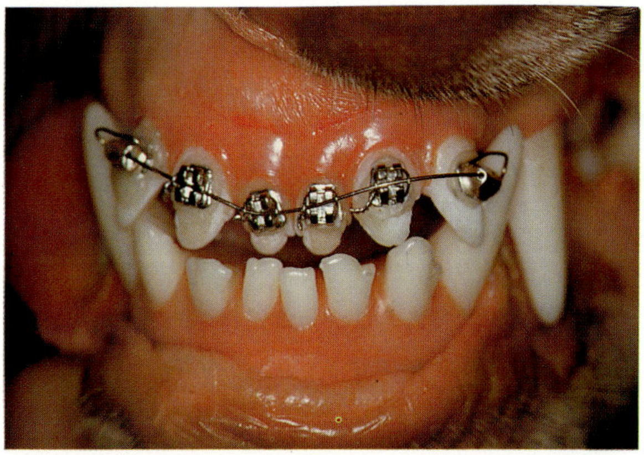

118 Fixed appliance on anteriors — Case 8a. A fixed appliance bonded onto the anterior teeth to correct the incisor relationship.

119

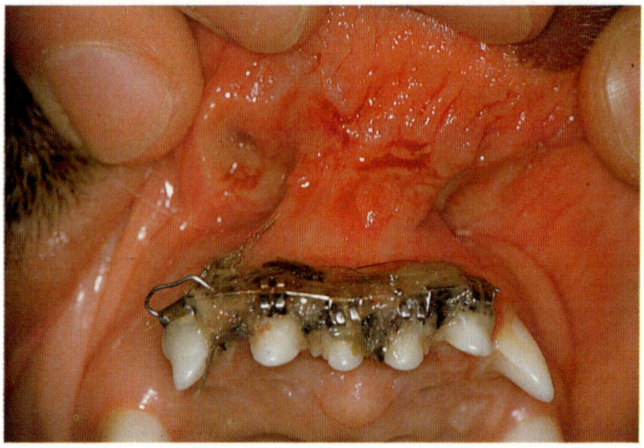

119 Food packing and ulcerated lip — Case 8b. The resultant food packing and the brackets ulcerated the labial mucosa.

6 Periodontal Disease and Treatment

Domestic pets, particularly cats and dogs, suffer from periodontal disease on an epidemic scale. Symptomatic of that is the high level of halitosis displayed by the animals. Indeed a cure for their bad breath is one of the most frequent demands pet owners make of a veterinary surgeon. Periodontal disease is best defined as the inflammation and/or degeneration and destruction of the soft and hard tissues which surround and support the teeth.

There is little doubt that the convenience diet that the domestic pet population is fed contributes to the build-up of debris on the surfaces of their teeth. The food is soft in consistency and requires little mastication, while its stickiness encourages it to cling to the teeth. The food also lacks the fibrous texture and form of a carnivore's natural diet, which would have to be chewed for a considerable time and therefore have a self-cleansing action.

A soft, light-coloured amorphous mass consisting of food debris, leucocytes, micro-organisms and desquamated epithelial cells is established on the surface of the teeth. This is the first stage in the formation of deposits which collectively are called dental or bacterial plaque. If allowed to mature, bacteria invade and proliferate within the matrix of the plaque. Mineralisation of the plaque may take place through the calcium and phosphorous salts present in the saliva. The deposits are then termed 'calculus', the rough surface of which encourages further build-up of plaque.

The aetiology of periodontal disease is complex and controversial. Some mouths have little evidence of inflammation or tissue breakdown in the presence of gross soft and hard dental deposits; by contrast, teeth that may appear relatively clean can be supported by rapidly degenerating periodontal tissues. While it is generally accepted that microbial activity plays a vital role in precipitating the disease, the variation in the individual's susceptibility to the periodontal pathogens, termed the host immune response (host response), is probably one of the most important aspects of the aetiology.

The progress of periodontal disease

The irritation from the endotoxins liberated from the bacterial plaque, depending on the individual's resistance or susceptibility, can initiate a level of localised inflammatory reaction at the gingivae which is termed gingivitis. The clinical picture is of red, swollen gingival margins which bleed easily to the touch. If the disease involves structures beyond the gingivae the name of the condition changes to periodontitis, although research indicates that periodontitis isn't a natural progression of gingivitis. In periodontitis the epithelial attachment migrates apically, and periodontal ligament and alveolar bone support will be destroyed. There is strong evidence that enzymes such as protease, collagenase and elastase play a major role in the breakdown of the periodontal tissues, as collagen is a primary component of periodontal ligament, and 50% of alveolar bone also has an organic component, much of it collagen. There is some controversy regarding the source of the enzymes. Many researchers support the theory that they are liberated by the microbes, while others argue that the infection induced response triggers the defensive action of the leucocytes, which depending on the host response, produce the enzymes that break down the periodontal tissues.

Once lost, alveolar bone will not regenerate, even if the inflammation is arrested. Spaces often develop between the teeth and gums, called periodontal pockets, which in turn harbour further microbial irritants. Periodontal abscesses can occur. Tooth mobility may be apparent and, occasionally, spontaneous exfoliation of the loose teeth occurs. Toxins will constantly be liberated into the bloodstream. Such a chronic bacteraemia can be an important contributing factor in the aetiology of endocarditis, nephritis, hepatitis or amyloidosis; hence, the systemic importance of eliminating periodontal disease.

120 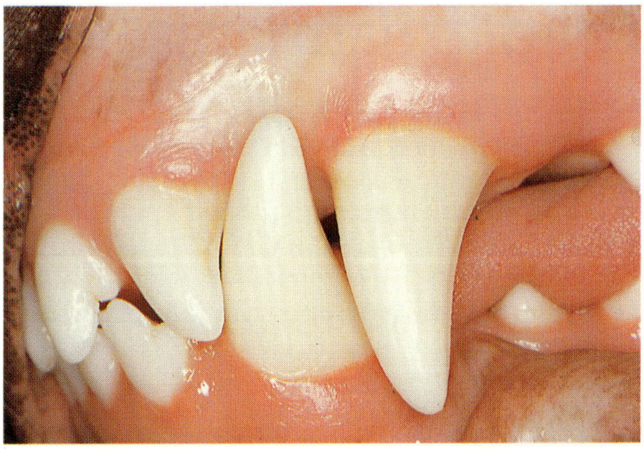

120 Normal gingiva. Healthy gingiva has a pale pink colour with natural pigmentation. The gingiva is not shiny, but has a matt 'orange peel' appearance. It is firmly attached to the teeth with no appreciable space other than a shallow gingival sulcus that exists between the teeth and the gums. No spontaneous bleeding occurs if the gingival sulcus is probed.

121 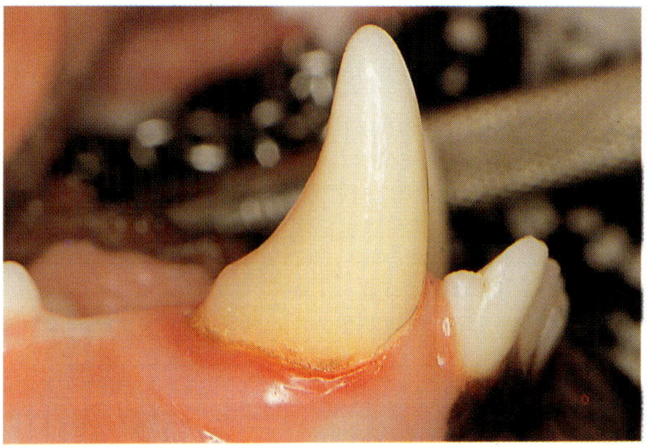

121 Gingivitis. In the first stage of periodontal disease the gingival margin becomes shiny, puffy and engorged with blood. Bacterial plaque or calculus deposits may be evident. Some false pocketing is usually present, and the gingival sulcus bleeds easily when probed gently. 'False' is the term used, as at this stage no apical migration of the epithelial attachment has taken place, and a decrease in the inflammatory condition would result in reversal of the defects.

122 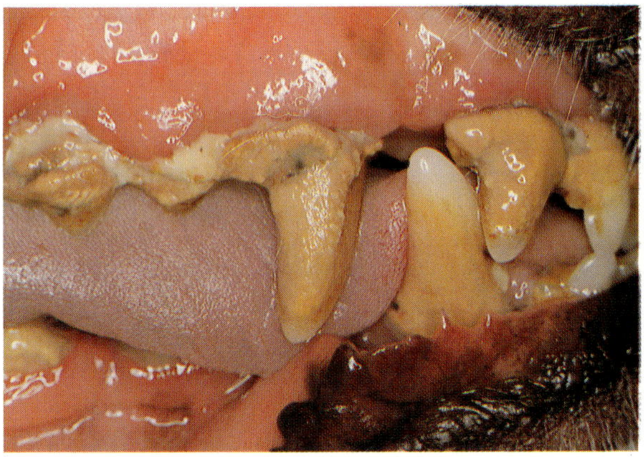

122 Chronic periodontitis — calculus deposits. At this stage the inflammation has progressed beyond the gingival tissues, the gingival margin has lost its natural congruence and a moderate degree of plaque or supragingival calculus may be present.

123 Chronic periodontitis. Heavy deposits of soft bacterial plaque are present. The level of halitosis may be very strong. The destruction has progressed to the deeper structures and true pocketing is present. This means that apical migration of the epithelial attachment has occurred and even if the level of inflammation was reversed the depth of the pockets would not revert to the shallow dimension of a healthy gingival sulcus. The pockets bleed easily on probing and some alveolar bone loss has taken place.

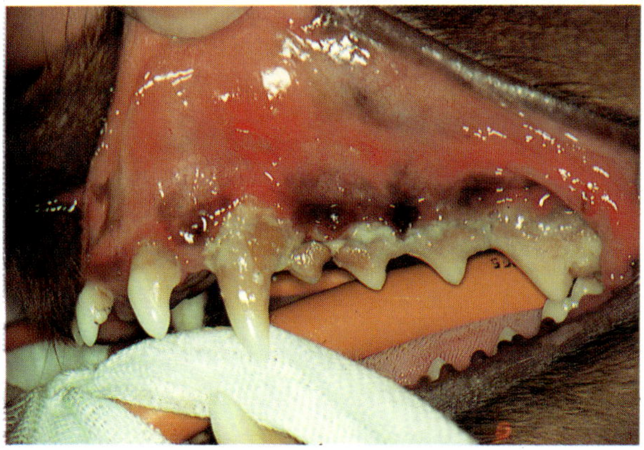
123

124 Calculus with hyperplastic gingivitis. Hyperplastic gingivitis occurs in some breeds more readily than in others. Although it can give the impression of severe periodontal involvement, the pocketing may be false with no alveolar bone destruction or apical migration of the epithelial attachment, but it is not reversible.

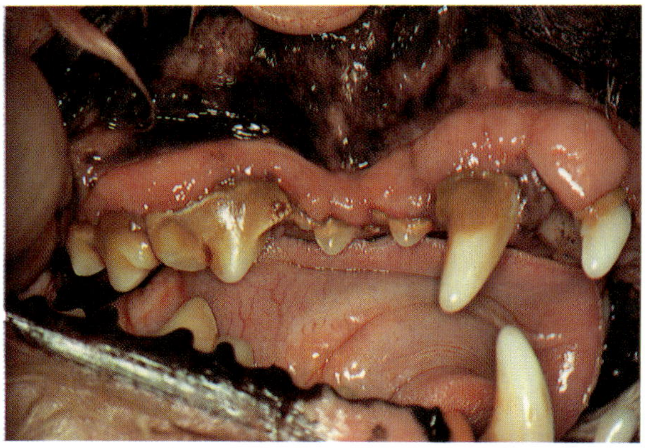
124

125 Advanced periodontitis. The gingiva has acquired a highly irregular appearance around the lower canine and bleeds profusely on probing. Deep pockets have formed and a considerable height of alveolar bone has been lost. Some mobility of the tooth may be present and periodontal abscesses may occur due to the stagnation of the bacteria in the dead space of the deep pockets. Extraction of the tooth is the treatment of choice.

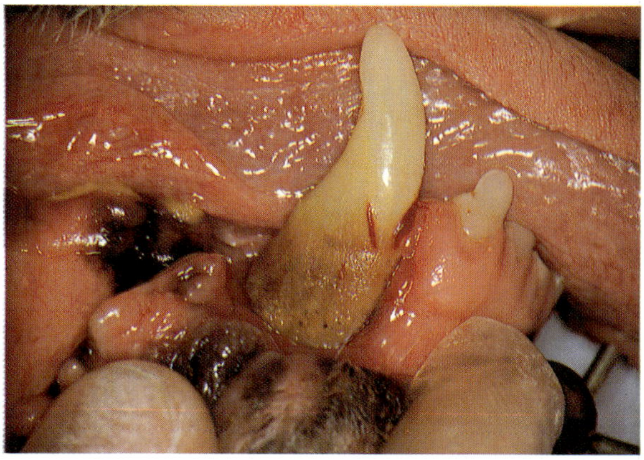
125

126 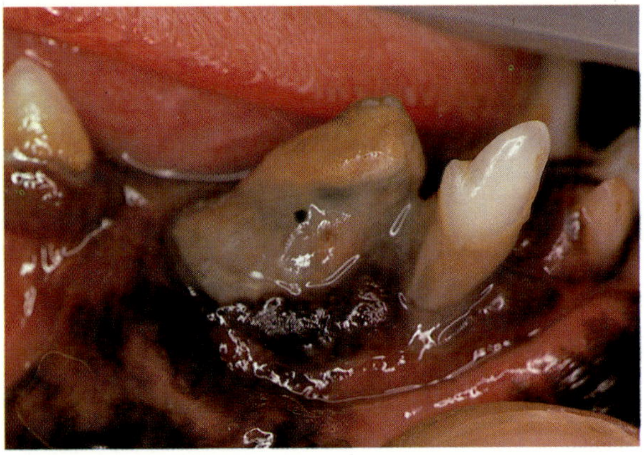

126 Terminal periodontitis. The gingival pocketing is virtually down to the root apices and no bone support remains to the affected teeth. The teeth are extremely mobile and there is a continuous discharge of purulent material from the pockets. Spontaneous exfoliation of the teeth may occur.

127 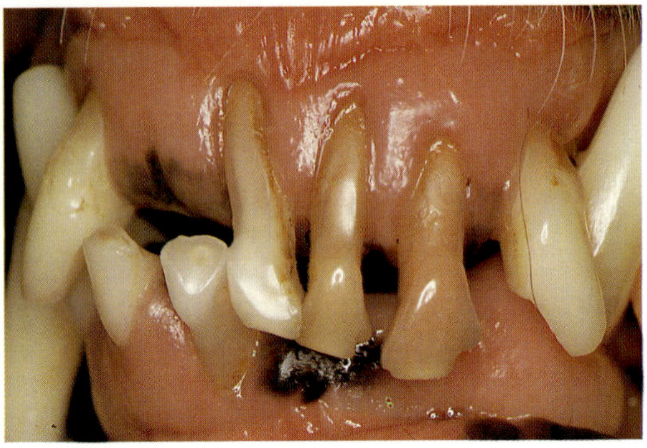

127 Severe recession. Gingival recession or alveolar bone loss does not necessarily lead to active periodontal disease and tooth loss. This aged animal demonstrated good gingival condition and the incisors were firm. No treatment was indicated.

128 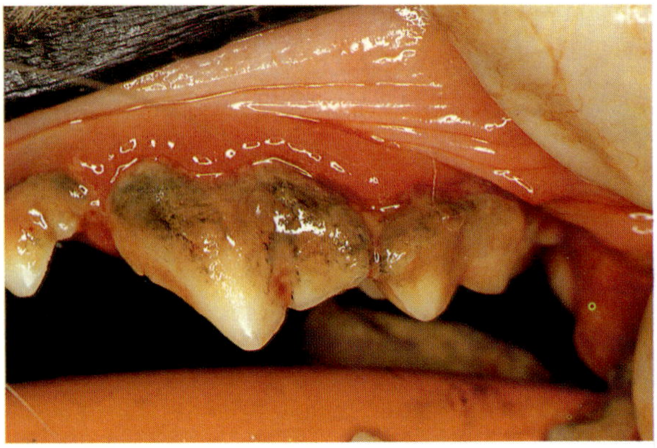

128 Severe periodontitis with no calculus deposits. This case illustrates severe periodontitis with minimal bacterial plaque or calculus, although some staining is present. The animal was suffering with severe halitosis, pocketing, alveolar bone loss and tooth mobility. Extraction was the only realistic treatment.

129 Heavy calculus deposits. Note the heavy calcified deposits on the teeth; also, the lack of inflammation of the gingivae. The bone support was good and there was no pocketing. Although calculus deposits may have a physically irritant affect on the gingivae, they do not necessarily contribute to destructive periodontal disease. The host response to the bacterial toxins is the key factor in the severity of the disease. The severity of the calculus deposits are partly determined by the self-cleansing properties of the diet and genetic factors that determine the calcium and phosphorus levels in the saliva.

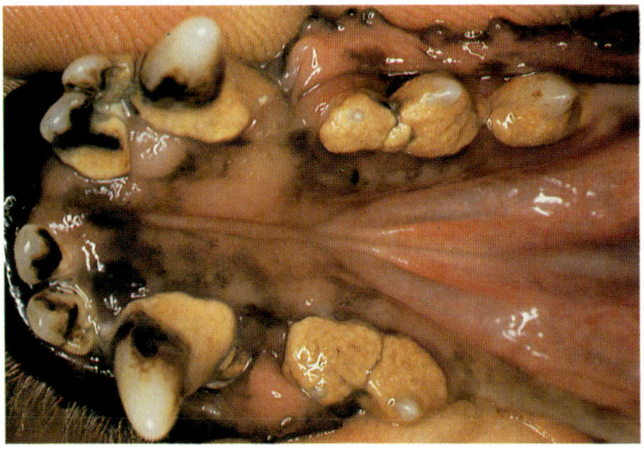
129

130 Acute ulcerative gingivitis. Acute ulcerative gingivitis usually occurs more frequently among small toy breeds of dogs. The organisms present in the lesions are usually teaming with the spirochaete *Borrelia vincenti* and *Fusobacterium vincenti.* A symbiotic relationship between the organisms has been put forward as a factor in the aetiology. The condition often has a strong level of halitosis and ulceration of the interdental gingival papillae occurs. Treatment with systemic metronidazole can be beneficial to control the acute phase. Once healing has taken place, however, the original shape of the gingivae will not recover and the flattened papillae will remain. An excellent long-term oral hygiene regime is required to prevent food and bacterial stagnation in the interdental spaces, or recurrences will occur.

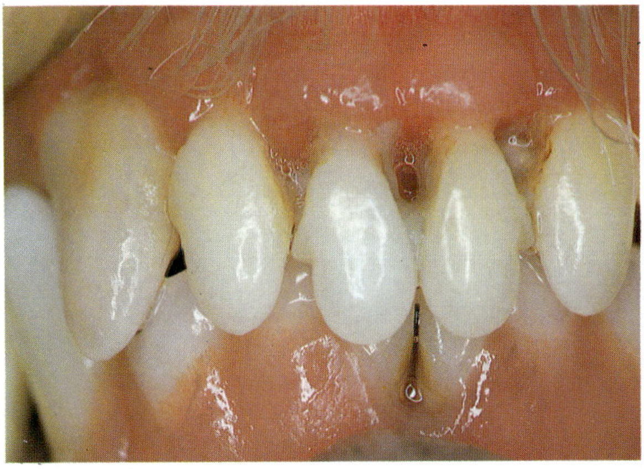
130

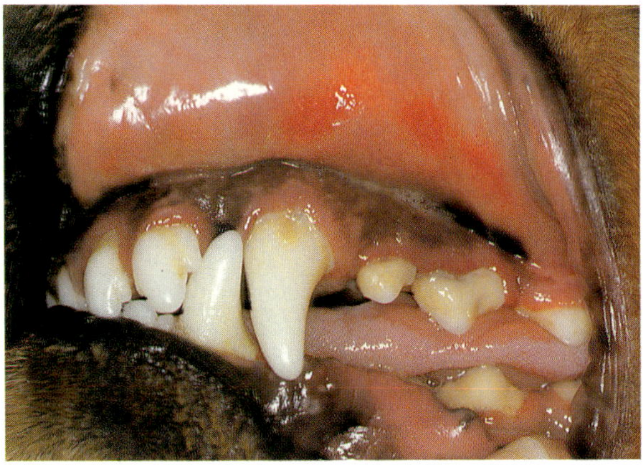
131

131 Labial and buccal ulcerations — ulcerative stomatitis. Certain breeds, such as spaniels and greyhounds, are more prone to the condition, even at a young age. Usually, it only affects the mucosa lying against the upper canines and premolars. Pressure against the teeth covered with bacterial plaque has a strong association with the condition. The aetiology is unclear, although uraemia and autoimmune conditions have been implicated.

132 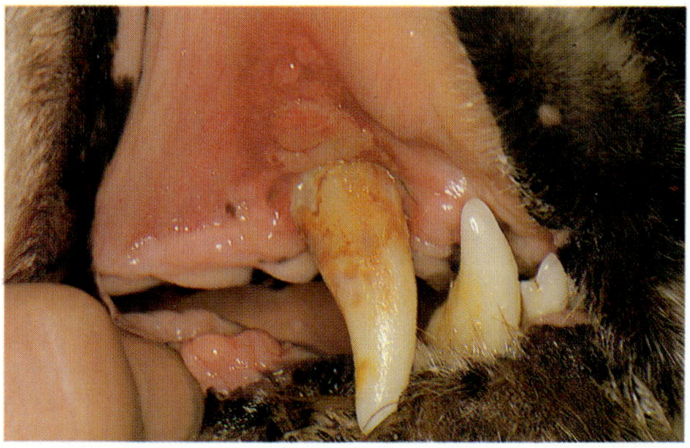

132 Severe labial ulceration. Ulceration of the labial mucosa is often mistaken for acute gingivitis. Usually, the level of halitosis is high. Antibiotic or antifungal therapy and rigorous oral hygiene regimes have not demonstrated a long-term improvement. Extraction of the teeth adjacent to the affected labial mucosa usually improves the condition and alleviates the symptoms.

133 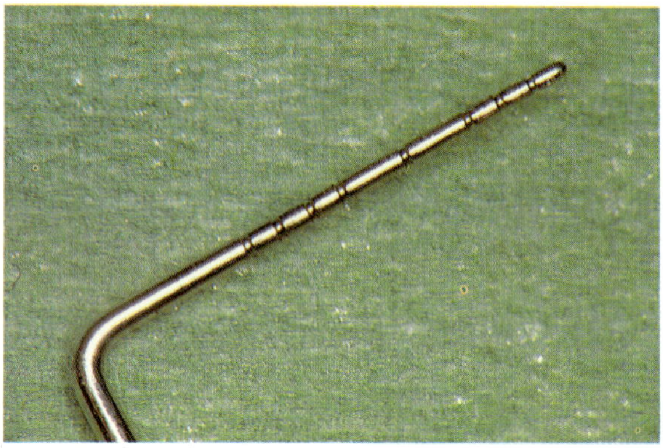

133 Pocket probe. Pocket probes, graduated in millimetres, are the most useful instruments for examining the periodontal condition and measuring the pocket depths.

134 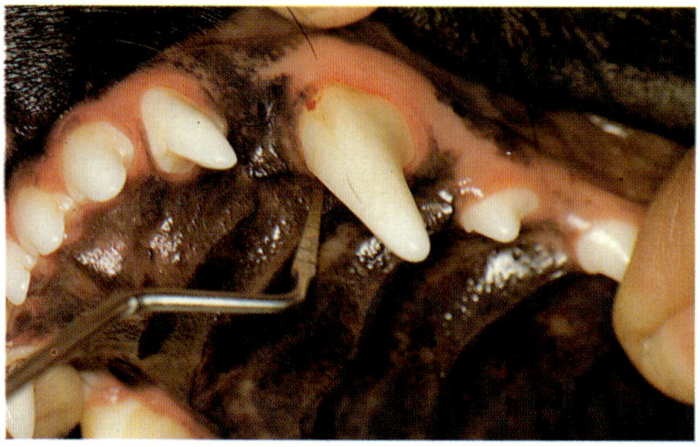

134 Measuring the depth of the defect. The normal depth of the gingival sulcus will obviously vary with the size of the animal. The yardstick of 2 mm for the normal depth in humans cannot be related to the veterinary environment. As a guide, the depth of the gingival sulcus in domestic carnivores with healthy gingivae will be negligible. Pocket depths less than one-quarter of the total root length are considered as clinically normal, while depths greater than one-quarter may be considered as pathological.

135 Gingival bleeding. The level of gingival bleeding that is elicited by gentle pocket probing is a reasonable indication of the periodontal inflammation present.

135

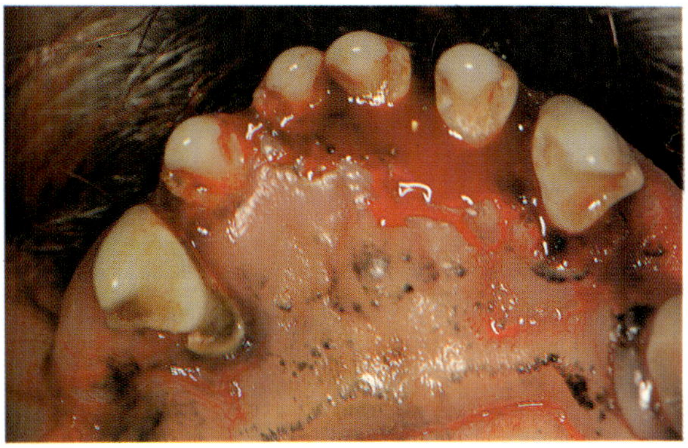

136 Subgingival calculus. It is important to investigate the level of subgingival calculus deposits that are not obvious to the casual observer. Their presence may be indicated by a dark line at the gingival margins, because they are darker in colour than supragingival deposits. They are also far more destructive than supragingival calculus.

136

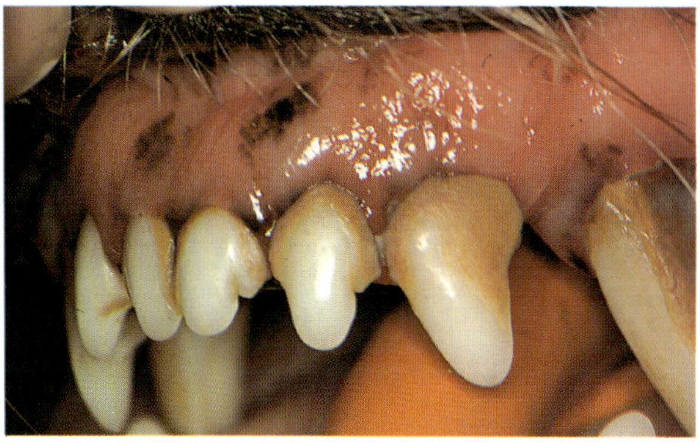

137 Subgingival calculus palatally. It is vital to investigate palatal pockets, especially around the canine teeth. These pockets, which may be extremely deep, occasionally extend to the apices of the teeth and cause oronasal fistulas, leading to chronic rhinitis, even when the teeth are still in situ.

137

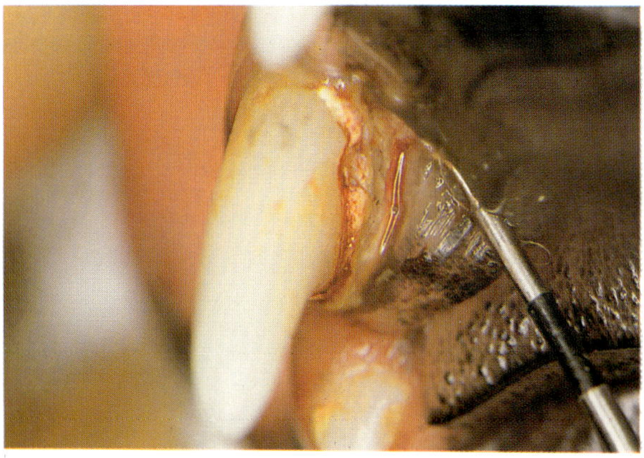

138

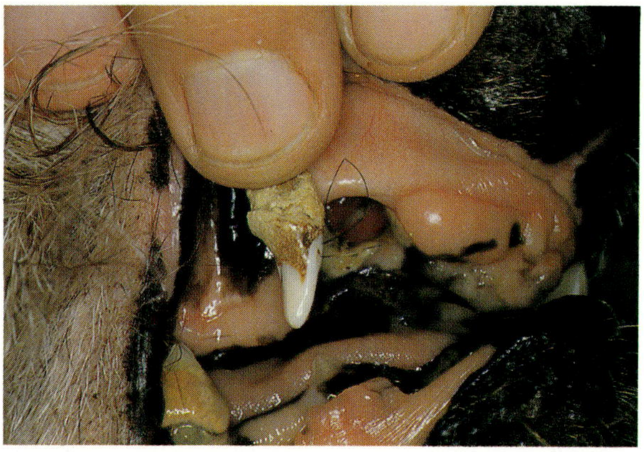

138 Oronasal fistula with exfoliated tooth — Case 1a. This upper canine was spontaneously exfoliated. Heavy deposits of long-standing subgingival calculi are evident. The periodontal disease has contributed to the destruction of the thin alveolar bone between the socket and the nasal cavity, resulting in the oronasal fistula.

139

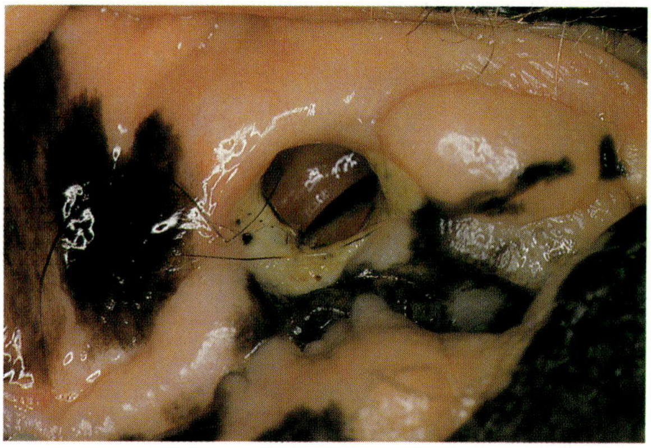

139 Close-up of fistula — Case 1b. The fistula contributed to chronic rhinitis.

140

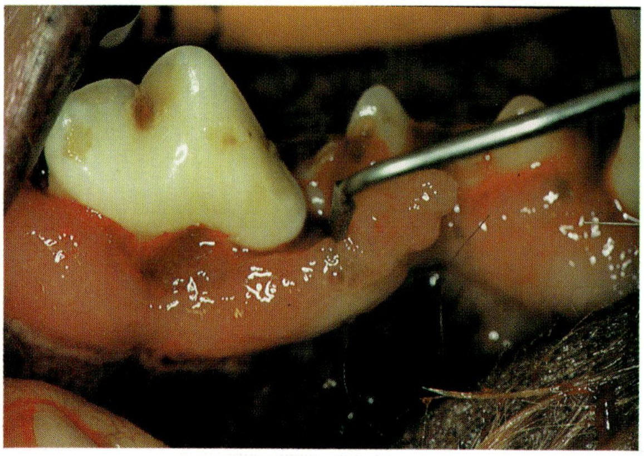

140 Deep pocketing. A pocket probe demonstrates the depth of a periodontal pocket. The treatment plan must be based on a number of factors: mobility, level of infection, bone loss and anaesthetic risks. In this case, extraction was the treatment of choice.

141 Palatal pocket. A deep infrabony periodontal defect was present at the furcation of the roots of the upper fourth premolar. Extraction was the treatment of choice.

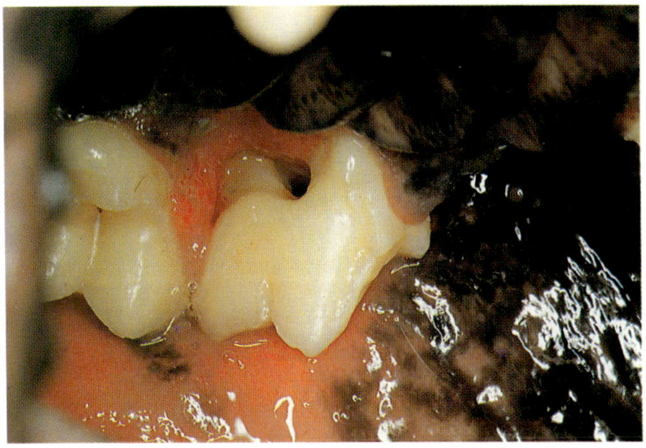
141

142 Bifurcations exposed. Although there had been some bone loss and food stagnation is taking place in this aged dog, these are not sufficient criteria for extractions. The teeth are firm and there is minimal pocketing: extractions would create considerable trauma in this brittle mandible, where the teeth may be ankylosed to the bone. The retention of the teeth is advisable in this case.

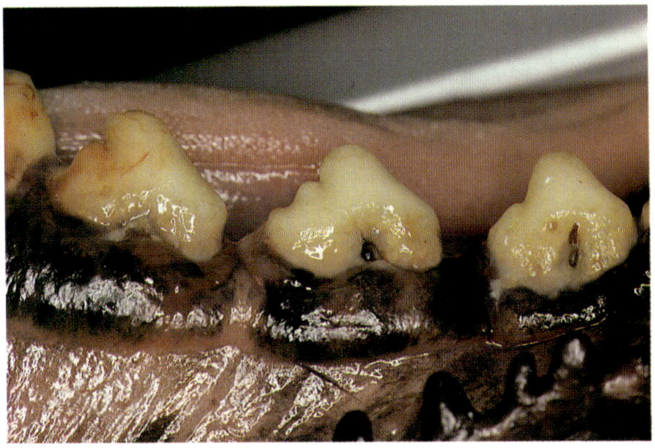
142

143 Haemorrhage from buccal sulcus — Case 2a. Occasionally, deep periodontal pockets may contribute to uncontrollable haemorrhages. In this case it occurred through the sinus tract evident in the buccal sulcus.

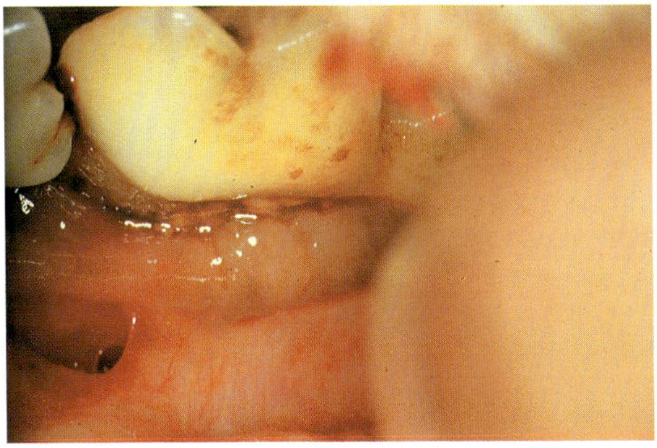
143

144

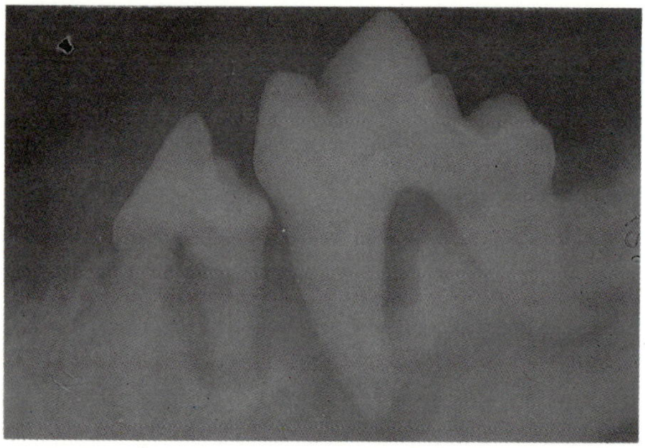

144 Radiograph of 143 — Case 2b. The depth of alveolar bone destruction associated with chronic periodontal disease is visible on this periapical radiograph. It contributed to the severe haemorrhage from the mandibular artery. The weakened mandible presented a risk of a pathological fracture, or one of iatrogenic origin during extraction. The teeth involved were carefully extracted through a flap procedure and the integrity of the mandible was maintained.

145

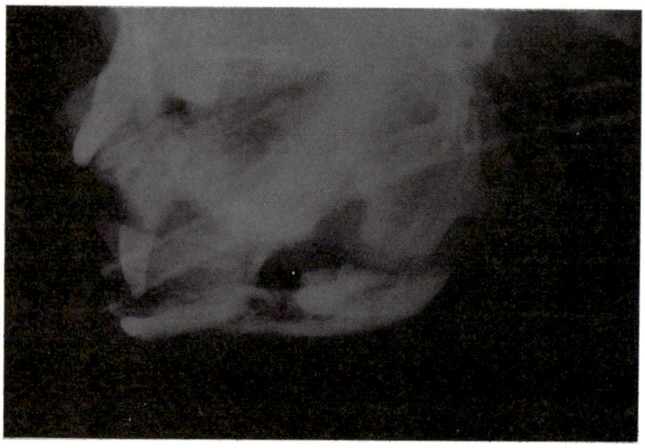

145 Pathological fracture of mandible. The animal presented with anorexia. This radiograph shows a pathological fracture through the socket of a periodontally involved lower premolar.

146

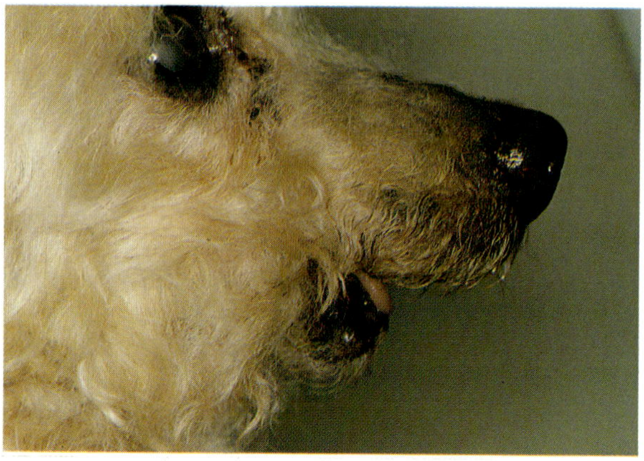

146 Rostral aspect of mandible destroyed. Chronic periodontal disease was responsible for long-standing osteomyelitis, which destroyed the rostral aspect of the body of the mandible. The dog was having difficulty in eating.

Feline periodontal disease

Chronic idiopathic feline stomatitis is a common condition characterised by halitosis, signs of oral pain, anorexia, hypersalivation, gingival ulcerations and haemorrhages. Because of the appearance of these lesions, it is important to bear in mind the differential diagnosis of oral neoplasms when chronic stomatitis is suspected. Feline viral diseases have been implicated in the aetiology of chronic feline gingivitis/stomatitis through immunosuppression. Although tests for viral diseases have been advocated, the prime objective of the dental treatment must be palliative.

Acute periodontal diseases in cats can become life-threatening under certain circumstances. The oral bacterial flora is strongly influenced by the presence of the teeth: the quantity and types of organisms found in the mouth are considerably reduced on the extraction of teeth adjacent to areas of inflammation. In a domestic situation these animals manage extremely well in a partial or fully edentulous state and operators must be realistic in conserving teeth in a mouth where periodontal disease or idiopathic stomatitis is rampant.

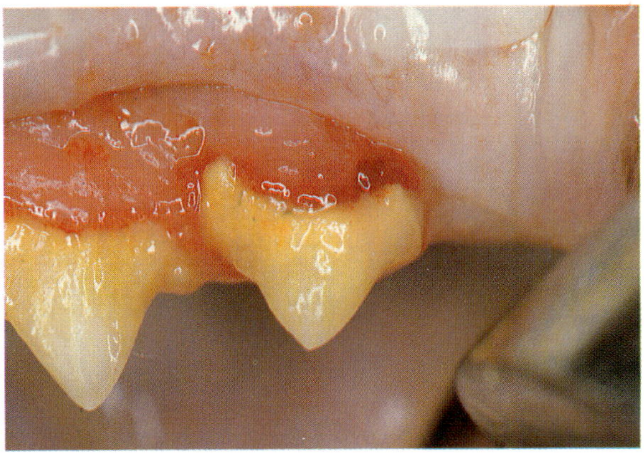

147

147 Marginal gingivitis. Marginal gingivitis in a cat with a minimal degree of calculus deposits present.

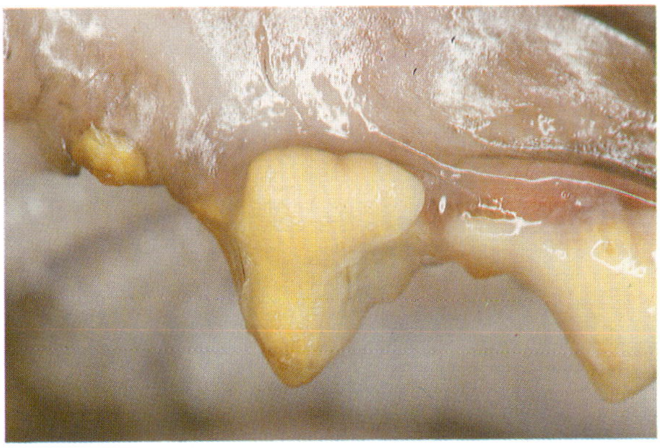

148

148 Heavy deposit of calculus — Case 3a.

149 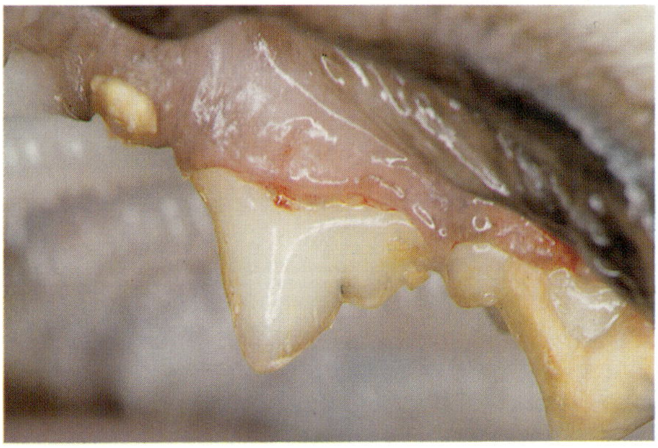

149 Calculus deposit removed — Case 3b. The removal of the deposit reveals a healthy gingival condition. As with canids, it is not the level of calculus that determines the state of the periodontal condition but the host response or the state of the immune defence system of the animal.

150 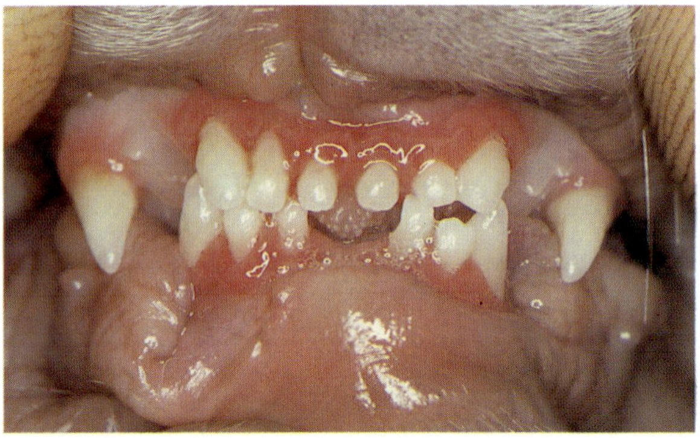

150 Periodontosis. A highly destructive form of periodontal disease where the teeth become mobile and are lost at a very young age due to rapid bone destruction.

151 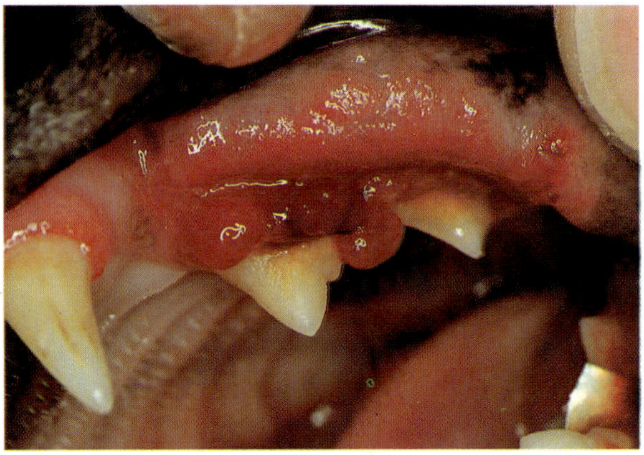

151 Hyperplastic gingivitis. With a compromised or suppressed immune defence system, a severe form of gingivitis and stomatitis are often seen. The gingivae are hyperplastic and haemorrhagic.

152 Purulent stomatitis — Case 4a. A more advanced stage, purulent stomatitis may extend into the oropharynx, with fatal results. The condition responds poorly to conservative treatment. The long-term prognosis must be guarded, but it appears that the extraction of the teeth adjacent to the gingivitis at an early stage of the disease and empirical treatment of the animal systemically with short-term antibiotics and anti-inflammatory medication encourages healing.

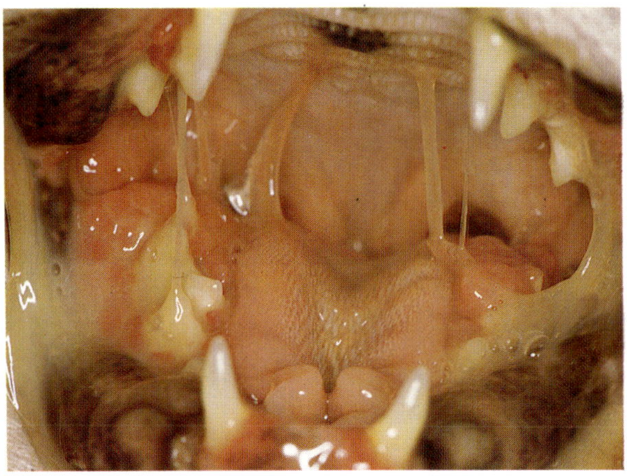

152

153 One month postoperative — Case 4b. Some improvement is seen in the oral condition after extraction of the teeth associated with the stomatitis and systemic treatment with corticosteroids and antibiotics.

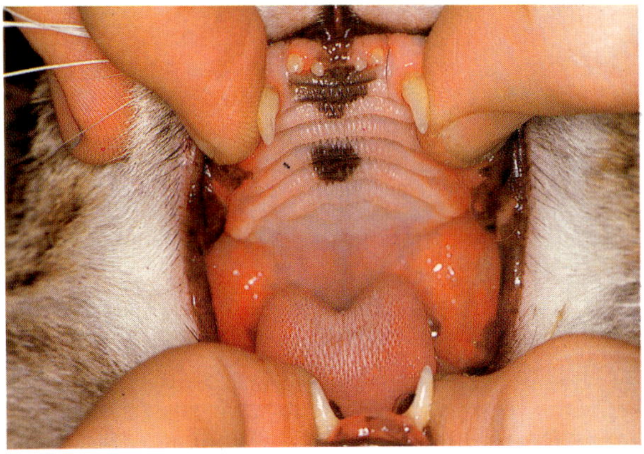

153

Periodontal treatment

Periodontal disease is a multifaceted condition. Usually there is no simple, single therapy to alleviate the condition. Treatment is often palliative, eliminating the signs and symptoms in tune with an accurate diagnosis. Periodontal treatment is divided into two equally important areas:

- *Professional treatment.* This involves scaling, polishing, elimination of any stagnation areas, extractions and motivating and instructing the client in oral hygiene techniques for their pets.
- *Home care and maintenance.* The utilisation of dietary and artificial oral hygiene aids by owners.

The importance of both areas must be stressed: they are strongly interrelated, so that failure of one will inevitably cause failure of the treatment as a whole.

Professional periodontal treatment (hygiene treatment)

This is usually understood to mean scaling, but it is much more than a haphazard removal of calcified deposits from the teeth. Dental hygiene treatment is a highly disciplined and skilled procedure. It must be carried out systematically, with a full understanding of the underlying pathology, objectives and limitations of the treatment. Without full knowledge of the underlying principles and the appropriate skills, irreversible damage may be done to the surfaces of the teeth through careless scaling, which will only exacerbate the periodontal disease.

Scaling and polishing involves the removal of the soft and mineralised pathogens from the surfaces of the teeth as atraumatically as possible; this leaves the surfaces smooth, which discourages the build-up of further deposits.

The underlying principle of scaling is that calcified deposits are fractured away from the surfaces of the teeth. It is usually performed with hand or ultrasonic instruments. These should go hand in hand as they both play an important role in achieving a first-class result in the minimum of time.

Hand scaling

Hand scaling involves placing the sharp edge of the instrument blade apical to the calcified deposits on the teeth and, while a finger rest is maintained, moving the instrument tip by a pulling action in a coronal direction. This action is repeated around the circumference of each tooth until all the deposits are removed. A large choice of hand instruments is available and they need to be used in sets so as to facilitate the correct angulation to the root surface during the scaling procedure.

Mechanical scaling

As hand scaling is a time-consuming and arduous procedure if a thorough result is to be achieved, there have been constant efforts made to automate the procedure. Ultrasonic instrumentation is often used for the rapid removal of gross deposits. The ultrasonic unit converts electromagnetic impulses into mechanical oscillations at the rate of 22,000–40,000 cycles/sec. The water spray is an important element in the ultrasonic scaling procedure as it not only cools the tooth and the instrument and irrigates the debris away from the site but it also has an important cavitating action. The underlying principle is that microscopic bubbles are created on the surfaces of the teeth and the bursting of these bubbles helps to loosen the deposits, hence the name Cavitron.

The principle of scaling is to fracture the calcified deposits away from the surface of the teeth through the power and nature of the vibrations of the instrument as well as the cavitation effect. The strength of attachment of the calculus to the tooth surface is not proportional to their thickness; hence, the futility of fracturing large deposits away with forceps and the potential damage such a procedure may create. Fine scaling would still need to be carried out with hand scalers, as only with these does one have the tactile sensation to eliminate stubborn subgingival deposits, which have the maximum potential to damage the periodontal tissues.

The choice of ultrasonic scaler should be made with care: there is variation in the power and efficiency of different makes and it is important to try the unit for efficiency and ease of operation before making a purchase.

In the author's experience, some of the human ultrasonic units have been designed with the conscious patient in mind, where maximum power is not usually desirable. Some very powerful, sophisticated units have proved to be unreliable when receiving rough treatment in a veterinary environment. On the other hand, some veterinary units have been found to be low powered, as they seem to have been designed with the cost factor in mind. In the author's experience, subsonic, air-driven oscillating scalers have proved to be less powerful than true ultrasonic units.

Rotary scalers are modified dental burrs operated in an air turbine drill. In the author's opinion these instruments are much more difficult to handle than oscillating units or hand scalers and potentially far greater damage can be inflicted on the teeth and the surrounding tissues with them.

154

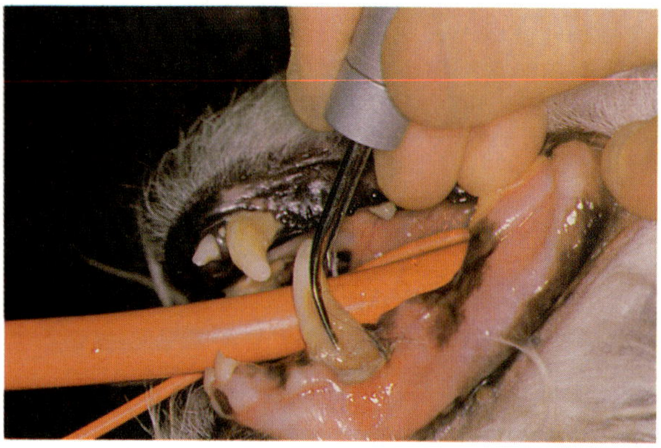

154 Instrument grip and fulcrum rest. The correct way to hold a scaler, be it a hand or powered instrument, is with a modified pen grip, between the thumb, first and third finger. Either the second and/or third finger of the hand should be used as a rest (fulcrum) on either the adjacent teeth or edentulous ridge: only in this way can the operator have complete control over the instrument. In a carnivore's mouth almost all the buccal and labial surfaces can be scaled through direct vision; at the same time, the contralateral palatal and lingual surfaces can be treated before the animal is turned for the opposite surfaces.

155 Hand scaling — Step 1. Using a hand instrument with the shape of the working tip that is most accurately adapted to the contours of the tooth surface to be worked on, the sharp blade edge is placed at the apical aspect of the calculus deposit to be removed.

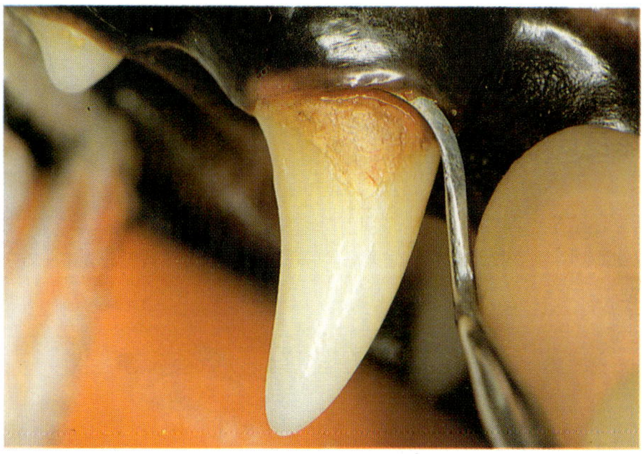

155

156 Hand scaling — Step 2. Maintaining the blade parallel to the gingival tissues and the fulcrum support to the hand, short forceful strokes are made in a coronal direction using finger movements only or using a short rotating action of the wrist, whereby the instrument blade is moved coronally to break away the calcified deposit. It is imperative to keep the angulation of the blade and its approximation to the tooth surface unchanged so the instrument does not damage the tooth surface by digging into it.

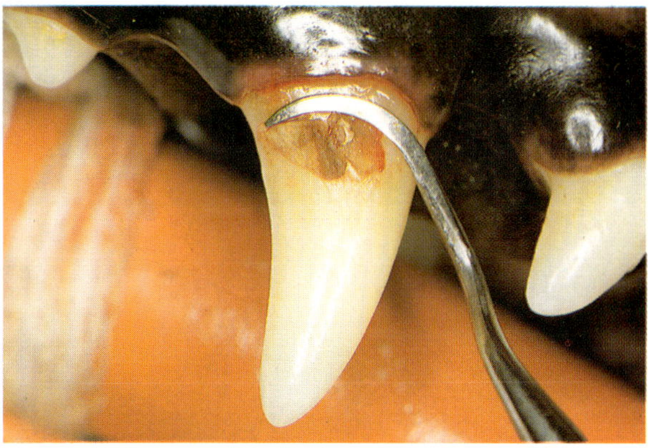

156

157 *Incorrect* use of scaler tip. The most serious error of scaling technique that untrained personnel make is to use the pointed tips of scalers to dig and scratch at the calculus. ***Do not do this under any circumstances,*** as it causes irreversible damage to the tooth surfaces, and the resultant roughness encourages a rapid build-up of new deposits.

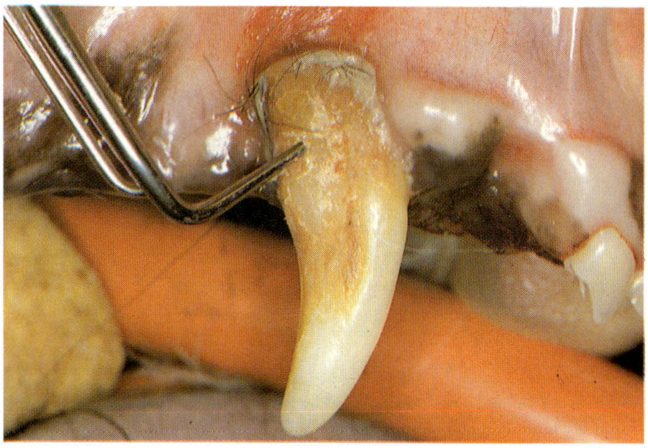

157

158

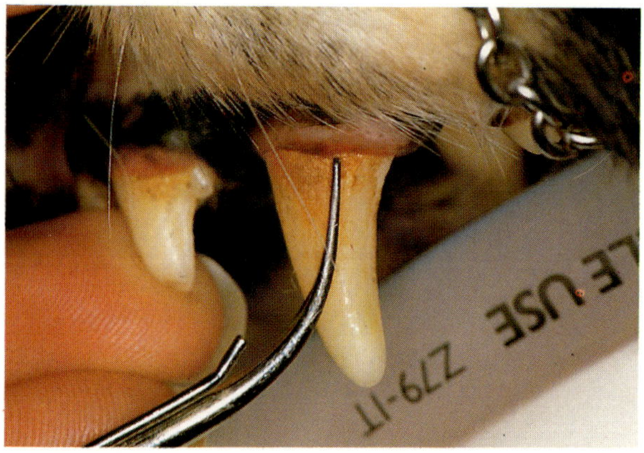

158 Correct use of ultrasonic scaler tip. The correct technique is to employ the side of the instrument and apply only moderate pressure through the ultrasonic scaler tip to the deposits being worked on. This way, the minimum of damage will be created to the teeth, leaving a relatively smooth surface. It is important to remember that increased pressure to the ultrasonic scaler tips will slow down the instrument, creating excessive heat at the point of contact to the tooth. This may cause irreversible pulpal damage to the teeth of the anaesthetised patient. All personnel engaged in the use of the ultrasonic scaler should apply the tip to their own fingernails to experience the level of heat that can be generated through excessive pressure.

159

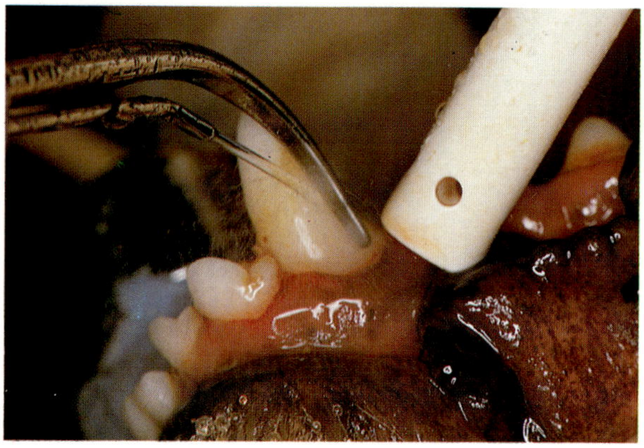

159 Irrigation and mechanical aspiration. Ultrasonic scalers, by their action, create considerable heat. The correct level of irrigation is vital: first, it prevents overheating of the instrument and the teeth; secondly, water irrigation is necessary for the creation of micro bubbles, the bursting of which is an integral part of the scaling procedure (cavitation principle). Aspiration equipment, if available, is invaluable in evacuating loose calculus, water and blood, thus minimising the chance of complications through inhalation.

160

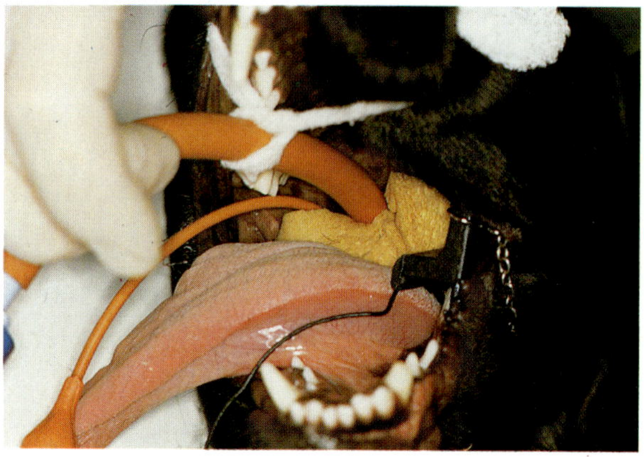

160 Throat pack. Water and debris are easily inhaled by the unconscious patient during general anaesthesia and can lead to serious consequences. One must protect the airway. Do not rely solely on endotracheal tubes: they may not be a close fit, or the inflatable cuff may be punctured. Use a properly designed sponge throat pack around the endotracheal tube, with a safety cord attached to it. Do not use cotton wool; as well as having poor water absorption properties, it can be lost or forgotten with fatal results.

161 Aerosol — mask and glasses. Ultrasonic scaling creates a bacterial aerosol. It is essential for operators to protect themselves with masks to minimise the dangers of aerosol inhalation.

161

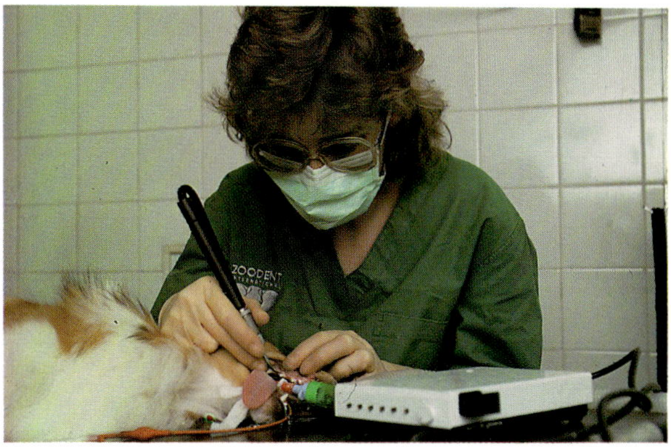

162 Curette — subgingival calculus. This model demonstrates subgingival deposits, which can be highly destructive and must be removed. Scaling at this depth cannot be performed efficiently mechanically, and manual instruments need to be used. However, the practicality of retaining teeth with very deep pockets needs to be carefully assessed, as home care and maintenance of such defects will be impractical. Progressive bone destruction at the base of a deep pocket may lead to oronasal fistulas in the maxilla or pathological fractures of the mandible.

162

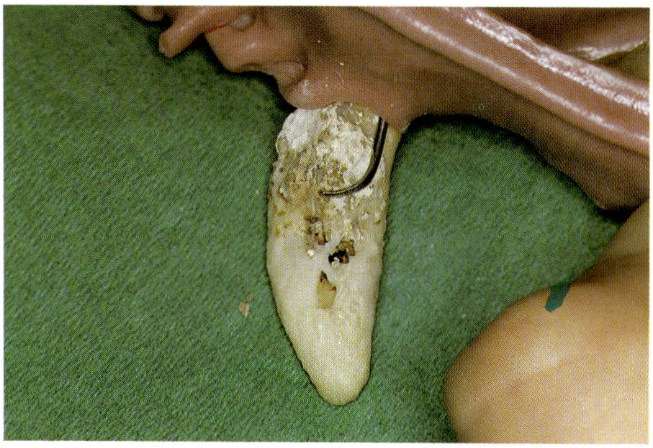

Periodontal surgery

Periodontal surgery in veterinary dentistry plays a very limited role. The long-term prognosis of periodontally involved teeth must be assessed in a practical way. The retention of such teeth for aesthetic, functional or social reasons is not a necessity and the maintenance of a moderate degree of periodontal disease would involve repeated general anaesthetics. Often, home care cannot be maintained to the high level necessary and in many cases of advanced periodontal disease extraction of the teeth is the treatment of choice.

163

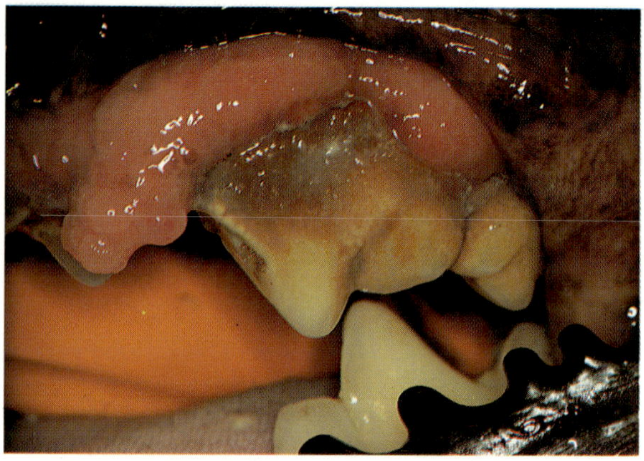

163 Hyperplastic gingivitis — Case 5a. Occasionally, simple gingival surgery in the form of a gingivectomy can be beneficial in eliminating false pockets as in the case of hyperplastic gingivitis. It is a useful procedure when a good support of alveolar bone is present. This simple form of surgery can eliminate the dead space of a pocket, which harbours debris of hair, bacterial plaque, etc.

164

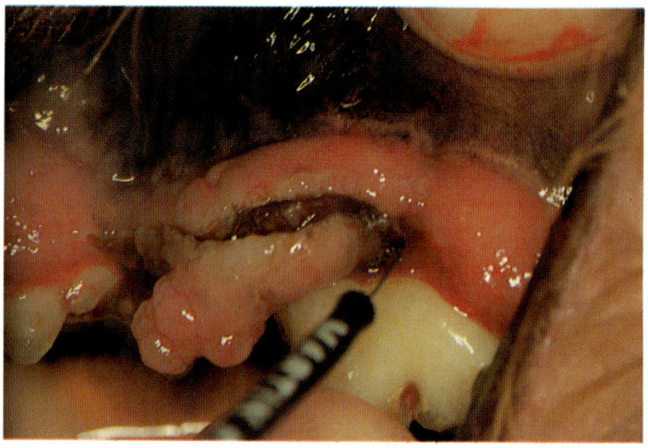

164 Gingivectomy — Case 5b. The underlying principle is to make a horizontal incision with either a scalpel or electrosurgery at the previously measured pocket depths, bevelling it into healthy gingivae.

165 Curetting resected gingivae — Case 5c. The resected gingiva is curetted away. Most non-dental operators are afraid to either scale subgingivally or aggressively curette the gingival tissues in case they cause damage to the soft tissues. Certainly, careless treatment is of no benefit, but the gingival tissues have great powers of healing. Careful and controlled elimination of granulation as well as hyperplastic inflammatory gingivae can help in improving the oral environment to aid in the maintenance of periodontal health.

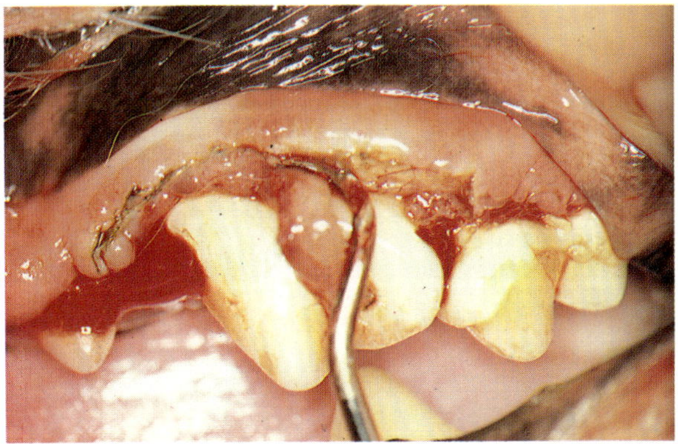
165

166 Postoperative appearance of gingivectomy — Case 5d. Once the hyperplastic gingiva is removed the previous subgingival defects are exposed. In this way, any home care can remove the bacterial plaque that would otherwise stagnate in the gingival pockets.

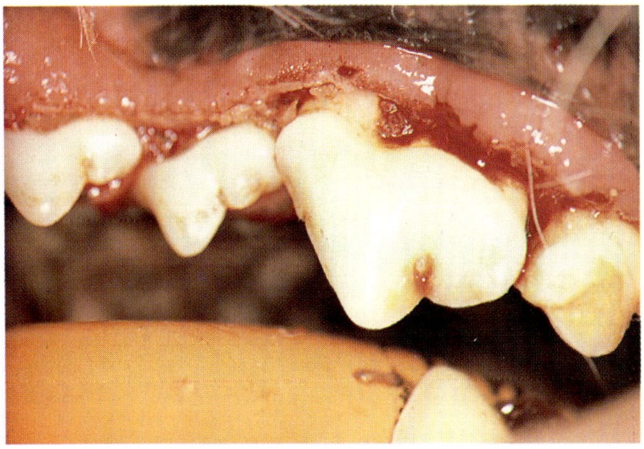
166

Polishing

167 Calculus — scanning electron micrograph (SEM). This SEM demonstrates the porous, rough surface of calculus deposits, which encourages further deposition of bacterial plaque.

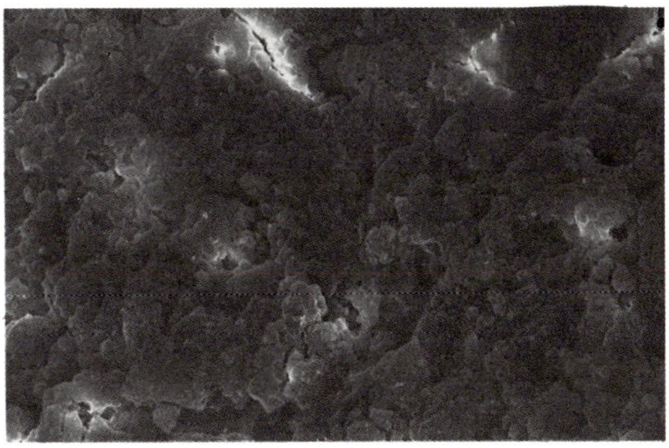
167

168 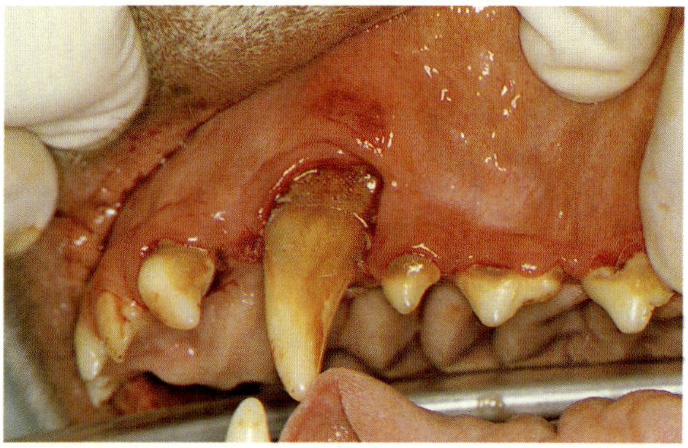

168 Rough dentine as a result of poor scaling technique — Case 6a. In some veterinary practices, owners of companion animals often complain that calculus deposits collect more rapidly on their animals' teeth since they have had regular prophylaxis. This is often the case, as poor scaling technique damages the dentine and enamel. Deep grooves and fissures are created that encourage the build-up of bacterial plaque, which in turn may mineralise to form calculus.

169 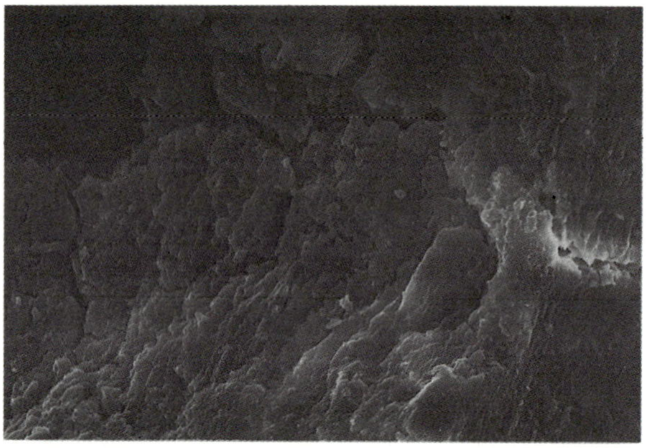

169 SEM of rough tooth surface. Scanning electron micrograph of enamel surface after moderate scaling and no polishing demonstrates the defects that can be created even with a careful technique.

170 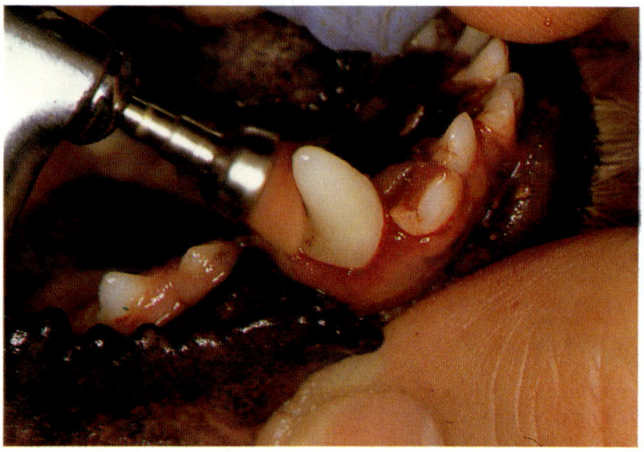

170 Polishing with a brush. Polishing after routine scaling is not for aesthetic reasons but to eliminate the microscopic scratches that have been created. The hold of a contra-angled handpiece is again a pen grip, with a fulcrum rest on the adjacent structure. A coarse or medium grit prophylactic paste is used with the brush. Care must be taken during the use of rotary instruments to retract the lips and the tongue and to avoid facial hairs of the animal getting entangled in the drills and brushes.

171 SEM after polishing. This micrograph illustrates the smooth surface that may be obtained through polishing compared with the rough surface after scaling **(169).**

171

172 Smooth tooth surface — Case 6b. The smooth root surface discourages the rapid build-up of bacterial plaque and calculus formation. Any home dental care will have a far better chance of succeeding.

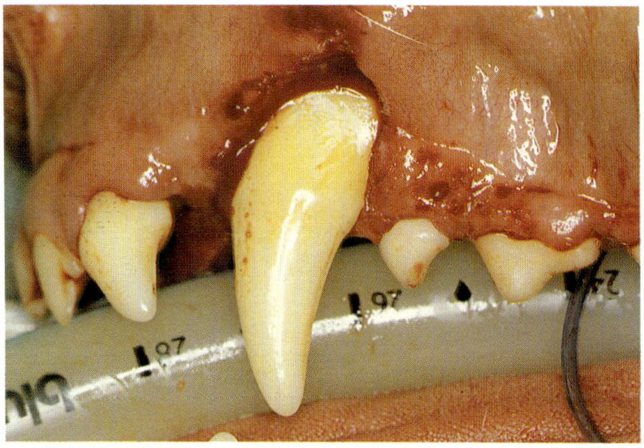
172

173 Close-up of rotary scaler. Rotary scalers are not ultrasonic scalers. They only rotate at the speed of the air rotor, which is usually about 350,000 rpm. These instruments have sharp points, which can easily damage the teeth.

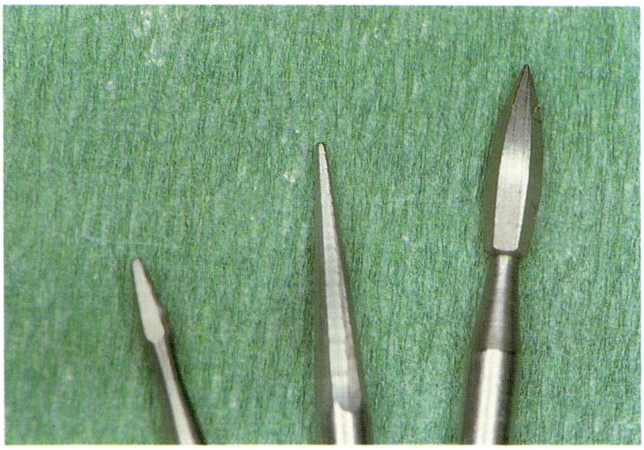
173

174

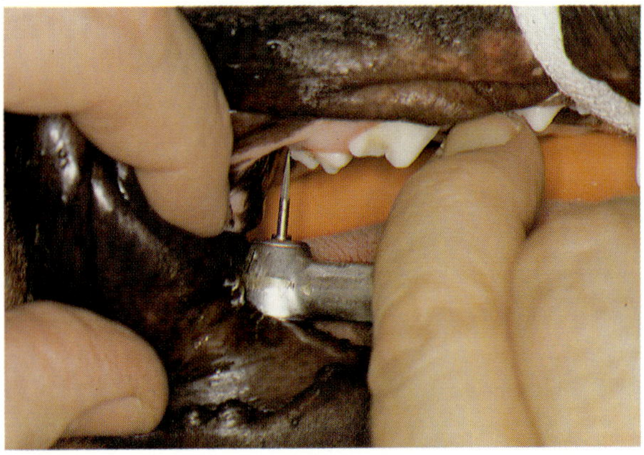

174 Rotary scaler in use. Rotary instruments are far less forgiving than oscillating scalers. The tongue and the buccal mucosa can easily be lacerated, especially when used in a confined environment by untrained personnel who often do not have proper grip and control of the instrument.

175

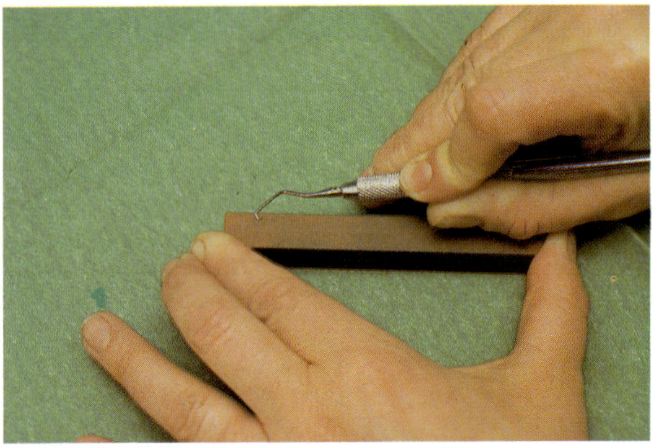

175 Sharpening instruments. For efficient use of hand instruments it is important that they are kept sharp and the correct angle of the cutting edges maintained. The sharpness of an instrument can be assessed by viewing the cutting edge: light is not reflected from the edge of a sharp instrument, but a blunt edge can be seen shining brightly. Simple oilstones can be used for sharpening, but a degree of skill is required for the freehand sharpening of precisely angled cutting edges. The operator must learn the principles of sharpening these instruments, otherwise the edges will be spoilt. The sharpness of an instrument can be confirmed by testing it on one's fingernail, an extracted tooth or a plastic rod.

176

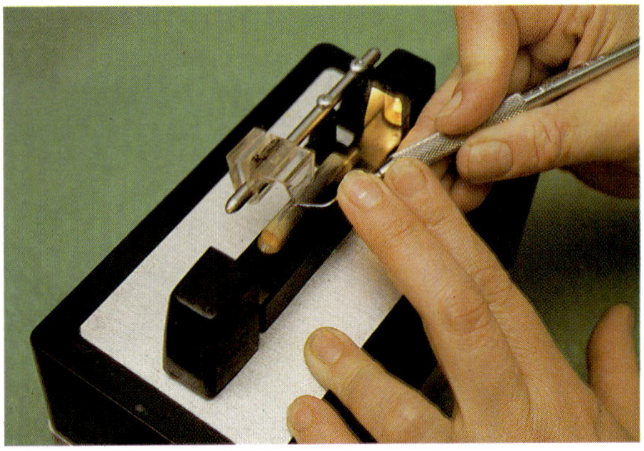

176 Mechanical sharpener. Sophisticated mechanical hones aid the sharpening of hand instruments and speed up the procedure. They also have built-in jigs, which help in the angulation of the appropriate cutting edges.

Prevention and diet

The purpose of professional periodontal treatment is to remove the irritants from the surfaces of the teeth and to create an environment that helps in the control of future build-up of these deposits. Unless positive steps are taken to control the accumulation of bacterial plaque immediately after scaling and polishing, a new pellicle will organise within 24 hours to reform the irritants.

As previously mentioned, there is little doubt that eating food of soft consistency plays an important role in the build-up of dental plaque, although the host response is the most critical factor in the level of periodontal disease seen in individuals. Pet foods are nutritionally balanced, but they lack the fibrous consistency that would have a natural self-cleansing action. Dry food does not appear to have a significant benefit in the control of destructive periodontal disease, although there are conflicting opinions as to whether it helps to control the calculus deposits on the teeth. When one examines the mechanics of carnivore mastication, it is difficult to see how 'dry hide' chewing can have a cleansing action at the important gingival margins, although it could be argued that the periodontal ligaments are 'exercised' and thereby strengthened by such chewing. Bone, contrary to popular belief, is not an ideal cleansing material when one considers its action; it is also not a natural food for most carnivores, being responsible for many fractured and infected posterior teeth. Carnivores will instinctively chew anything if they do not have the mental satisfaction of extended chewing activity through their food.

In recent years the diet of zoo carnivores in North America has largely consisted of convenience food, which is stored frozen in manageable blocks. It is composed of ground meat, with all the nutritional supplements added. Many of the animals on such a diet have developed periodontal disease similar to that seen in the domestic pet population.

The successful periodontal treatment of domestic animals lies with their owners, who have to be motivated to take an active step in the care and maintenance of the animal's oral health. Working with human patients and owners of animals, the author fully understands the difficulties involved in motivating people to change their habits and improve their level of oral hygiene. Many want to actively delegate their responsibilities to the professionals responsible for the hygiene treatment. When working with animals, the owner is the third party and the task becomes even more difficult.

It must be stressed that motivation is the key. People will not necessarily carry out instructions unless they attach great importance to the benefit they will gain from their actions. With the periodontal treatment of domestic pets, the motivational factors may be one or all of the following:

- *Cost.* Not having to meet the expense of another anaesthetic and scaling.
- *Smell.* By diligent home care, the obnoxious level of halitosis would be reduced.
- *Anaesthetic.* By daily maintenance, the bacterial plaque and inflammation level would be controlled, and the pet would not be subjected to the risks associated with further general anaesthetics.
- *Tooth conservation.* Some owners identify strongly with their pets and desperately want them to avoid loosing teeth.

Very few people are motivated to carry out a task or action on their first exposure to it. It is generally accepted that it may take 7–10 repetitions before the majority of people respond positively to such suggestions.

Diet

The great majority of owners feel that their pet's food needs to be finely chopped, as if the animal was unable or did not need to masticate. This attitude is carried over from commercial products to which they are constantly exposed, which are highly convenient to dispense. When they do make the effort to feed fibrous meat, many owners very closely identify their pets as part of the family and subconsciously feel that the food needs to be cut up as it would be for children who could not use a knife and fork. It is difficult to change dietary habits in today's fast, highly processed food trends, where the owners do little chewing themselves. Tinned or dry pet food may be nourishing and nutritionally balanced with vitamins and minerals, but if a large piece of fibrous meat, in the form of an ox heart or ox tail, is added to the daily rations of domestic pets, this can have a considerable self-cleansing action on the teeth.

It is best to start the regime at an early age, as once the bolting of the paste-consistency food is acquired, many animals will try and do the same with lumps of meat, especially if it is not presented as large pieces that have to be masticated before swallowing can be attempted.

Artificial cleaning technique

Brushing teeth is an important way of reducing bacterial plaque, especially if the diet contains a high proportion of soft convenience food. If the regime is commenced at an early age, all pets can be trained to accept it as part of the daily routine. Dogs can be trained at a later age as well, but cats at that stage will not usually tolerate it.

The toothbrush used for animals should be of a size that is compatible with the size of its mouth and of a texture that will mechanically loosen the attached soft plaque. In the author's experience, cotton buds, gauze squares and soft-textured brushes are useless in cleaning teeth. Many people are worried that they will be creating damage. It should be explained to owners that bleeding gums are an indication of inflammation. It is not an excuse to stop the cleaning procedure, and only with regular cleaning and removal of the irritant deposits can this inflammation subside. Also, it must be explained that brushing is not going to remove mineralised deposits; that requires professional scaling and polishing.

The choice of toothpaste should be made carefully. In the author's opinion, it should be used as a vehicle for animals to accept the cleaning procedure. A number of products have been formulated, especially for the pet market, that contain meat flavour additives which make them particularly attractive to carnivores. Human toothpastes are too strongly flavoured and too frothy for most animals to accept: they are not usually digestible and, as animals are unable to spit them out, they can upset their digestion. Salt most certainly should not be used as its ingestion can easily upset the electrolyte levels of these relatively small animals, with fatal results. Hydrogen peroxide solution can have an irritant localised effect on the oral mucosa. Chlorhexidine and sanguinarine have been shown to be effective in the removal and inhibition of bacterial plaque and in encouraging the healing of inflamed oral mucosa. The use of chlorhexidine as a long-term agent in animals has been disputed due to its flavour, occasional localised irritation, changes that occur to taste, staining potential, some evidence of resistant strains of bacteria and the danger of the animals developing digestive complications as they are unable to spit out the chemical and inevitably ingest it.

177

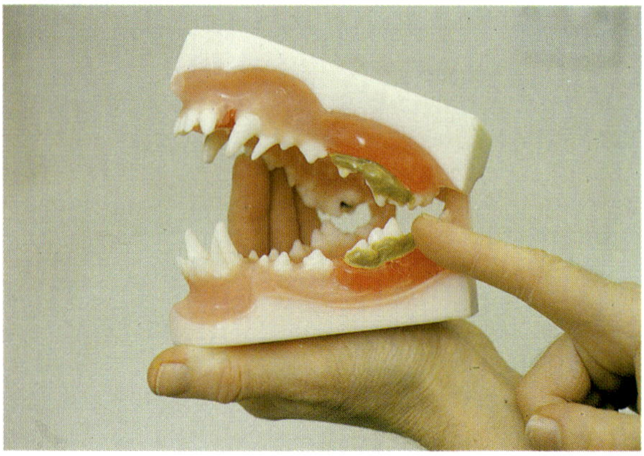

177 Demonstration models. Prevention in the form of home dental care is the key to the success of periodontal treatment. Specially made demonstration models, such as 'Canis' and 'Felid', are ideal for demonstrating to owners the need for dental treatment as well as for motivating them in the importance of their involvement.

178 Selection of toothbrushes. Dogs can be trained easily to accept regular oral hygiene maintenance: the earlier training is commenced, the better. Any size toothbrush that is compatible with the size of the dog is acceptable. Nylon is the preferred material as it is more hygienic — it does not have a central canal, like natural bristle, and does not putrefy as easily.

178

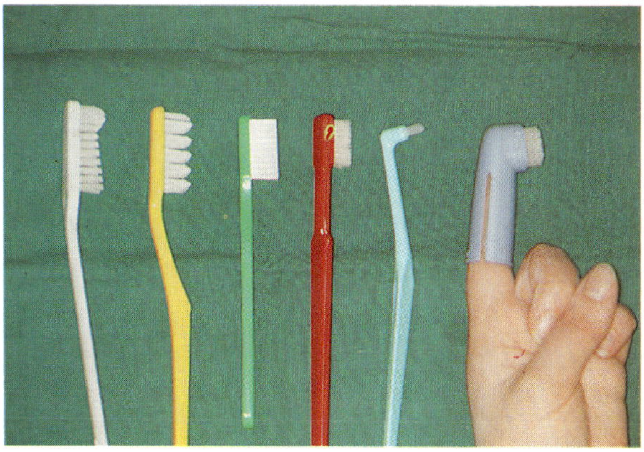

179 Toothpaste for dogs. Avoid the use of human toothpastes: they are too frothy, can be an irritant when swallowed and have an unpleasant flavour to animals. A specially designed dog toothpaste that is completely digestible is desirable. Introduced in 1975, DVM claims to be the first veterinary toothpaste. It has a meat flavour to encourage dogs to accept the oral attention.

179

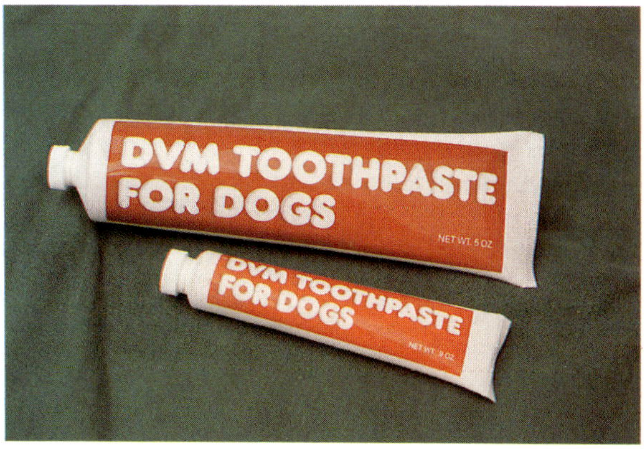

180 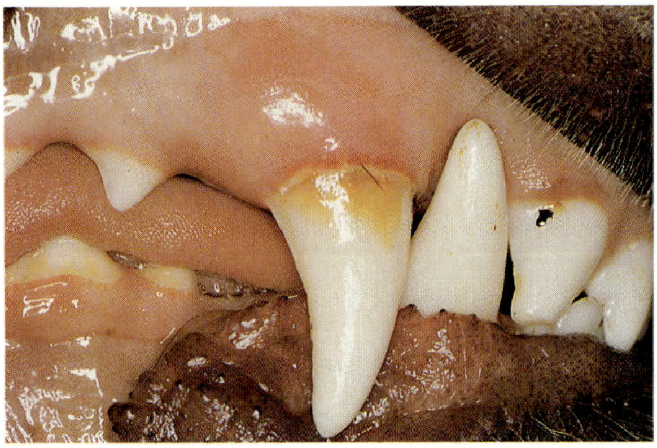 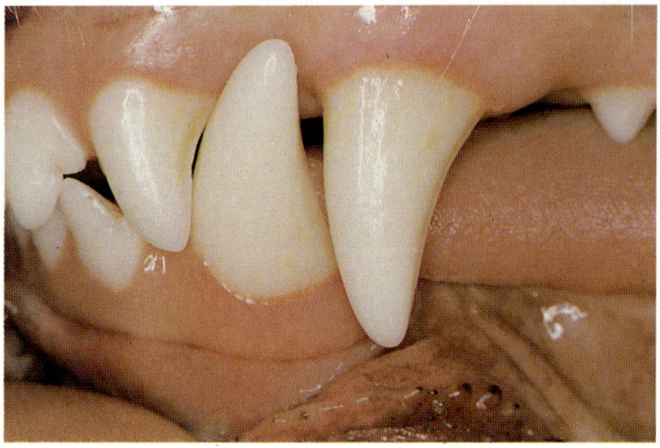 181

180,181 Comparative pictures — animals from the same litter, aged 10 months — Cases 7a & b. It is interesting to compare the periodontal condition of two dogs from the same litter, therefore having a very similar genetic background and host response, over a five-year follow-up period. The animals were on the same diet. Case 7a received no home dental care while Case 7b had the teeth brushed two or three times a week, for approximately 30 seconds on each occasion.

182 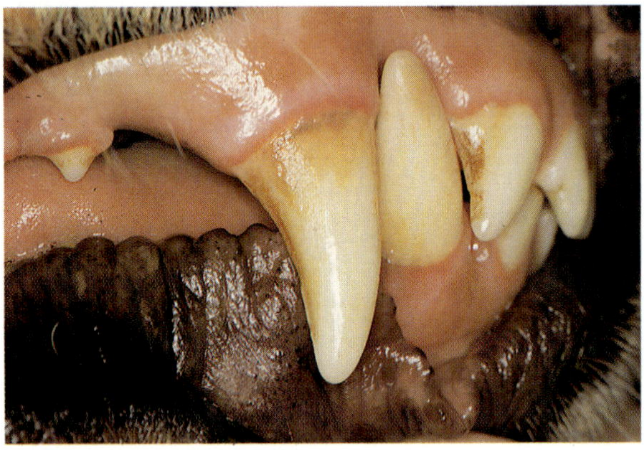 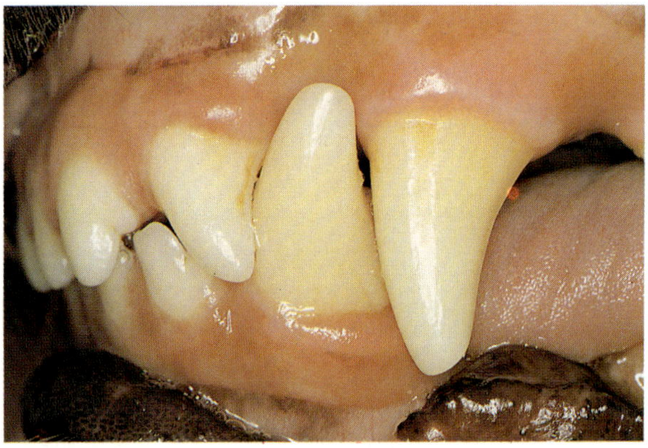 183

182, 183 Five years later — Case 7c & d. The same two animals (**180, 181**) — five years later. Both were on a diet free of self-cleansing fibrous material and neither of them had any professional scaling or polishing performed. Again, Case 7c had no home dental care, while Case 7d had her teeth cleaned for about 30 seconds twice a week. (**182** is the opposite side to **180** but reversed for layout purposes.)

The above demonstrated that regular attention will control the soft and hard deposits on the teeth as well as reduce the inflammatory gingival response. It illustrates the periodontal condition in individuals with very similar immunological backgrounds and suggests that destructive periodontal disease does not necessarily occur in a neglected mouth. Although halitosis and some marked marginal gingivitis was present in the animal that did not receive home dental care, the host response was relatively mild when the periodontal tissues were examined.

184

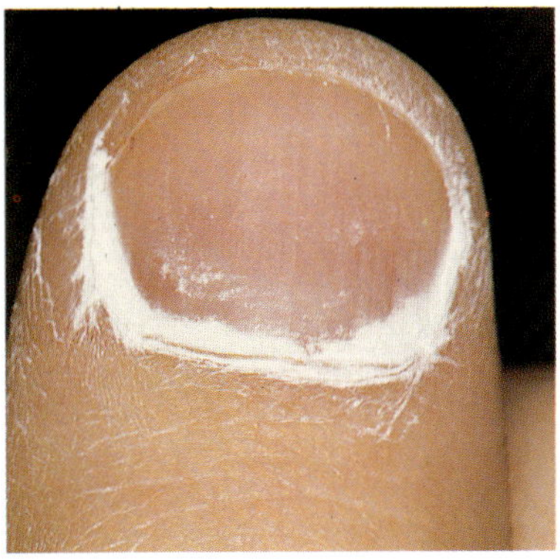

185

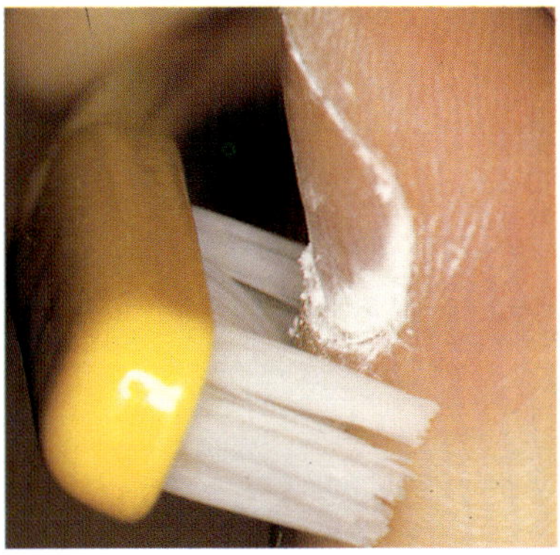

186

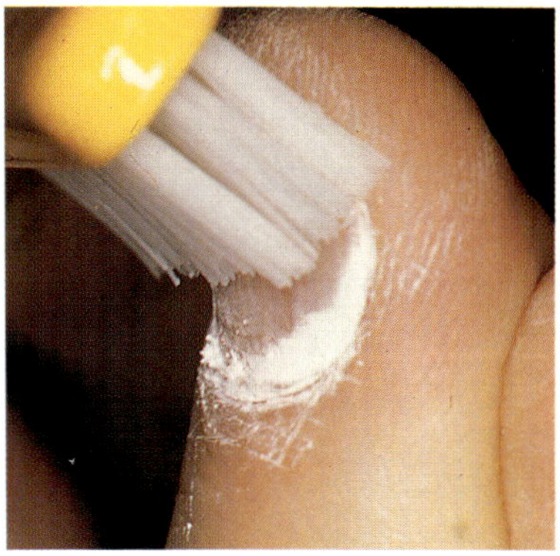

184 Brushing demonstration (after Kilpatrick). An excellent way to demonstrate to clients the efficiency of different brushing techniques is to use ones own thumbnail. The nail represents the tooth and the cuticle the gingival sulcus. A white powder sprinkled around the cuticle represents the bacterial plaque.

185 Brushing demonstration — gum to tooth. It is often suggested that a toothbrush should be used in a coronally sweeping motion (from gum to tooth). The movement is unnatural and many people find it difficult to execute.

186 Brushing — powder remaining in sulcus. If this action is used, especially if the gingival margins are swollen as they often would be in the presence of periodontal disease, the bristles miss the vital sulci and the deposits remain.

187

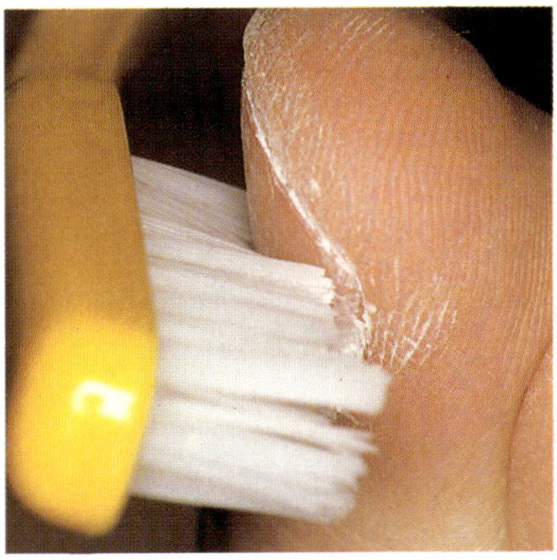

188

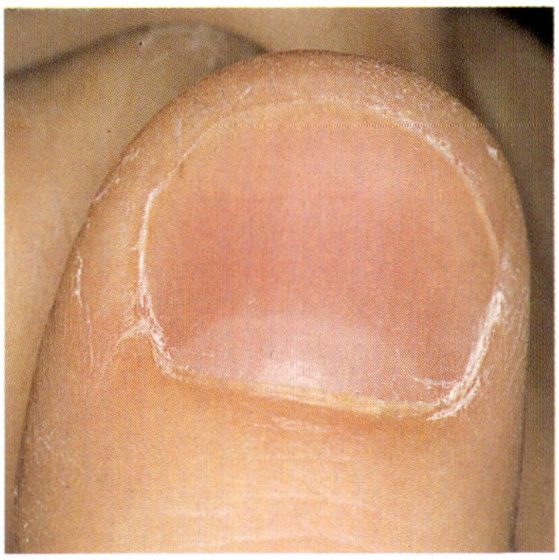

187 Brushing — bristles pointing into sulcus. If the bristles are aimed into the gingival sulcus and are vibrated gently from side to side with moderate pressure, the deposits are loosened and removed.

188 Brushing — deposits removed. The bacterial plaque is removed from the gingival sulcus.

7 Diseases of the Calcified Dental Tissues and Conservative Dentistry

Conservative treatment plays a major role in restoring the ravages of dental caries in human dentistry. In veterinary work the clinical needs are quite different. Therefore, it is important to carefully analyse the necessity or advisability of restoring developmental defects or retaining diseased teeth.

Developmental abnormalities

189 Enamel hypoplasia. Amelogenesis imperfecta affecting the permanent dentition. The dentine is prone to discoloration but is resistant to smooth surface caries. The lesions usually remain symptomless throughout life and the restorative treatment of enamel hypoplasia in animals cannot be justified for aesthetic reasons. The defects can be covered with bonded composite material, but as the attachment of the enamel to the dentine is usually poor in cases of enamel hypoplasia the quality of bond of the restoration will also be unpredictable.

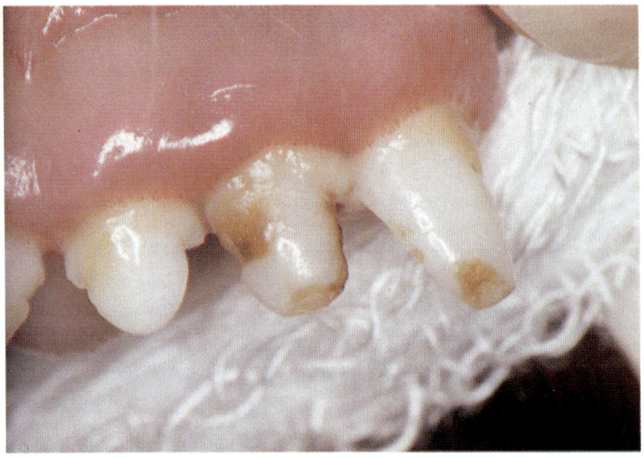

189

190 Enamel hypoplasia — Case 1a. Occasionally, large areas of dentine are denuded of enamel protection. The condition is usually symptomless but, rarely, owners report that young animals suffering from such defects avoid hot food and cold water. The large areas of exposed dentine and the proximity of the pulp may be responsible for increased thermal sensitivity.

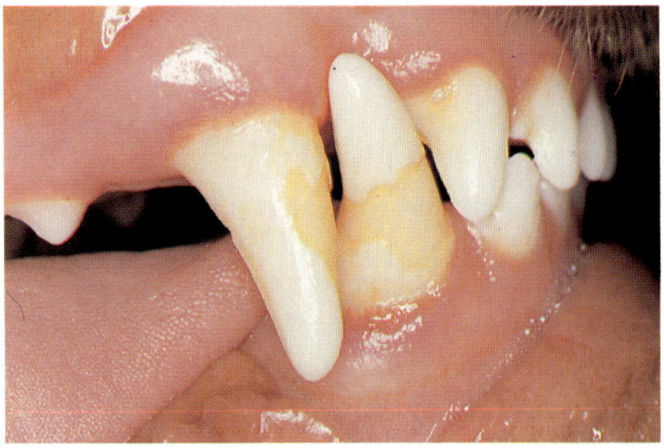

190

191 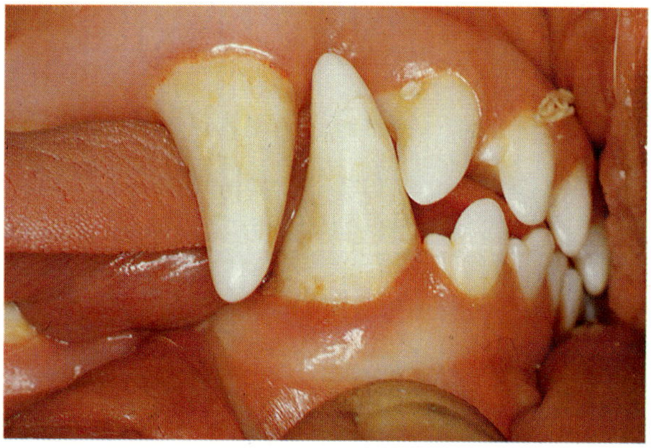

191 Restoration with glass ionomer cement — Case 1b. Covering the dentine with glass ionomer cements can protect the sensitive dentine. It must be appreciated that due to their anatomical position and the destructive environment, the restorations can only be of a temporary nature. Any mechanical preparation to improve the retention of the restorative material to the enamel and/or dentine by grooving it is positively contraindicated. This can create unnecessary trauma to the immature tooth and in the event of restoration failure, which will inevitably occur, the tooth will be in a far worse condition than before treatment.

The use of self-tapping pins to increase the retention of restorative materials is contraindicated in animal dentistry. The risk of pulpal perforation and the resultant complications outweigh the imaginary benefit any such modalities may offer in a veterinary environment.

Dental caries

Carnivores are much less prone to dental caries than humans, who universally suffer from the disease. A number of anatomical, physiological and dietary factors play vital roles in the rate of caries:

- Salivary pH.
- Food stagnation areas between teeth.
- Occlusal anatomy.
- Dietary refined carbohydrate level.

The mechanism of caries follows a sequence:

1 Food debris stagnates:
(a) between the teeth at the contact points;
(b) in the pits and fissures of the biting surfaces;
(c) in the gingival sulci.

2 The bacterial plaque, especially streptococcal mutants, breaks down the stagnating dietary refined carbohydrates (e.g. glucose, lactose), creating a highly acidic by-product that decalcifies the enamel.

3 Once the enamel is perforated, caries can progress rapidly in the dentine, destroying tooth substance and eventually creating pulpal irritation and pain. The undermined, unsupported enamel may fracture.

4 Eventually, the pulp is exposed by the caries, a stage which is associated with acute pain. The pulpitis thus created is followed by pulp necrosis, which can lead to periapical infection.

Dogs

The pH of dog saliva is usually between 7.5 and 8.5. Food packing between the teeth of carnivores is uncommon and is rarely seen as a contributing factor in caries. Caries of the smooth surfaces and cervical margins is also rare in dogs.

The occlusal anatomy of the posterior teeth, which have pits and fissures, encourages food stagnation. Dogs fed on a natural diet that contains no refined carbohydrates will not develop caries despite these danger areas. If products containing sugar are introduced to the diet, however, the anatomically prone areas may be attacked and rampant caries can develop.

Cats

The pH of cat saliva is usually between 8.0 and 9.0. Cats are not prone to dental caries. They are unique in suffering extensively from resorption lesions that most often arise at the necks of their teeth, at the cemento-enamel junction.

Caries in the dog

192 Occlusal caries — upper molar. In some of the posterior teeth of dogs, anatomically normal pits and fissures exist. These areas harbour food particles and bacteria. In the presence of refined carbohydrates, such as chocolates and sweets, the danger areas are much more prone to caries than smooth enamel. Once the dentine is penetrated, the carious lesion can rapidly increase in size and depth and undermine the enamel.

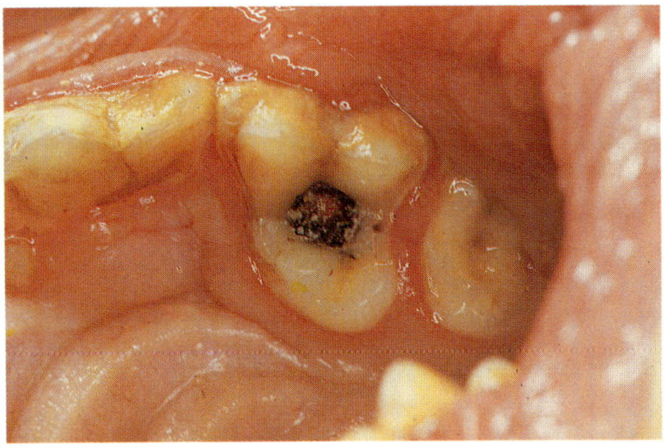

192

193 Radiograph illustrating pulp horns. The anatomy of dogs posterior teeth is such that even in older animals the pulp horns extend well into the cusps. This feature makes pulpal exposure common, even in cases of moderate caries.

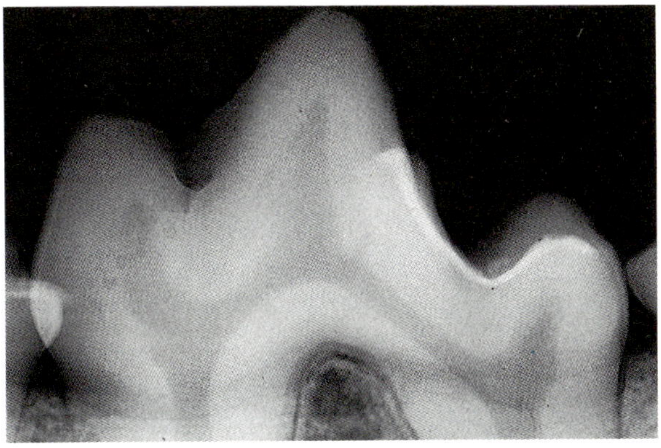

193

194 Large occlusal carious cavity — Case 2a.

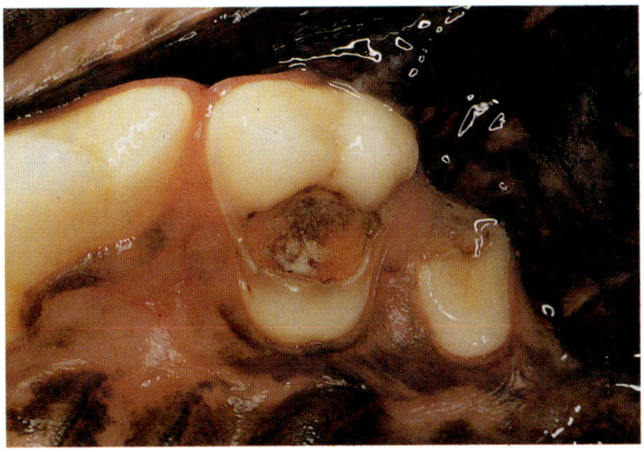

194

195

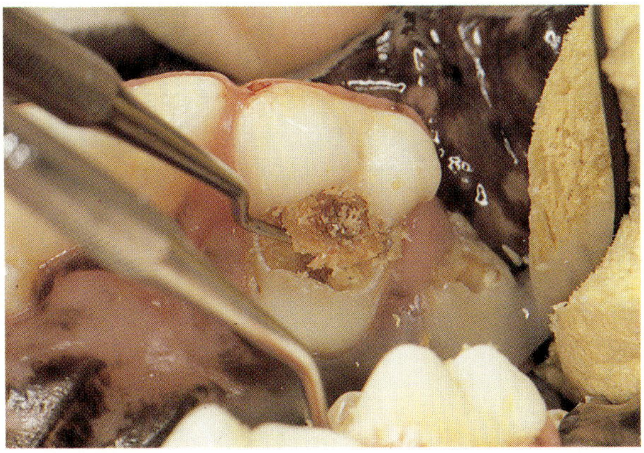

195 Excavating caries — Case 2b. The caries has a leathery or hard cheese-like consistency, which can be easily curetted with a spoon excavator.

196

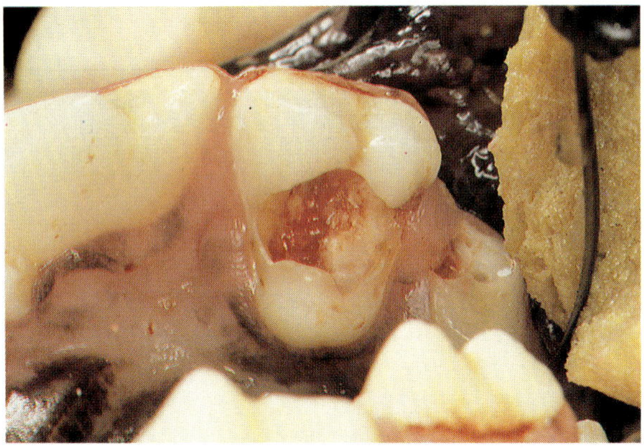

196 Pulp exposure — Case 2c. Often, the dentine is carious to a depth where it invades the pulp chamber.

197

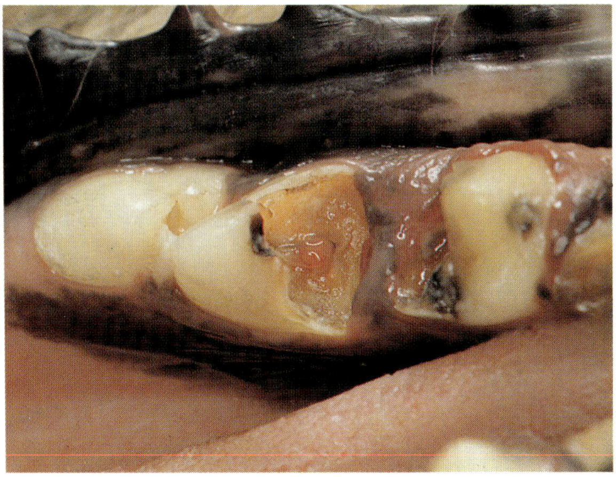

197 Extensive cavity. Occlusal caries has bisected the lower first molar at its bifurcation. A pulp polyp can be seen extruding from the large exposure of the mesial root canal. It is interesting to note that adjacent to such a large lesion, food packing at the contact point between the lower fourth premolar and the first molar has not brought about dental decay.

198 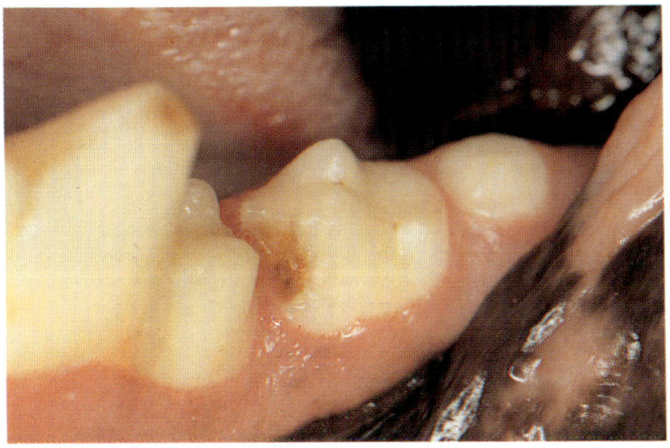

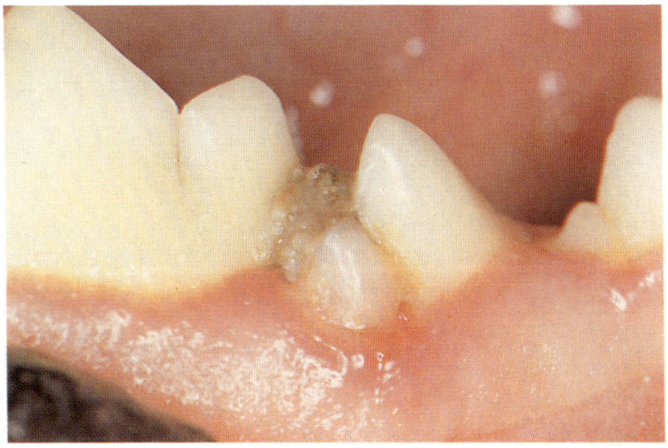 199

198 Interstitial caries. In dogs it is unusual for caries to occur in areas other than the occlusal danger areas. This animal had no food packing in the interdental area and the aetiology of the bilateral lesions only in the lower second molars was unclear.

199 Interdental food packing. In cases of dental irregularities, which can contribute to food stagnation, interstitial decay can occur. The photograph demonstrates the typical grey translucent appearance of caries. Note that the lesion had perforated the tooth from the lingual to the buccal surface.

Guidelines for the conservative treatment of caries

The restoration of carious cavities in animals must be assessed on the long-term prognosis of the tooth in question and the benefits gained by its retention. As in other aspects of veterinary dentistry the guidelines are to provide the most predictable and least traumatic treatment to establish oral health and avoid repeated anaesthetics. In conservative dentistry factors that must be taken into consideration are the size of the lesions, pulpal involvement, periodontal condition and anticipated length of anaesthesia. Generally speaking, the posterior teeth of carnivorous domestic animals do not play a functional role, and with extensive lesions extractions are the treatment of choice. Prevention can play an important role if the cavities are small and shallow — where single surface amalgam fillings can halt the progress of the dental decay. In a veterinary environment, topical fluoride gel applications are highly questionable in their efficacy in preventing or arresting active caries and their use cannot be justified on clinical grounds.

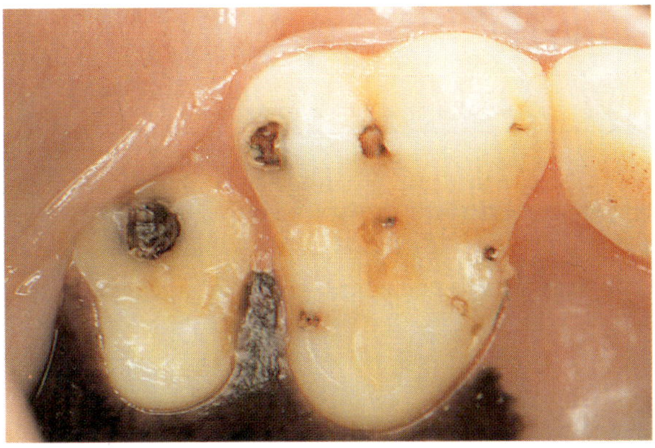 200

200 Smooth surface caries. In dogs, occlusal caries rarely occur on smooth enamel. This animal suffered from rampant caries of the posterior teeth. Enamel defects in the form of pits may have been a predisposing factor of the condition. Restorations of the early lesions arrested the caries, while the second upper molars were extracted.

201

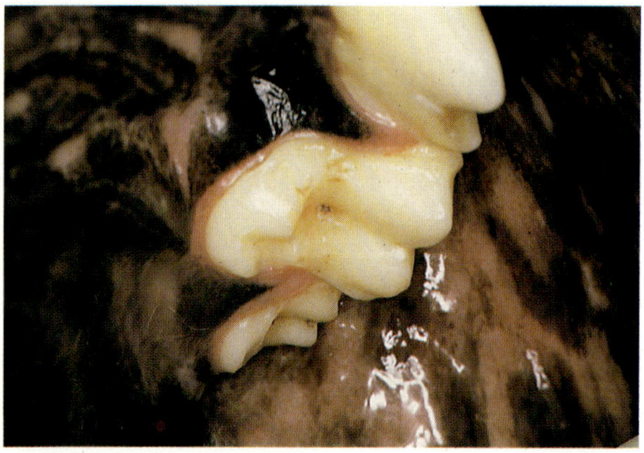

201 Small cavity — Case 3a. Small carious central pit of the upper first molar.

202

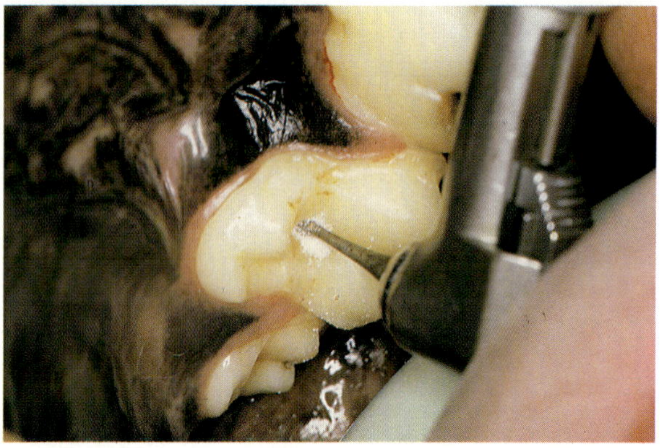

202 Removal of caries — Case 3b. Early carious lesions can be easily eliminated through minimal cavity preparation.

203

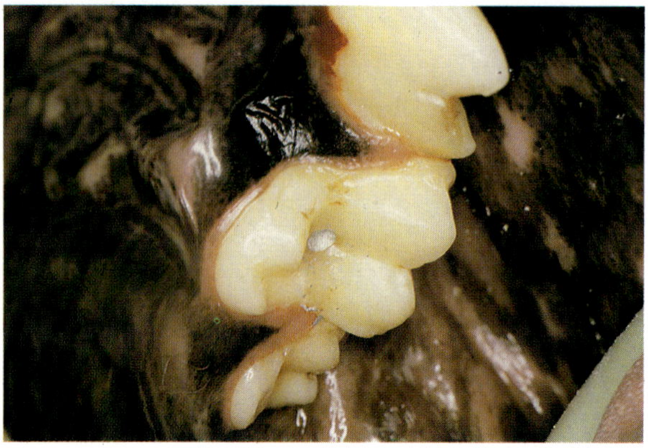

203 Small amalgam restoration — Case 3c.

204 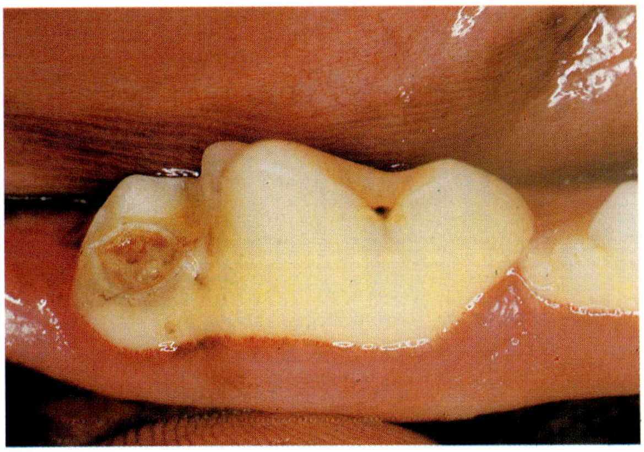

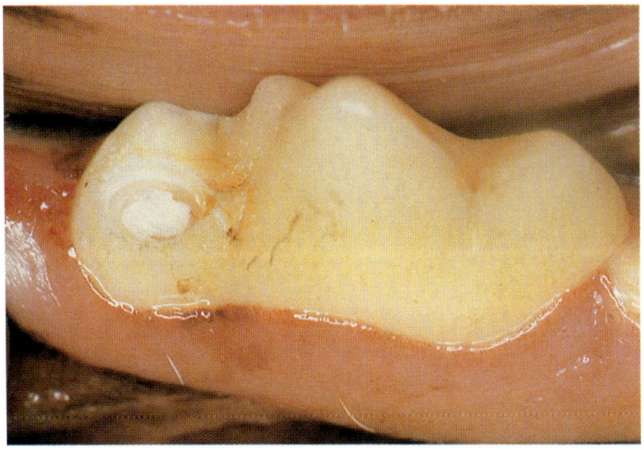 205

204 Occlusal caries of lower first molar — Case 4a.

205 Prepared cavity lined — Case 4b. No carious exposure of the pulp was encountered; the floor of the cavity is lined with an insulating material.

206 Five-year follow-up — Case 4c. Amalgam restoration five-years postoperatively. Occlusal prematurities need to be checked on placement of the restorative material, depending on the interdigitation of the teeth.

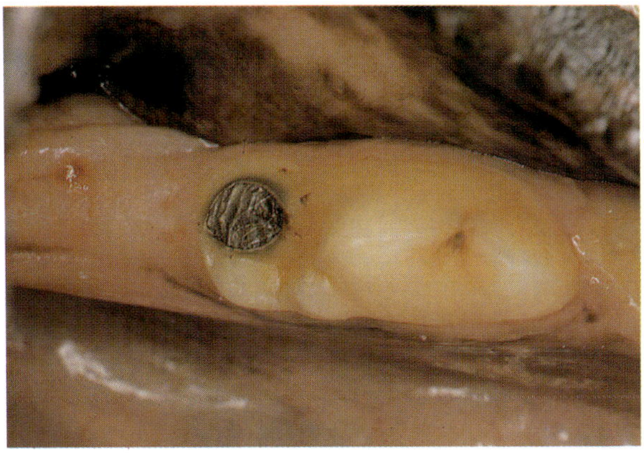 206

Degenerative lesions to the teeth of felids

Domestic cats often suffer from destructive lesions to their teeth at the cemento-enamel junction. The cavities are not the result of dental caries but of the activity of odontoclasts, which are inflammatory multinuclear cells identical to osteoclasts. The aetiology of the condition is unclear, but chronic periodontitis associated with bacterial plaque stagnation appears to be an important factor. It may be seen in some animals associated with even sub-clinical levels of gingivitis.

A dietary link with processed food cannot be dismissed. It is interesting to note that these lesions did not exist in the skulls of domestic cats examined by Sir Frank Colyer early in the 20th century. It is recognised that zoo felids fed on a natural self-cleansing diet rarely suffer from cervical lesions, although ones fed on soft, processed commercial diets often exhibit similar lesions to those seen in domestic cats.

The clinical appearance of resorptive lesions in cats may be classified into two main groups:

- External resorption of the crown and root, usually originating at the cemento-enamel junction.
- External resorption of the root only.

207

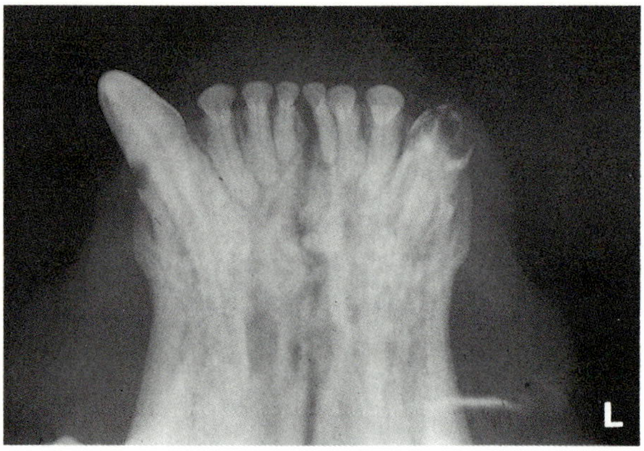

208

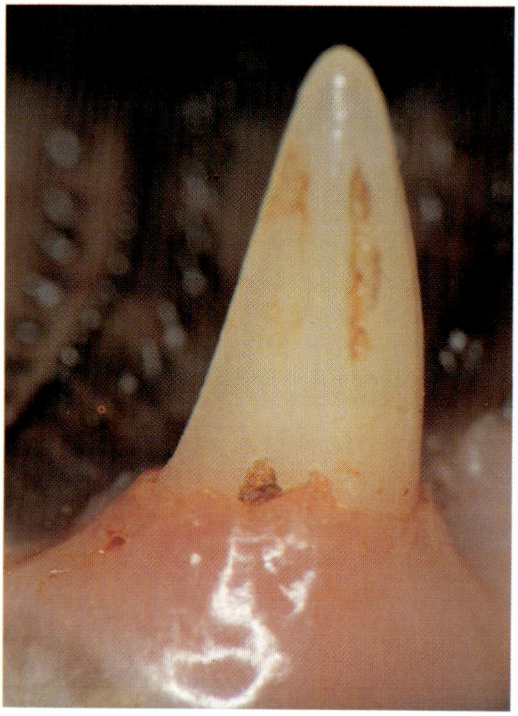

207 Radiograph of cervical cavity — canine — Case 5a. Radiograph of a mandible, illustrating the cervical cavity in the lower right canine of a cat. Note the fractured lower left canine; this often occurs as a result of horizontally invasive cervical cavities which weaken the structure of the tooth.

208 Intra-oral view of lesion on lower right canine — Case 5b. The coronal extremity of the subgingival cavity can be seen at the gingival margin.

209

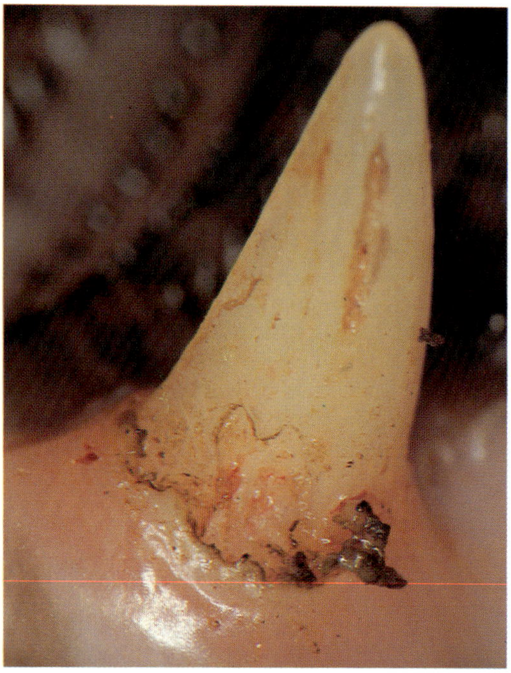

210

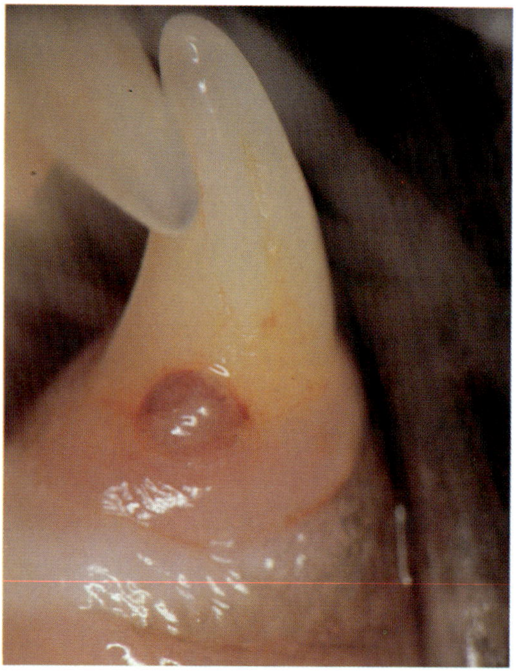

209 Close-up of cavity — hyperplastic tissue resected — Case 5c. The irregular margins and the rough surface of the cavity are clearly demonstrated. A pulp exposure at the floor of the cavity can be seen.

210 Early external resorption. Localised gingivitis is often the first clinical sign associated with cervical resorptive cavities. The confirmation of a cavity should be made by subgingival probing. The lesions have a rough, irregular texture and are extremely painful for the animal. When the cavities are probed the animals exhibit hypersensitivity, even under a moderate degree of general anaesthesia.

211

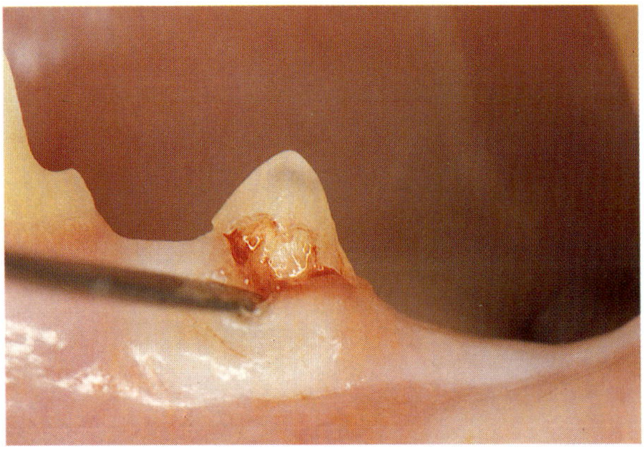

212

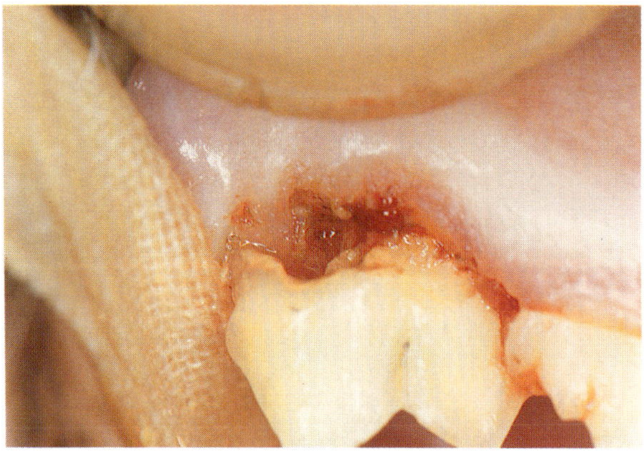

211 Cervical cavity in lower premolar. A large cervical cavity is visible by retracting the gingiva that has granulated into the defect.

212 Deep cervical lesion. An extensive cervical cavity that amputates the distobuccal root from the crown of the upper third premolar.

213

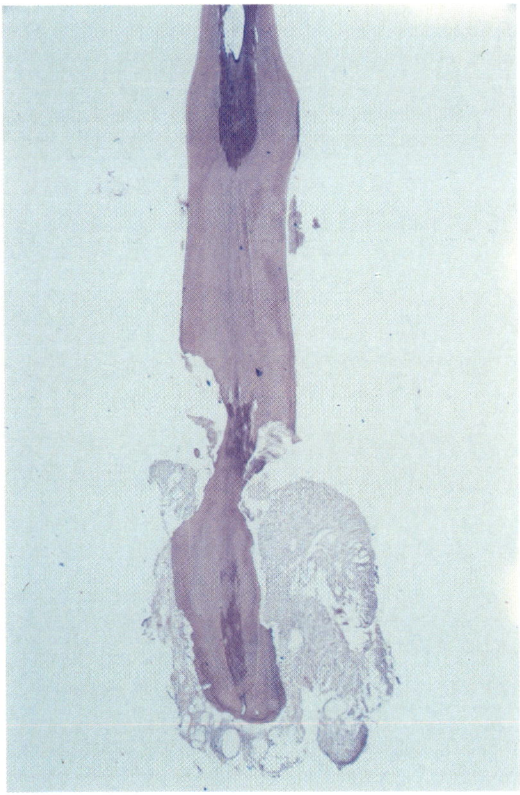

214

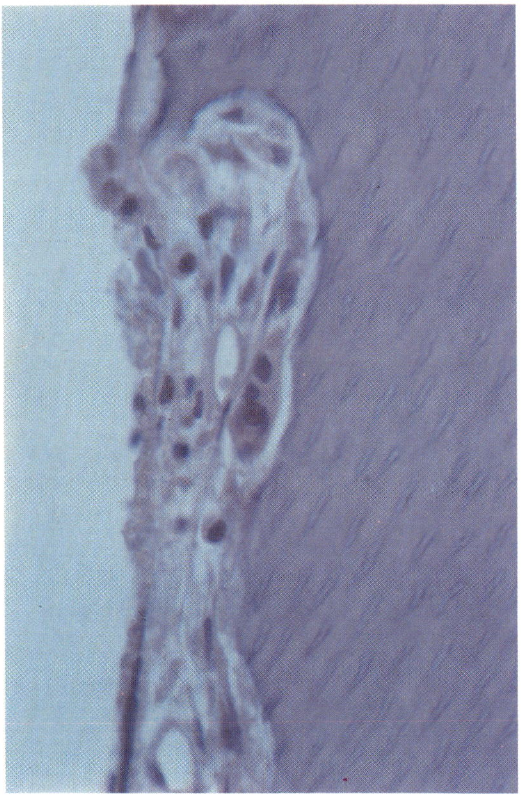

213 Histopathology (×*12*). Longitudinal section through a lower permanent molar of a domestic cat includes the crown and one root. There are extensive cavities that also involve the apical part of the root. The outlines of the lesions are irregular, although they are fully mineralised, hard and no evidence of caries is visible. Calculus and bacterial plaque are seen lining the cavities. Granulation tissue with a chronic infiltrate of inflammatory cells is seen around the roots and in the cavities.

214 Histopathology (*× 750*). An odontoclast is seen in a shallow lacuna with associated inflamed granulation tissue in the cavity.

215 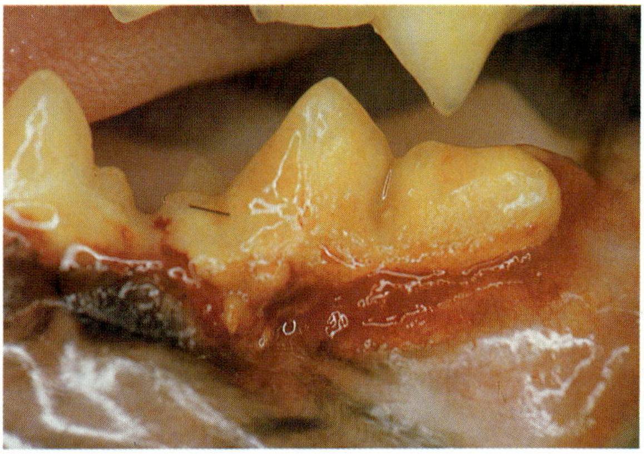

216 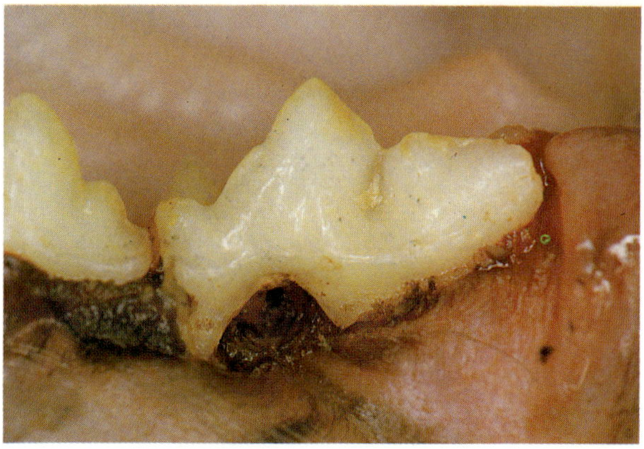

215 Cervical concavity — Case 6a. Marginal gingivitis and cervical concavity in tooth was suspected to be a cervical resorptive cavity.

216 Close-up, confirming bifurcation — Case 6b. When examining feline cervical cavities, the diagnosis between pathological lesions and normal anatomy is made through the close inspection of the surfaces for integrity and texture. Inspection of the area once the gingival seepage had been controlled with ferric sulphate solution clearly demonstrated that the lesion was a normal root bifurcation, associated with some loss of alveolar bone height, and not a resorption cavity.

Coronally migrating resorptive lesions

Occasionally, feline resorptive cavities do not follow the classical pattern of invading in a pulpal and apical direction: some cavities extend coronally, destroying enamel, with associated migration of hyperplastic gingiva.

It is interesting to note that the gingivae in these cases usually demonstrate a keratinised response, rather than the frail inflammatory granulation tissue that is often associated with horizontally invasive lesions at the cemento-enamel junction.

2 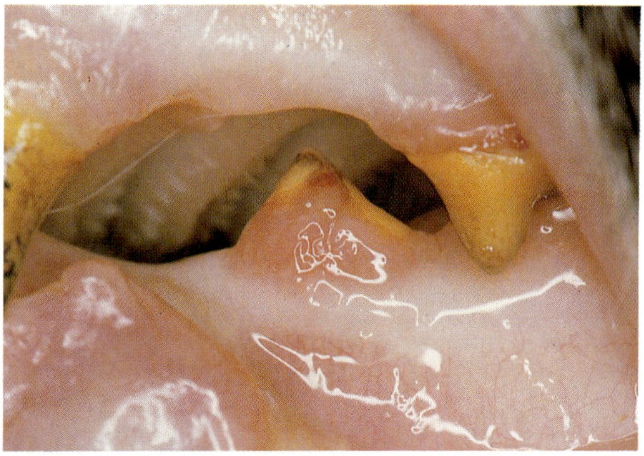

2 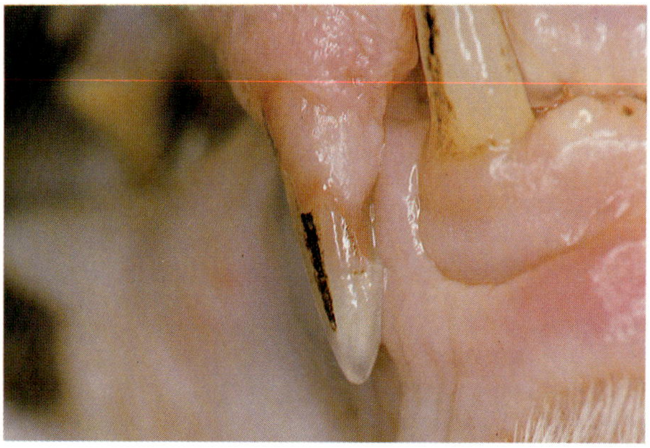

217 Lower premolar, with coronally invasive lesion. Hyperplastic gingiva covers the coronally invasive resorptive lesion and extends almost to the tip of the crown.

218 Gingiva extending coronally. Coronally invasive resorption destroyed the enamel of the crown of this upper canine. The granulation tissue, of gingival origin, had migrated into the lesion. It was firmly bound to the tooth, unlike horizontally invasive lesions, where it may be easily teased away from the underlying dentine.

219 Histopathology *(×9)*. The cells associated with the lesions indicate that there is no difference in the histopathology of apically, horizontally or coronally invasive resorption. The significant feature of one specimen that demonstrated both apically and coronally invasive resorption was the extensive deposition of reparative trabeculae of cementum in the resorptive cavity to the extent that the root was almost completely formed of cementum.

219

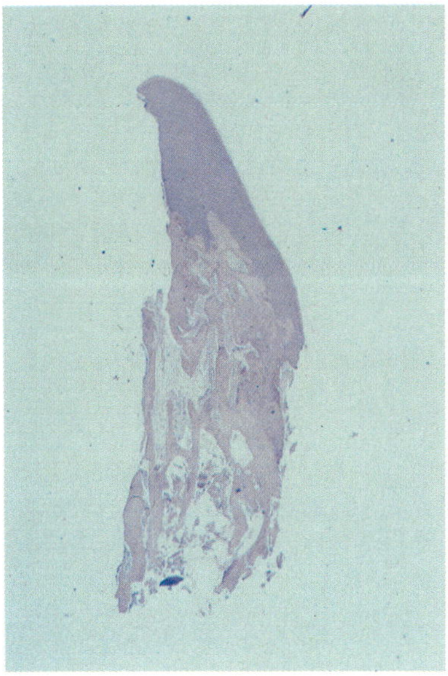

Root resorption

220 Root resorption of canine. External resorption of the root caused destruction of the entire surface, which resulted in spontaneous exfoliation of the tooth. The aetiology was unknown, but periodontal disease or trauma to the tooth may have played a contributing role.

220

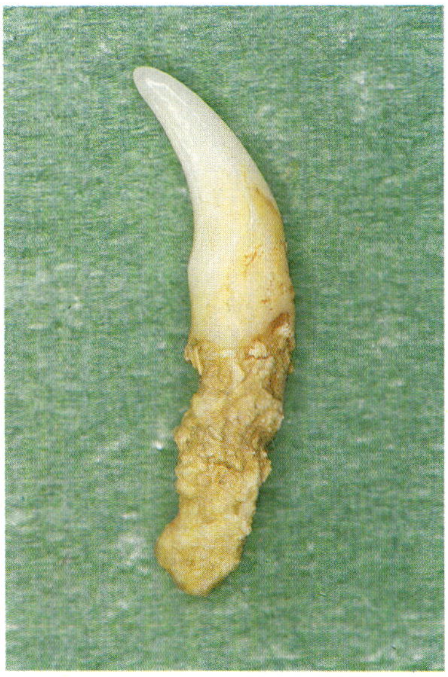

The treatment of feline resorptive lesions

Feline cavities are extremely painful. Usually, animals tolerate and control the pain, although observant owners notice changes of behaviour. This may manifest itself in a lower level of social activity, increased aggression — pawing at the mouth and nose — or a decreased appetite. A thorough investigation of the oral cavity should be performed, for which a general anaesthetic is usually required.

The treatment plan of resorptive lesions must be realistic and in line with the animal's age, general health and anaesthetic risk. Operators in veterinary dentistry must appreciate that most of these animals are fed a convenience diet and that restoration and retention of the teeth are unnecessary for functional or aesthetic reasons, in contrast to human dentistry. The treatment objectives should be to eliminate pain and the source of infection in the most predictable and least-traumatic way, so that the animal does not need to be subjected to repeated anaesthetics.

The restoration of feline cervical cavities seems an attractive treatment option as it involves the minimal amount of trauma. But it must be appreciated that the pathology of the lesions is not that of dental caries. Therefore, topical fluoride gel treatment or varnishing the resorption cavities, as advocated by some writers, does not have any logical or scientific basis. There is also no scientific basis for the restoration of feline cervical cavities and no studies have yet demonstrated long-term clinical success with these procedures. On the contrary, many workers have noted rapid breakdown of restorations and recurrence of resorptive cavities postoperatively. Posterior teeth with cervical lesions should be extracted. This may be difficult, as the small divergent roots are extremely well retained in the alveolar bone. The approach to the extraction of the roots should be performed in a practical way, not putting the integrity of the mandible or the life of the animal at risk for the sake of small root apices. Infected roots should be extracted in their entirety. If small apices with vital pulp contents fracture, and are difficult to retrieve, it is acceptable to suture the gingivae over them. The healing potential of these animals is good, and the blood supply from the alveolar bone and periosteum can maintain the vitality of the pulp in the root fragments, which will remain symptomless.

Canine teeth can be difficult and traumatic to extract. It is acceptable to root fill the teeth affected by resorptive lesions and amputate them subgingivally. The gingivae will granulate over them and the inert roots isolated from the oral environment will remain symptomless.

221

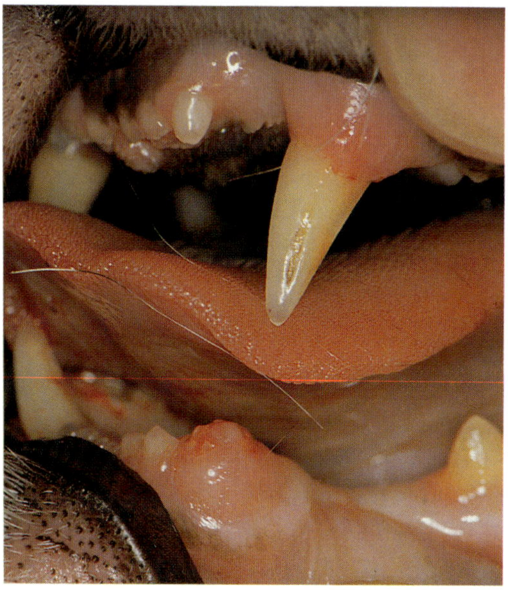

221 Fractured canine due to resorptive lesion with pulp granulating out of root canal — Case 7a.

222 Radiograph, with endodontic file in root canal illustrating length of root — Case 7b.

222

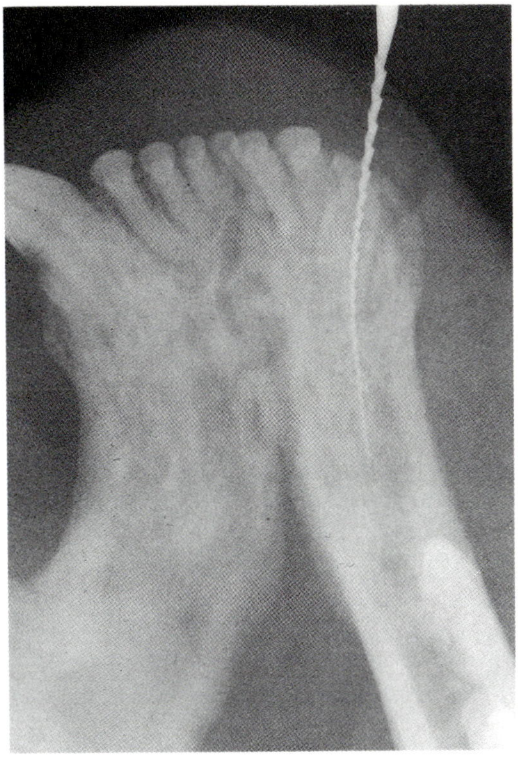

223 Amalgam filling in place over root filling — Case 7c. The root was amputated to the level of the alveolar crest.

223

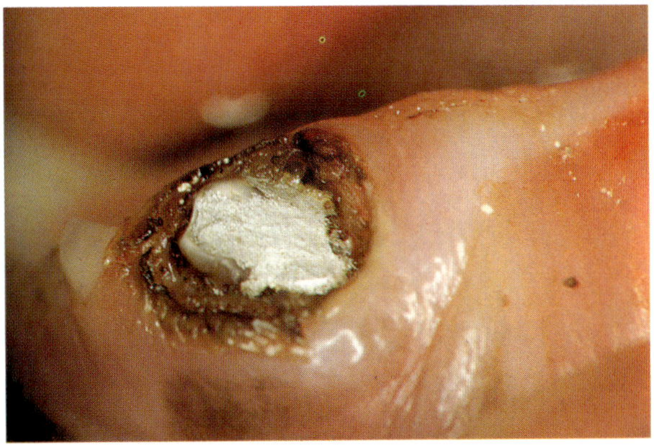

224 Two weeks postoperatively — Case 7d. Excellent gingival healing over buried root. Tooth remained symptomless for the life of the animal.

224

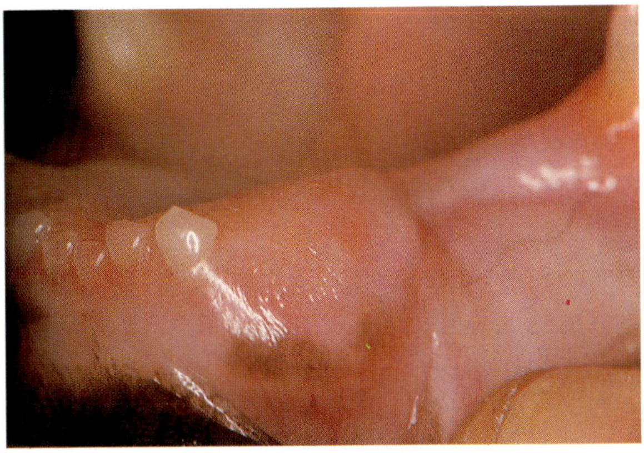

8 Dental Trauma and Endodontics

The consequences of dental trauma can present themselves in a number of ways. It is important to have an understanding of the development of the teeth, pulpal physiology and pathology, so that an accurate diagnosis of the condition can be made and the correct treatment plan implemented to ensure a high degree of predictability and success.

The pathogenesis of the dental pulp

The primary function of the pulp is the formation of dentine to constitute the bulk of the tooth. Once the root development of the anelodont tooth is complete through the deposition of primary dentine, the apical foramen of the root canal becomes constricted, which in turn decreases the blood supply to the pulp and reduces the activity of the odontoblasts. Secondary dentine is normally produced at a slow rate throughout the life of the animal, which in turn reduces the size of the pulp cavity. The secondary function of the pulp is one of defence. It supplies dentine with its sensory supply, but whatever the stimuli the sensation is one of pain. Through this property, which increases the activity of the odontoblasts, the pulp has a limited self-protective mechanism.

Any chronic stimulation of the pulp, such as attrition caused by rock or habitual bone chewing, can encourage a defensive mechanism which lays down a reactive type of secondary dentine in the pulp chamber in an attempt to wall off the irritant as long as the pulp is not exposed. Sometimes, root canals can be completely obliterated through the response to chronic pulpitis.

If the pulp of an anelodont tooth is exposed to the environment, it does not possess the mechanism to naturally repair or wall off with secondary dentine this highly sensitive area. There may be acute pain, but usually only on physical contact with the pulp, which may occur when biting into food. Bacteria will eventually invade the pulp cavity and multiply and chronic or acute pulpitis will occur. Like other connective tissue in the body the pulp will undergo inflammatory changes. Chronic or acute pulpitis — the inflammation of the pulp while it is still vital — will result. Antibiotic therapy cannot prevent or halt the onset of pulpal inflammation and degeneration in the confined environment of the pulp cavity. If the exudate is unable to drain, as in the case of a small exposure, or foreign matter occludes the exposure site, pressure necrosis of the pulp takes place. This is a painful condition, but once the pulp is gangrenous, no further symptom will arise from inside the tooth.

It is important to note that exposure of the pulp does not need to take place for pulp necrosis and periapical abscess formation to occur. Direct trauma to a tooth can displace the root apex beyond the physiological limit the pulp tissue will stretch. This action severs the blood supply to the pulp at the apical foramen which causes the contents of the pulp cavity to degenerate. Even though the contents were originally sterile and uncontaminated by the oral environment, the devitalised tissue devoid of blood supply becomes invaded by bacteria through a haematogenous route via the apical foramen.

Irrespective of whether the pulp necrosis was caused by exposure or not, bacteria will multiply in the pulp cavity. As pulp death has taken place, there is no blood supply to fight the bacterial invasion and multiplication in this dead space. The bacteria will spill eventually into the periapical region and cause inflammatory changes, which can lead to chronic or acute periapical abscesses. Acute pain may not be present unless there is a build-up of pus in the bone, and the exudate is unable to discharge. Once the exudate has broken through the cortical plate of the jaw, the pressure is released, acute cellulitis may form, or a chronic sinus tract, discharging either intra- or extra-orally. Antibiotic therapy of lesions arising from pulpal necrosis can only offer a temporary resolution. Any permanent therapy is either through extraction of the affected tooth or root filling the infected canal(s).

225
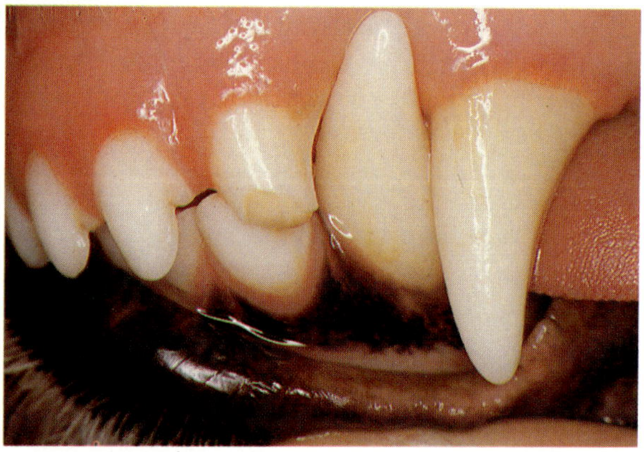

225 Simple fracture no exposure. Fracture of the enamel and dentine with no pulpal involvement. No restorative treatment is indicated, but it is advisable to occasionally examine the tooth and the adjacent teeth for pulpal death through trauma.

226
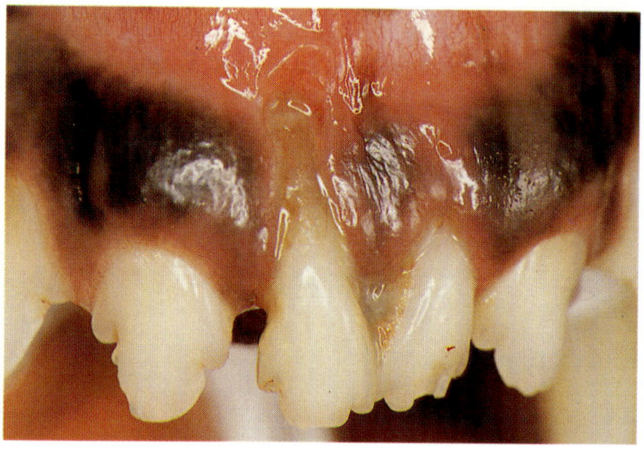

226 Fractured enamel and adjacent tooth damage. Occasionally, trauma to the mouth is dissipated among a number of teeth. Where no coronal fracture has occurred, root damage or pulp necrosis can develop from the force being transmitted to the deeper structures. As the photograph illustrates, the upper-left first incisor has received enamel damage, but in the adjacent upper-right first incisor, where no coronal damage is apparent, the force had been transmitted to the root apex, which has resulted in pulp death, periapical abscess, labial bone and gingival destruction. At this chronic stage, loss of the mobile tooth is inevitable.

227
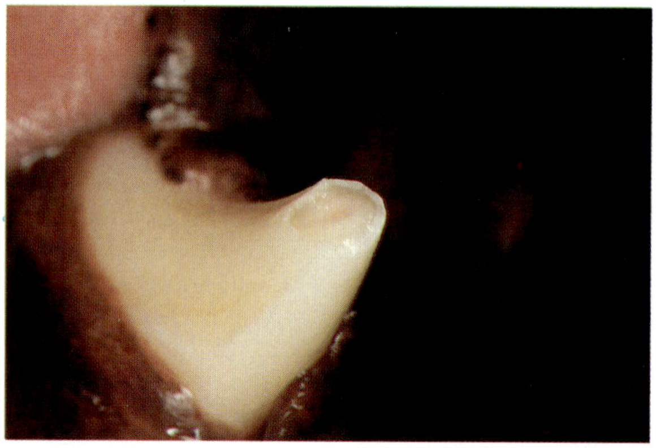

227 Simple fracture — pink dentine — Case 1a. Fracture of the canine tooth, with a thin layer of dentine (which is seen as a pink area showing through) still covering the pulp. Although no exposure of the pulp was elicited with a probe, microscopic exposures, which may eventually contribute to pulpitis, can not be dismissed. Review of the fractured surfaces should be performed three–four months after the initial trauma.

228
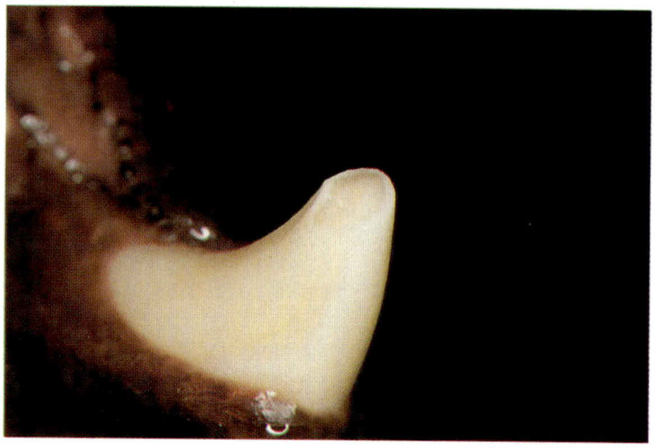

228 Three months later — Case 1b. Three months after the incident, no indication of the pink area or a discoloured spot is visible. Deposition of secondary dentine in the pulp chamber has taken place. No symptoms of discomfort were noticed by the dog's owner. There are no clinical benefits or indications for these shortened teeth to be restored and operators must resist such requests from owners. Bonded materials and pin-reinforced restorations will inevitably fail. Self-tapping dentine pins can also cause pain and irreversible damage to the pulp through traumatic exposures.

229 Fracture of premolar with no obvious exposure but discoloured spot — Case 2a. Occasionally, fractured or worn-down teeth do not present with obvious pulp chamber exposures, although discoloration of the centre of the tooth can indicate pulp necrosis.

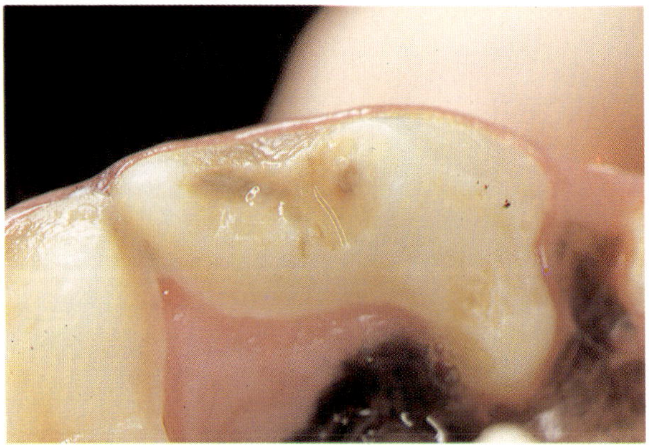

229

230 Osteomyelitis — buccal sinus — Case 2b. This apparently normal tooth had become devitalised through a microscopic pulp exposure that could not be elicited with a sharp explorer. The buccal osteomyelitis and sinus tract were the result of pulp necrosis. The tooth was extracted.

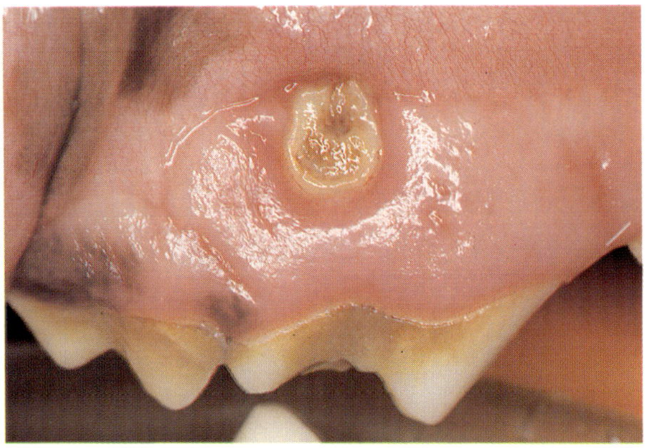

230

231 Discoloured secondary dentine. It is easy for the inexperienced operator to mistake normal attrition/abrasion and secondary dentine as a clinical sign of pulp necrosis. Secondary dentine is deposited inside pulp cavities through age and is enhanced by chronic external stimuli. It is a darker colour than primary dentine and no treatment is required unless there are positive indications for endodontics.

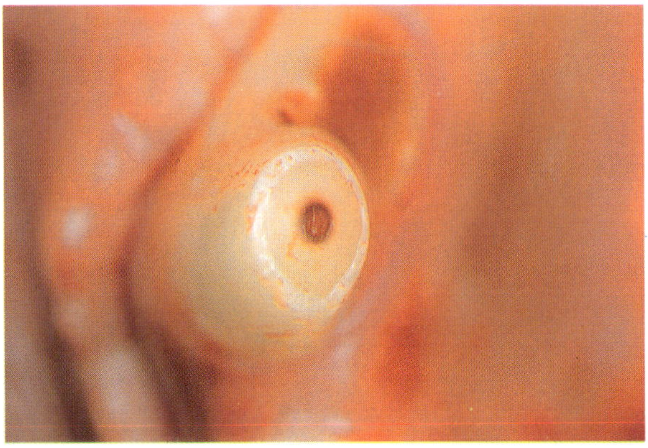

231

232

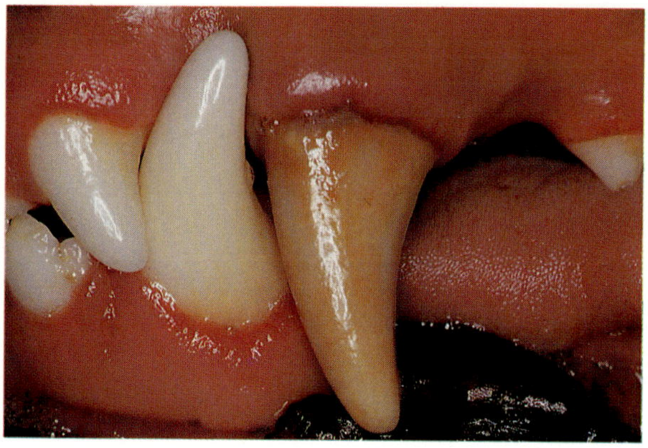

233

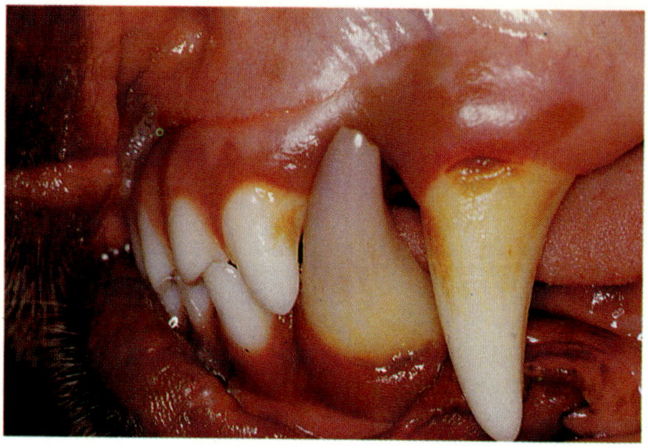

232 Discoloration indicating pulp necrosis. Pulp exposure is not the only cause of pulp damage and necrosis. Trauma, in this case, has severed the blood supply to the tooth. Discoloration of the tooth is the indication of such pulp necrosis. The whole crown may have a brown, grey or pink hue. The discoloration is caused by the breakdown products of haemoglobin penetrating and staining the dentinal tubules.

233 Tip discoloration. Occasionally, only the tip of a single tooth has a lilac or brown discoloration. The tooth would have received some form of trauma, with internal haemorrhage taking place. Many of these 'bruised' teeth remain vital and endodontics should not be performed on them routinely unless clinically indicated. With cooperative animals it is possible to test the vitality of teeth with cotton pellets soaked in ethyl chloride. It is important to compare reactions with the normal tooth on the opposite side of the arch. Radiographic examination can be useful, but the absence of a radiolucent periapical lesion is not a definite proof of a healthy tooth. The comparison of root canal sizes of contralateral teeth in young animals can be revealing as non-vital teeth cease deposition of secondary dentine in the pulp chamber and the root canal.

234

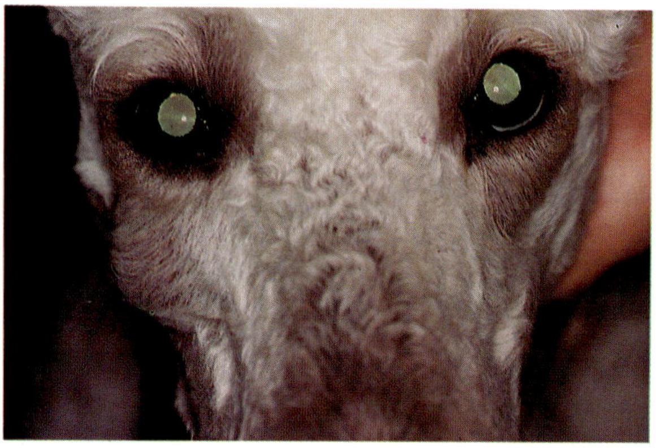

23

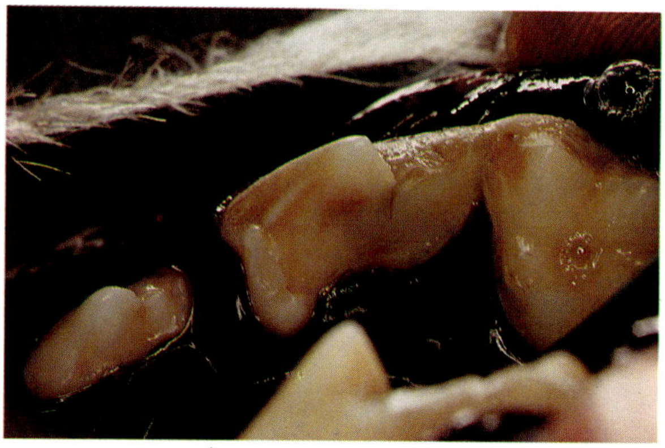

234 Facial swelling — Case 3a. Malar abscesses are usually of dental origin. Intra-oral and radiographic examinations showed no dental cause.

235 Undisplaced crown fracture — Case 3b. The teeth usually responsible for these abscesses are the upper fourth premolars. Close examination with binocular scopes revealed a hairline fracture in the tooth. This undisplaced fracture obviously penetrated into the pulp chamber, which allowed bacteria to invade and cause irreversible pulpal inflammation and necrosis. The pink spot is a confirmation of this. Extraction was the treatment of choice of this acute condition.

236 Fresh vital exposure. The pink spot associated with the exposed pulp chamber at the centre of the fracture line is the common appearance of a vital pulp exposure. Touching the pulp tissue will cause acute pain at this stage.

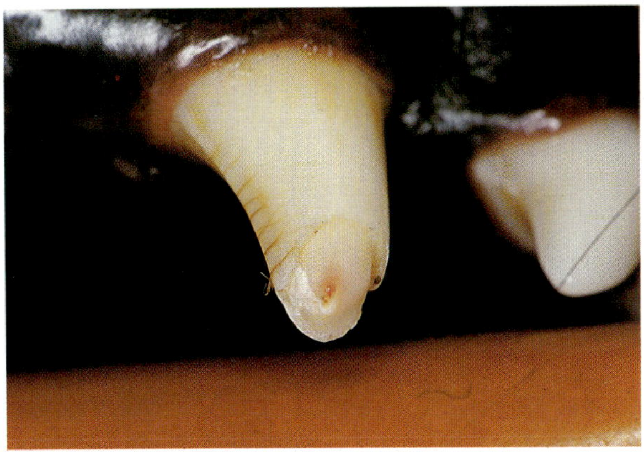

236

237 Pulp polyp — Case 4a — cat. A 'pulp polyp' may rarely develop after pulp exposure. The pulp has epithelialised over. Certain criteria must exist for this to occur. The animal must be young, with wide root canals, and the blood supply to the pulp must be profuse. The exposure must also be large, so that any exudate that may develop at the early stages can escape and not cause pressure necrosis. The condition is unstable and endodontic treatment should be considered. The large diameter of the pulp polyp gives the false impression of an extremely wide immature root canal, which may be ideal for a coronal pulpectomy procedure.

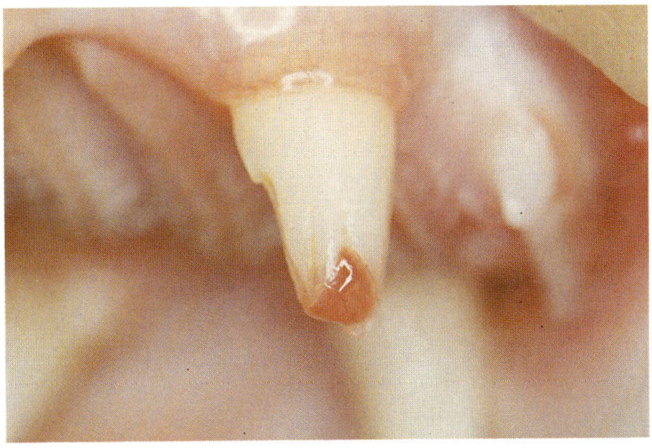

237

238 Resected polyp — Case 4b. Once the extruded polyp is resected, the true diameter of the pulp chamber is visible. Conventional root filling was the treatment of choice.

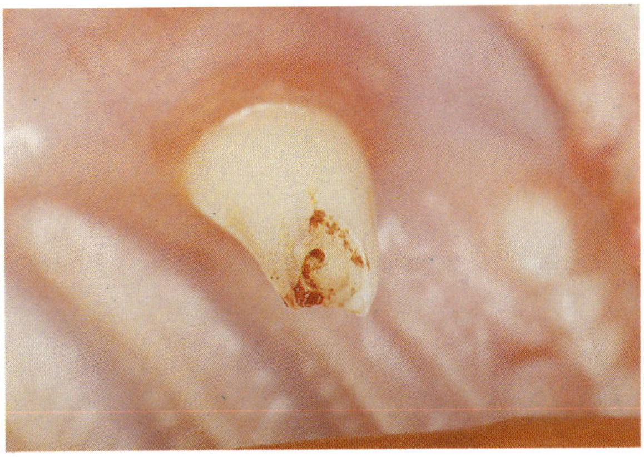

238

239

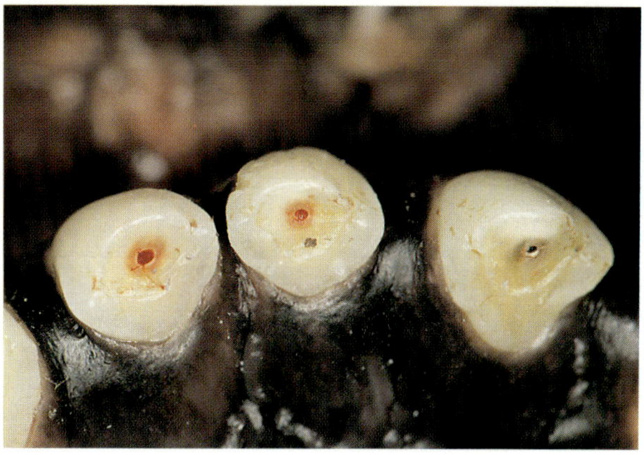

239 Incisors exposed. Stone chewing has exposed the pulp chambers of the upper incisors. In two of the teeth the pulp was still alive, while in the third tooth it had already suffered necrosis. This is confirmed by the black spot at the centre of the tooth.

240

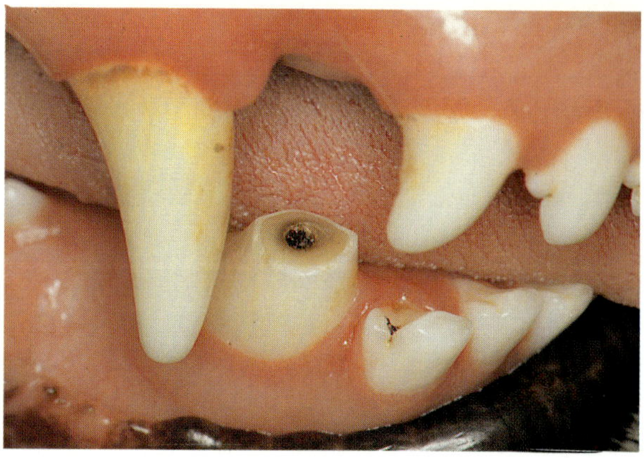

240 Infected pulp chamber. The final sequel of tooth fracture and pulp exposure is total pulp necrosis. The opening to the infected pulp cavity is usually brown or black in appearance and it may become occluded with necrotic material.

Endodontic treatment

Endodontics is defined as the treatment of the innermost part of the tooth, that is the pulp, pulp chamber and the root canals. The objective of endodontics is to eliminate painful, infected or potentially unstable pulpal conditions by employing techniques that conserve the teeth.

Root canal treatment is probably one of the most predictable areas of dental surgery, but also one that has received the greatest amount of abuse since its conception. This discipline has also had the most numerous techniques advocated, and a variety of materials used to obtain superior results, speed up procedures or, inevitably, to cut corners. Endodontics in veterinary dentistry should remain conservative in its approach, simple and predictable.

Endodontic treatment can be subdivided into:

- Pulp therapy. Usually this implies treatment to maintain the vitality of the exposed vital pulp tissue.
- Root filling. Treating root canals by eliminating all their contents, irrespective of whether this is vital or necrotic material.

Nomenclature

Pulpotomy

The term 'pulpotomy' is universally used for the partial amputation of the exposed and living pulp from the pulp chamber, which is the 'coronal' aspect of the pulp cavity. It is a misleading and inaccurate name for the treatment modality as the suffix '-tomy' means 'to cut' by definition and does not indicate the removal of any tissue. The precise term in this instance would be *partial coronal pulpectomy*, while removing all the pulp from the pulp chamber, leaving the pulp to remain undisturbed in the root canal(s) should strictly be termed *total coronal pulpectomy*. These terms will be used throughout this atlas to indicate such procedures.

Root filling

The total elimination of pulp tissues from a tooth is correctly termed 'pulp extirpation' or 'pulpectomy'. The expression *root filling*, which accurately describes the completed treatment, is used throughout this atlas to indicate such procedures.

Pulp therapy

Pulp capping

This technique involves the covering of exposed vital pulp tissue with a lining, usually calcium hydroxide, without any other form of invasive action. It is usually confined to the treatment of very small, sterile, accidental pulp exposures related to cavity preparation in human dentistry. It is probably the least-predictable form of pulp therapy and should not play a role in veterinary dentistry.

Partial coronal pulpectomy

Partial coronal pulpectomy involves excision of a part of the exposed coronal pulp and covering the stump of the amputated tissue surface with materials to maintain pulp vitality, and encouraging secondary dentine bridge formation, to wall off the exposure. This in turn allows continued root development and dentine deposition, to complete the formation of the walls of the roots to normal thickness and length, as well as the maturation to normal root apical anatomy.

This procedure should only be considered in:

- immature teeth in young animals, where the blood supply to the pulp is high and the apices are dilated. The large pulpal volume and apical foramen provide a relief mechanism, enabling any intrapulpal inflammatory exudate that might form during the operation to dissipate; thus, pressure does not build up inside the pulp cavity and cause pressure necrosis and pulp death.
- The second set of criteria for a successful partial coronal pulpectomy are that the exposed pulpal tissue should exhibit no sign of purulent exudate and should bleed easily when probed.

The time limit of one hour after exposure for performing the technique, as advocated by some writers, is unacceptably rigid and is not supported by clinical evidence. Experience and clinical judgement must be used to assess the suitability of each case.

Pulp mummification

(a) The procedure involves the total removal of the coronal pulp and the treatment of the healthy vital pulp of the canals with products that contain paraformaldehyde as an active ingredient. The rationale of the original technique was to mummify the pulp tissues in the apical half or one-third of the root canals so they would act as an inert filling material. 'N2' (second nerve) was one of the first proprietary materials used for this type of treatment. The use of the technique is controversial, and in humans there are numerous reports of severe postoperative pain and paraesthesia if the material is accidentally introduced into the periapical space. There is no clinical indication for the use of this technique in veterinary endodontics.

(b) The use of the formol cresol technique in conjunction with a total coronal pulpectomy can only be justified in rare instances in the treatment of traumatically or cariously exposed primary teeth of great apes.

Root filling

Vital pulp exposures in mature teeth or infected root canals are most predictably treated through the removal of any remaining vital pulp tissue, or the removal of pus and necrotic pulp tissue, and the obturation of the whole pulp cavity.

The underlying principles of root fillings are:

- *Access.* Complete access must be obtained to the contents of the root canal(s) for proper debridement and obturation.
- *Debridement and instrumentation.* All the contents of the canal(s), whether it is vital tissue, necrotic pulp or frank pus, must be removed. Canals must be prepared, to eliminate irregularities and infected dentine from their walls, and widened to a practical diameter, so that proper obturation can take place.
- *Disinfection.* The walls of the canal are disinfected to reduce the remaining microorganisms to the minimum. Sterilisation of root canals to bacteriological standards cannot be performed.
- *Obturation.* The canal must be hermetically sealed with a permanent, biocompatible, filling material. Thereby, no organisms are able to penetrate the canal, either from the periapical tissues or the oral environment, and multiply in a dead space.

By fulfilling the above criteria an ideal healing environment is created for periapical infections to resolve.

Endodontics

Pulp therapy — partial coronal pulpectomy

241
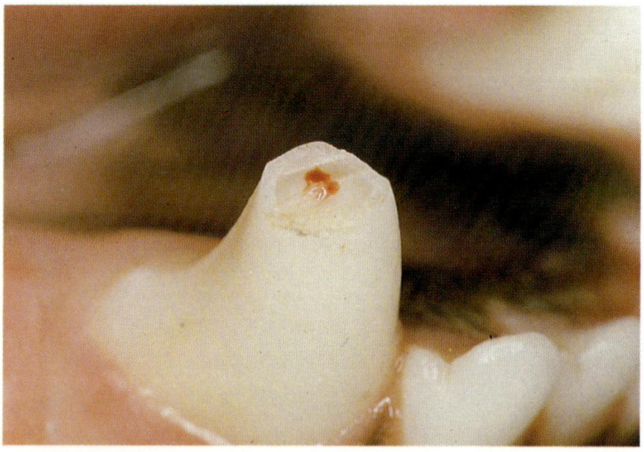

241 Fresh exposure — Case 5a. The least-invasive form of endodontic treatment is a partial coronal pulpectomy. This modality is reserved for relatively fresh pulp exposures of immature teeth where no infection is present. At the same time it must be appreciated that this form of treatment carries a greater element of failure than orthograde root fillings of mature teeth.

242
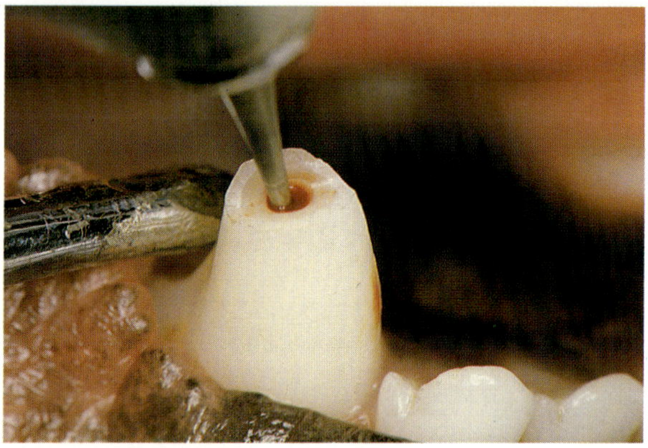

242 Drilling into pulp chamber — 5b. Although the water coolant spray of the drills and the proprietary cements, sealers and gutta percha points are not sterile, as with all aspects of endodontics an aseptic technique should be employed wherever possible. Part of the coronal pulp tissue is removed with a sterile high-speed tungsten burr, using profuse irrigation so as not to overheat the pulp. The depth of penetration depends on the size of the tooth. It should be of the minimum depth practical but deep enough to be able to retain the medicinal and restorative materials. As a rule of thumb three times the diameter of the access cavity is a desirable depth.

243
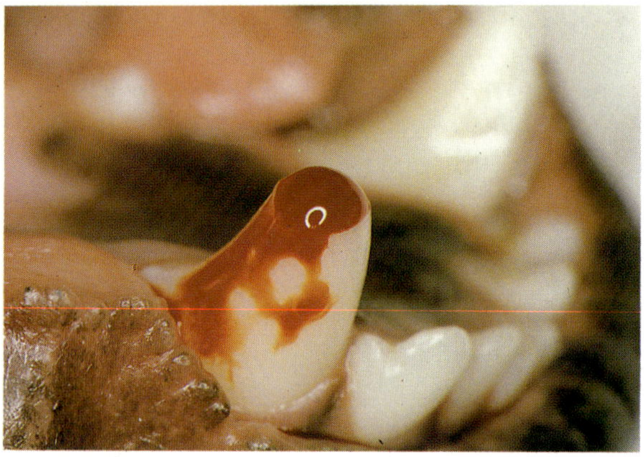

243 Haemorrhage of pulp — Case 5c. The drilling procedure produces haemorrhage of the pulp. It is mandatory that this is completely arrested before proceeding with the treatment any further.

244 Paper point arresting haemorrhage — Case 5d (mirror image). Applying very gentle pressure with the blunt end of a paper point for a few minutes may control the haemorrhage. Haemostatic agents, such as adrenaline or thrombin solution, have proved disappointing in the control of pulpal haemorrhage. Proprietary ferric sulphate solution, applied very sparingly on the blunt end of a paper point, can be a help in cases of difficult haemostasis. Any coagulum should be rinsed away with a 5% solution of hydrogen peroxide followed by saline.

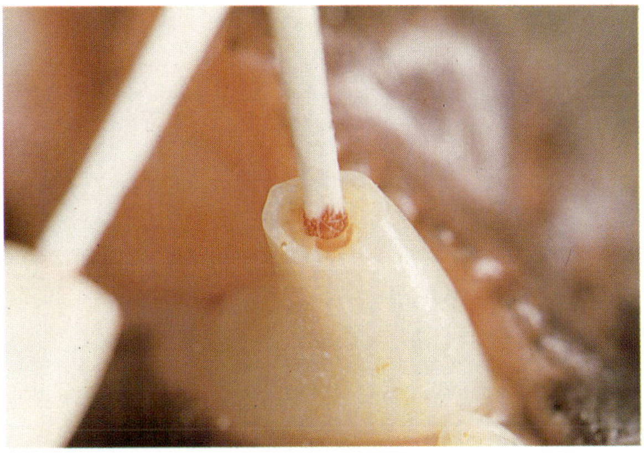

244

245 Dry pulp — Case 5e (mirror image). Haemostasis and the absence of a clot should be confirmed. If even the slightest ooze exists, the procedure of haemostasis must be repeated. Success of the treatment very much depends on attention to detail at every stage.

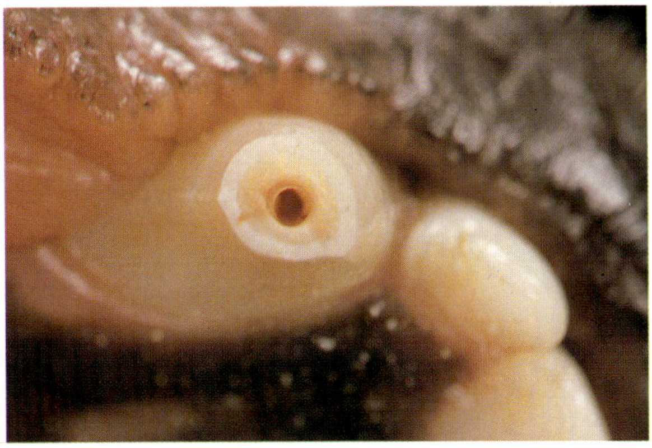

245

246 Applying calcium hydroxide — Case 5f. Calcium hydroxide powder should be applied directly to the dry pulp surface. The blunt end of a paper point is a useful tool to aid distribution of the material at the base of the preparation. The layer should be thin but completely cover the pulp. At the completion of this stage it is important to again check for haemostasis as even the slightest trauma to the pulp may start an ooze.

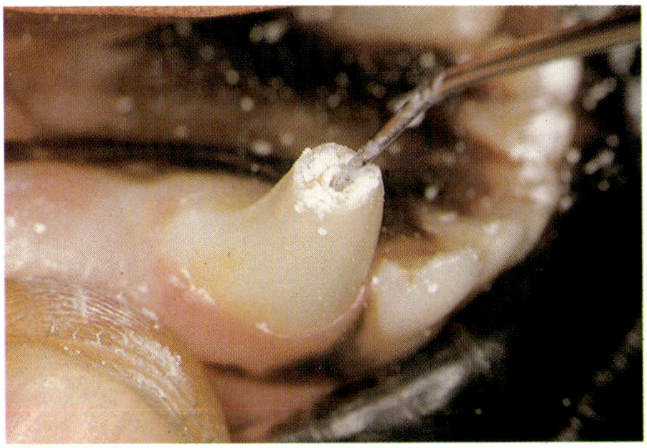

246

247

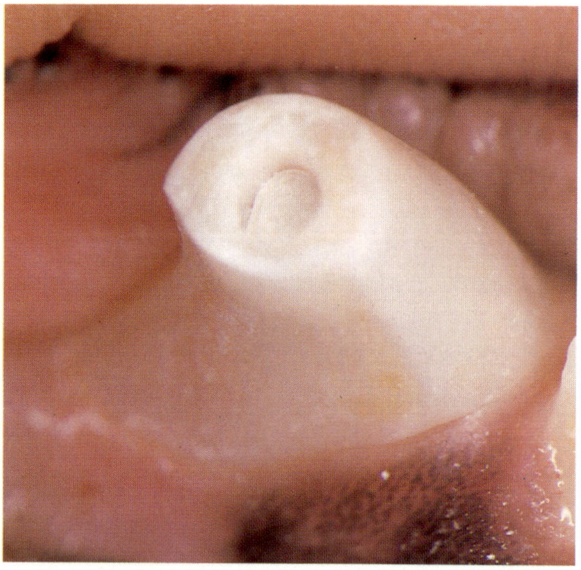

247 Sublining applied — Case 5g (mirror image). A compatible cover to the powder layer, a calcium hydroxide lining material, is used in moderate thickness. A material with a long working time is preferable as it can be difficult to apply the material accurately in a deep cavity. It is also important not to disturb the powder layer and to have no voids in this material. Once fully hardened, an inverted cone burr can be used to remove excess material from the walls of the pulp chamber and create an undercut for the retention of the coronal filling.

248

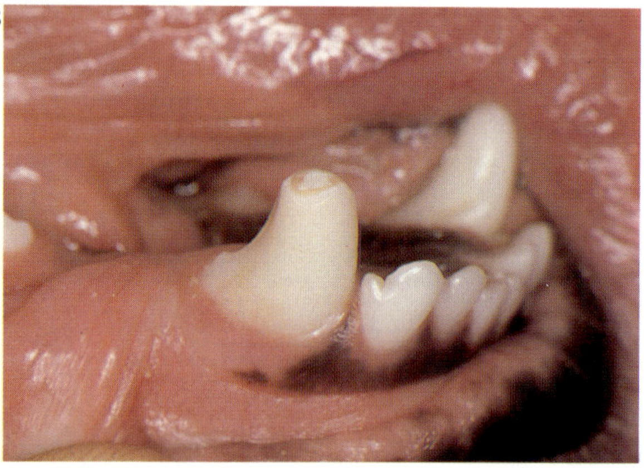

248 Composite filling — Case 5h. Any permanent material may be applied to fill the cavity.

249

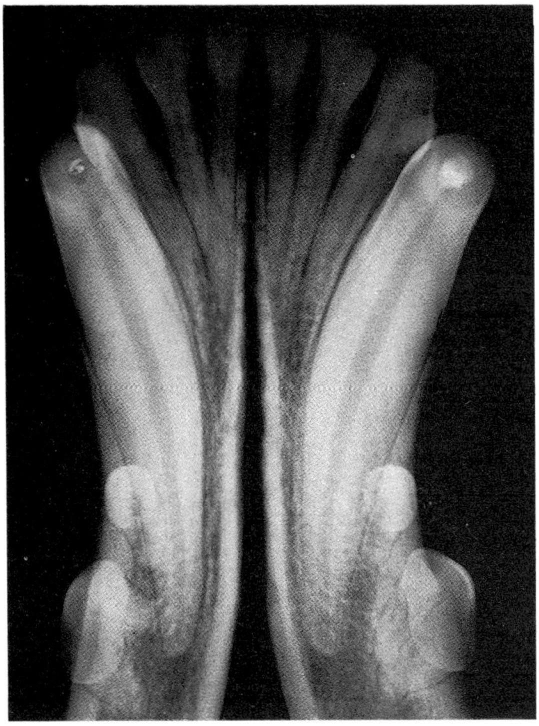

250

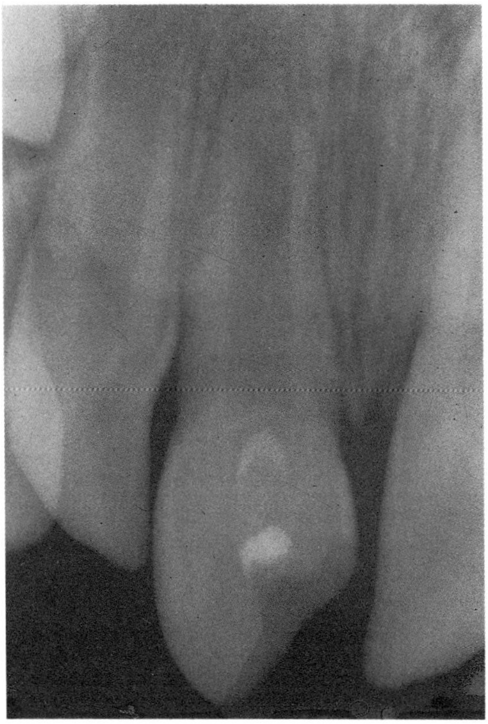

249 Postoperative radiograph. It is considered unethical to routinely re-anaesthetise animals soleley for the purpose of radiographic examination, to confirm the success of endodontic treatment. In veterinary endodontics often the absence of active infection, clinical judgement and the observations of the owner regarding the lack of symptoms must be used as criteria for success. If an animal is to be anaesthetised for other reasons the tooth/teeth in question may be radiographed. In this case the animal was castrated at the age of two years, one year after the partial coronal pulpectomies were performed on both the lower canines. It illustrates root canal dimensions to those teeth which are consistent with the age of the animal and the absence of periapical radiolucencies. The presence of dentine bridges cannot be elicited due to the thickness of coronal tooth substance that is superimposed on the radiograph at the points of restorations.

251

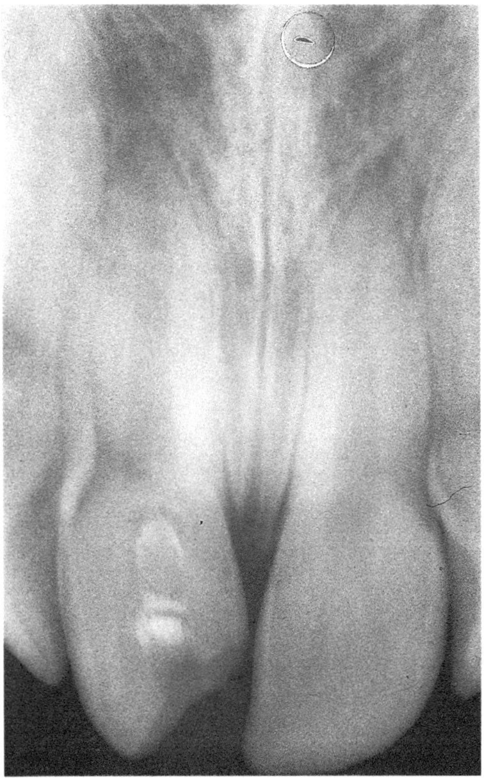

250 Radiograph of human tooth eight weeks after partial coronal pulpectomy — Case 6a. A human example is used to demonstrate the sequel to successful partial coronal pulpectomy. Note that the apical foramen is still dilated and the walls of the root are relatively thin, but there is already a thin bridge of calcified material under the radio-opaque calcium hydroxide dressing.

251 Postoperative radiograph at 16 months — Case 6b. The apex of the tooth is more mature and the apical foramen has become constricted; the root walls are thicker, in line with the development of the adjacent tooth. A well-defined calcified bridge is evident.

252 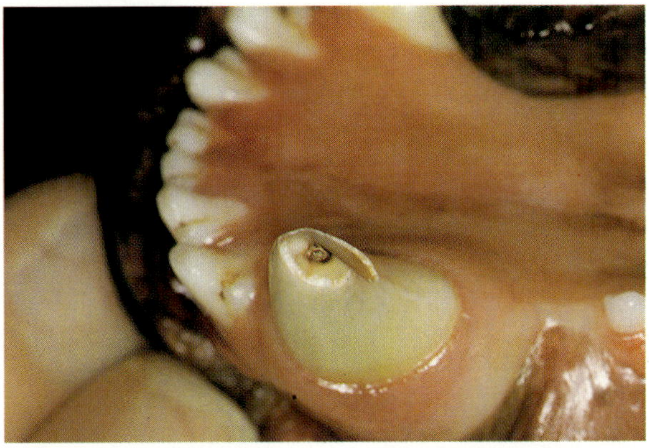

252 Lower canine of a middle-aged dog with an infected root canal — Case 7a.

253 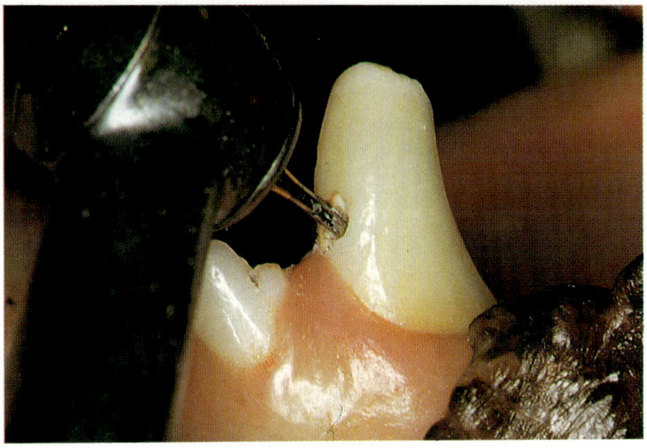

253 Accessing the canal — Case 7b. If the fracture of a tooth is close to the gingival margin, direct access can often be gained through the exposure. If only the tip of the crown is fractured, access to the full length of a canine root canal with endodontic files through the exposure is very difficult because of the curvature of the root and the narrow diameter of the exposure. To ease preparation of the canal and minimise the binding and possible fracture of the files, access is gained to the canal via a mesial point close to the gingival margin. A straight-line approach is gained by this procedure.

254 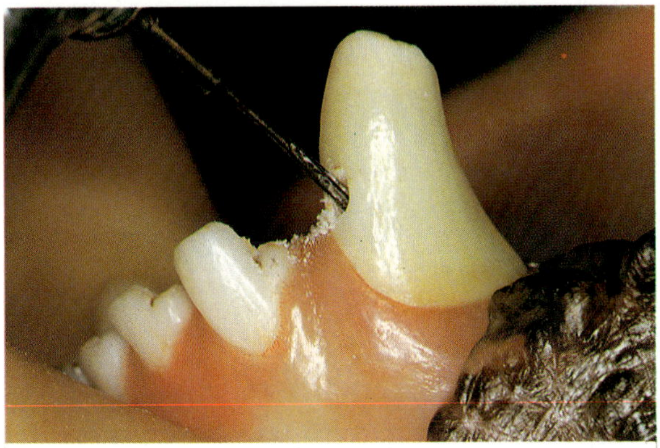

254 Enlarging access cavity with engine reamer — Case 7c. For proper debridement access must be gained to the maximum diameter of the pulp cavity, which is apical to the gingival margin. Only in this way can any remaining pulp tissue be removed intact. Peeso engine reamers are useful instruments for this procedure, but careless technique can cause fracture of the instrument inside the canal. Once the access cavity to the pulp chamber has been prepared, fine endodontic files can be used to determine the length of the root canal.

255 Extirpating pulp — Case 7d. Occasionally, the vital or necrotic pulp may be removed whole, with the aid of one or more barbed broaches, as long as the access cavity is wide enough. In narrow canals, one usually relies on piecemeal debridement, using files, for complete removal of the pulp.

255

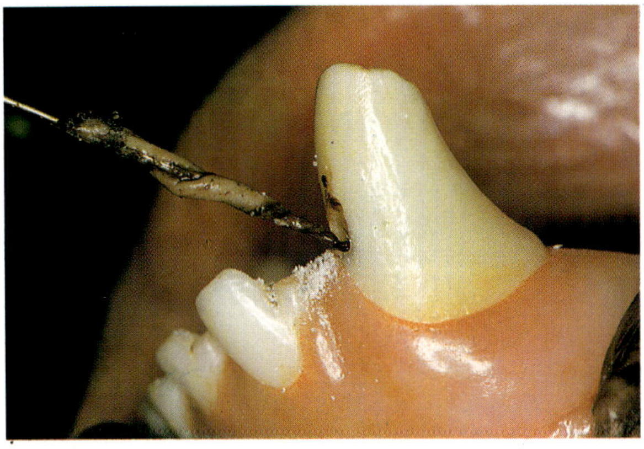

256 File in the canal — Case 7e. It is imperative to prepare the root canals to their full lengths without penetrating into the periapical tissues. Only by having endodontic instruments of the appropriate lengths and the complete range of diameters can thorough debridement be performed. Mature carnivores' root apices usually have a delta formation, which does not allow root canal instruments to pass into the periapical space unless through carelessness or by the use of excessive force. An experienced operator is usually able to estimate canal lengths by judging the lengths of the crowns of the undamaged teeth and tactile feedback through the files. The operator should be skilled and experienced enough, through specimen or phantom head training in endodontics, to eliminate the need to waste valuable anaesthetic time on routinely confirming root lengths with radiographs. The extent of instrumentation is determined by such factors as the severity of the infection, the diameter of the canal, pulpal haemorrhage and the quantity of necrotic debris in the canal. It requires experience and judgement and cannot be conveyed fully in the format of a general atlas. As all veterinary endodontic therapy requires a general anaesthetic, the procedure must be completed in a single session.

256

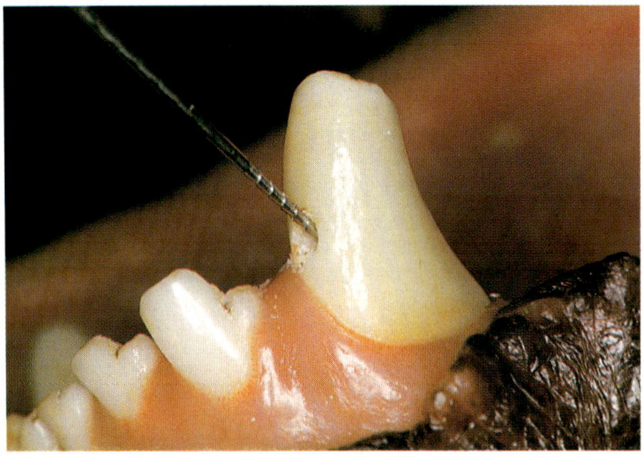

257

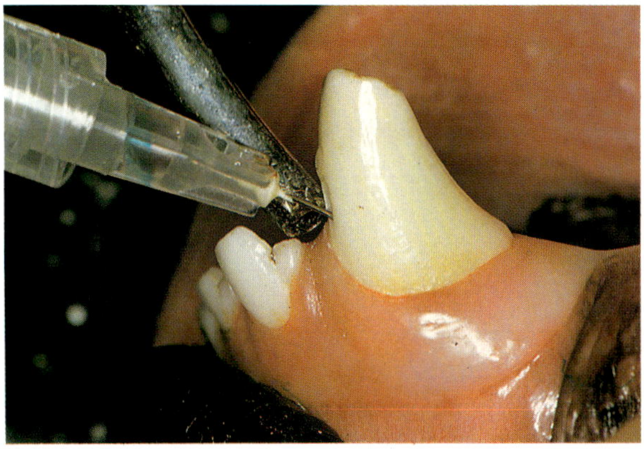

257 Irrigating the canal — Case 7f. During debridement, the root canal needs to be frequently irrigated to remove the 'dentine mud' that is created by the filing process. The alternate use of a 5% solution of hydrogen peroxide and 2% sodium hypochloride as irrigating fluids is an excellent combination. The solutions must be used in that sequence, so that any residual peroxide is neutralised.

258

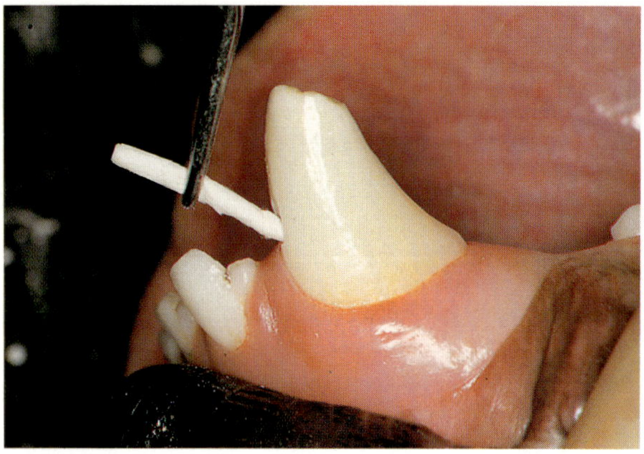

258 Drying the canal with a paper point — Case 7g. Sterility cannot be obtained in the root canal. Once the operator is satisfied that optimum cleanliness has been obtained, the canal is dried with the aid of the appropriate length paper points. Occasionally, it is necessary to arrest a persistent apical haemorrhage by applying pressure to the apex of the canal with paper points, the tips of which have been impregnated with ferric sulphate solution. The drying of root canals with compressed air is prohibited: it can result in emphysemas.

259

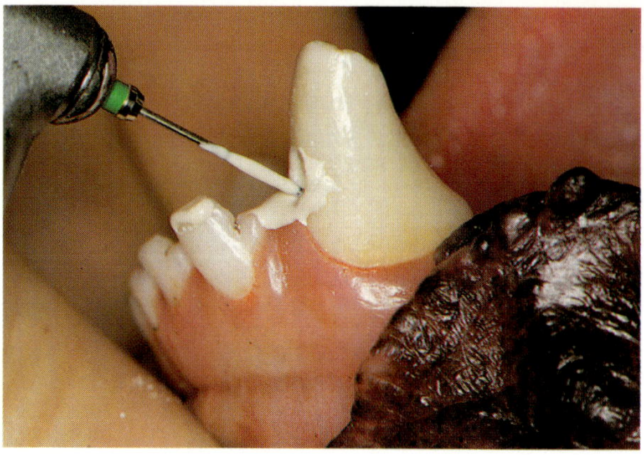

259 Filling with sealer — Case 7h. Once the canal has been fully debrided, enlarged in diameter to a size which is practical to fill, irrigated and dried, it is filled with the root-filling sealant of choice, using a rotary paste filler; then, a master and accessory gutta percha points are inserted. Root canals of large volume can be more easily filled with sealer using a syringe and a wide-bore needle.

260

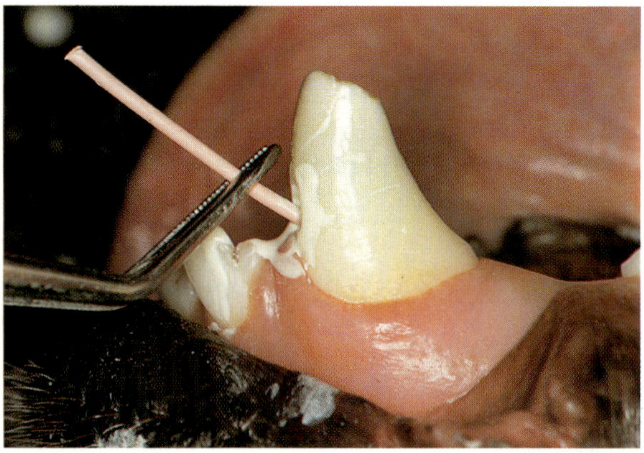

260 GP point in the canal — Case 7i. The master point, which matches the largest size of endodontic file used to prepare the apical portion of the root canal, is first placed in the full length of the canal.

261

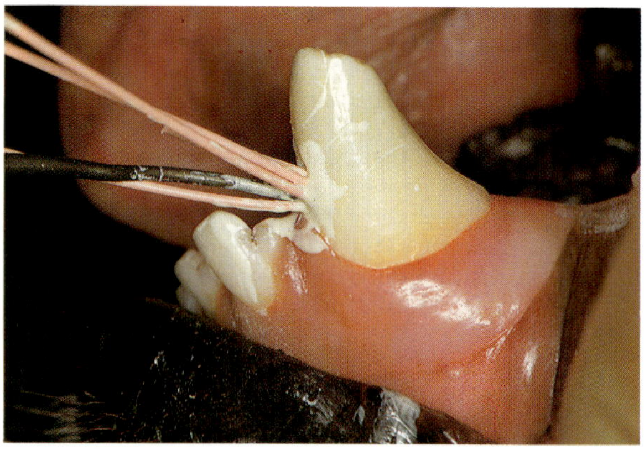

261 Accessory points — Case 7j. A root canal spreader or plugger is used to create lateral space in the canal. This space is filled with accessory points to eliminate the dead space and to obturate any lateral canals that may be present.

262

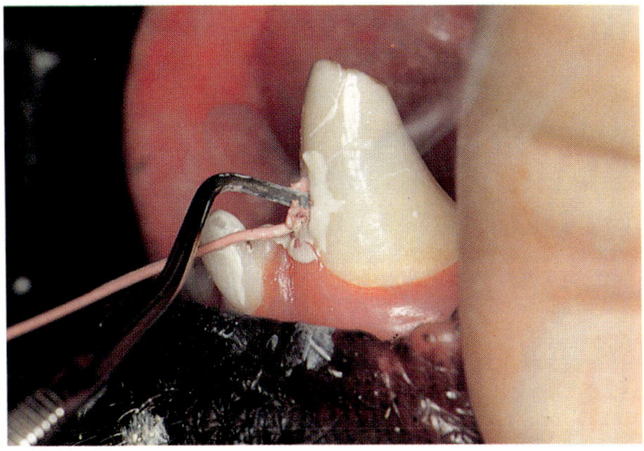

263

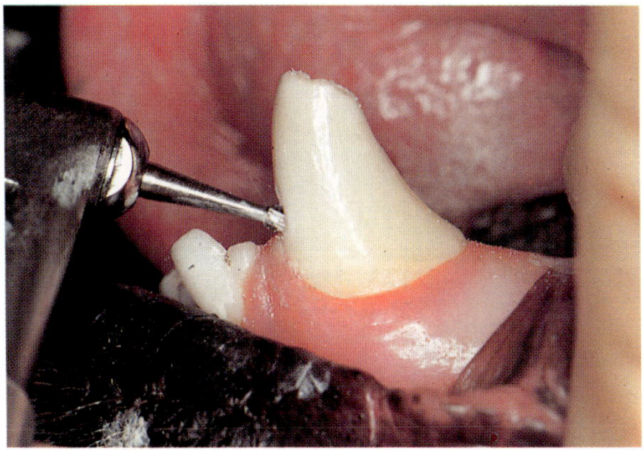

262 Burning gutta percha out — Case 7k. Once the canal is fully obturated, gutta percha is burned out of the pulp chamber with heated instruments.

263 Preparing the cavity — Case 7l. The gingival access cavity and the original exposure are prepared with an inverted cone for retention.

264

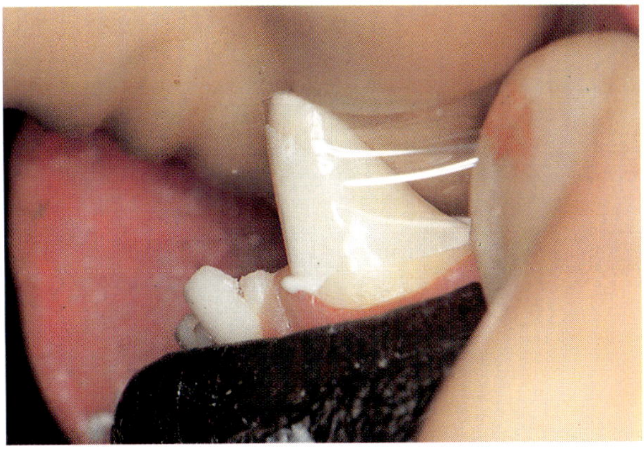

265

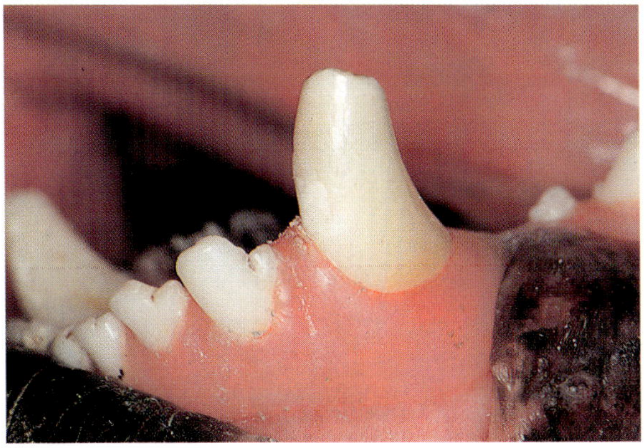

264 Strip placed around composite material — Case 7m. The cavities are filled with the restorative material of choice. Filling the pulp chamber and the coronal aspect of the root canal with a restorative material, be it a composite resin or amalgam, can act as a reinforcing structure. The author believes that chemically activated composites are more practical than 'light cured' materials, where only certain depth can be hardened at a time. A celluloid strip is used to shape the material until it is set. Traces of oil of cloves-based root-filling materials must be cleaned from the cavities as they act as a retarding agent to chemically activated composites.

265 Completed composite restoration — Case 7n. Finally, the excess material is polished off.

266
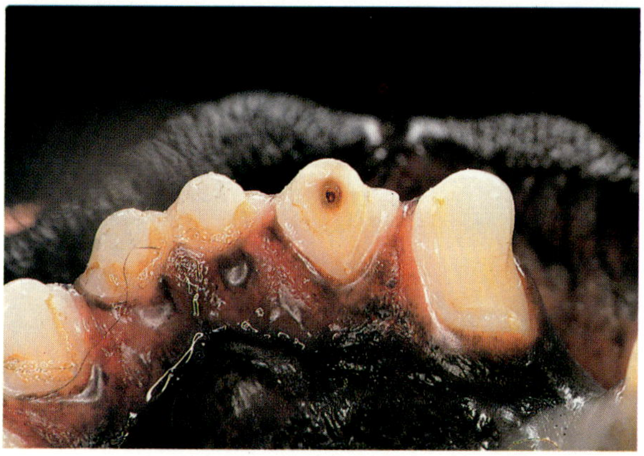

266 Palatal exposure — Case 8a. Mirror image of a fractured upper incisor with an infected root canal.

267
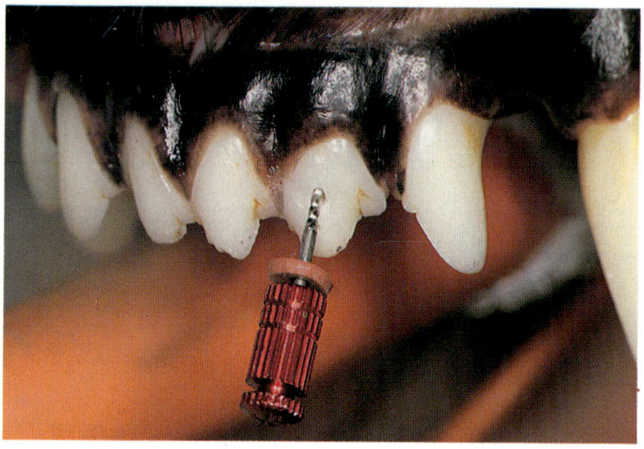

267 Labial access cavity — Case 8b. Approach to the root canal is not necessarily through the surface of the exposure. The root morphology and curvature must be considered for the most direct approach. Access cavities in line with the root canal greatly facilitate canal debridement. In this case a labial approach and a final white filling allowed for an acceptable restoration.

268
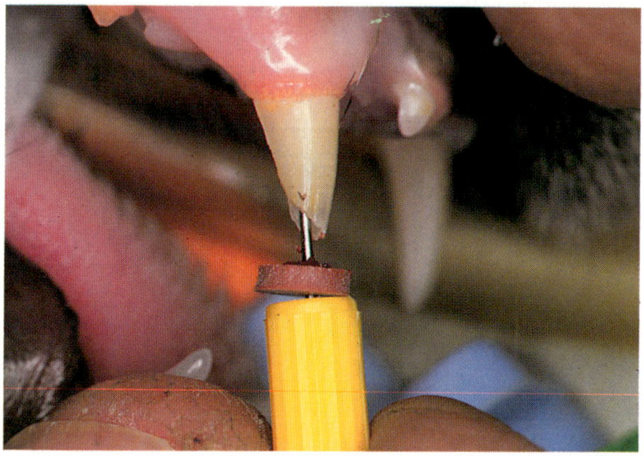

268 Feline canine. The pulp cavity of the cat's canine tooth is usually straighter than that of the dog. Often, even with pulp exposures that are close to the coronal tip, direct access to the full length of the canal can be gained through the exposure hole without having to make a separate cavity.

269 Buccal abscess — Case 9a. This police dog was reluctant to perform duties that involved the use of its teeth. Purulent exudate from a non-vital lower canine of this young animal (18 months of age) was seen discharging into the buccal sulcus, adjacent to the first permanent premolar.

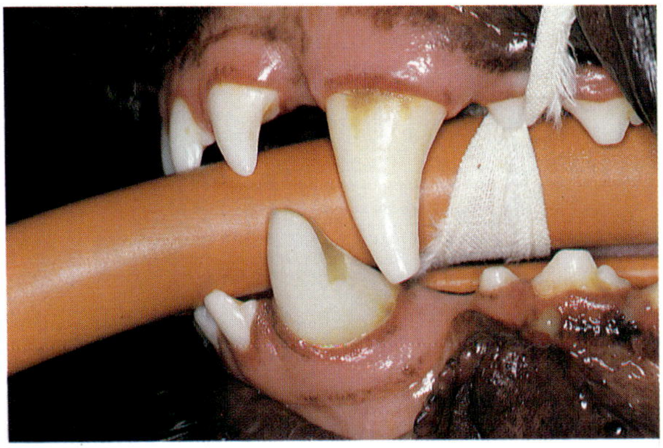

269

270 Radiograph of lower canines — Case 9b. A large radiolucent area was visible at the apex of the lower canine. The relatively thin walls of the root and the large-diameter canal, compared with the other permanent lower canine, indicate that the fracture and pulp necrosis must have occurred at approximately one year of age.

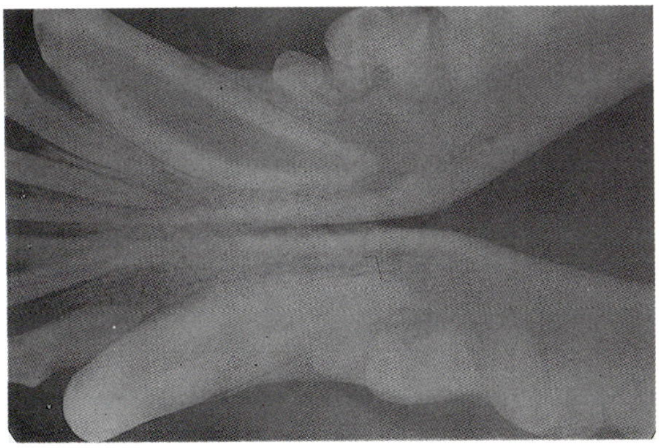

270

271 Radiograph with a file in the root canal — Case 9c. The largest-diameter endodontic file demonstrates the immaturity of the tooth. The apex of the tooth seems to be well formed and the apical foramen constricted. Orthograde root filling would not be predictable had root formation ceased at the dilated stage.

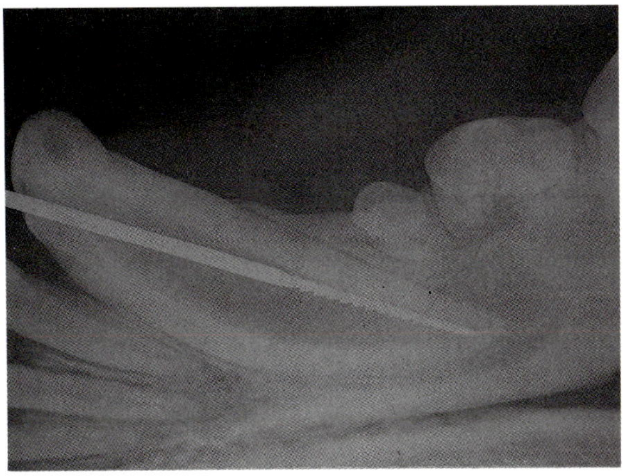

271

272

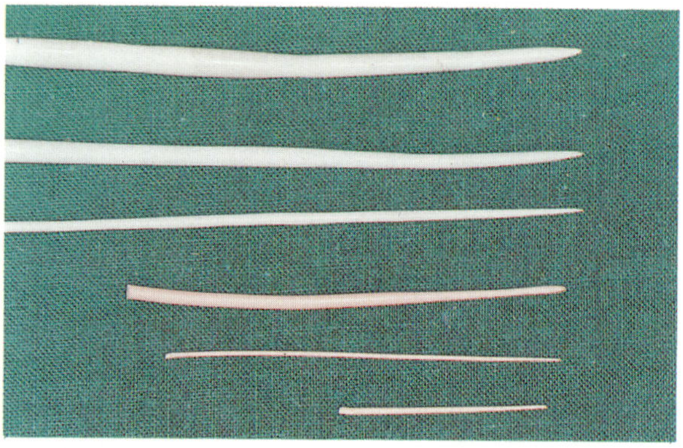

272 Selection of gutta percha points — Case 9d. Root canal sealer on its own is not a reliable root-filling material. It is often resorbed with time and the empty canal can give rise to a recurrence of periapical infection. Gutta percha is an excellent non-resorbable root-filling material. Some manufacturers have developed diameters and lengths that are suitable for the majority of small animal endodontics, but there are situations when larger points are required. In the illustration standard human length is at the bottom, two veterinary points in the centre and three custom-rolled points are at the top.

273

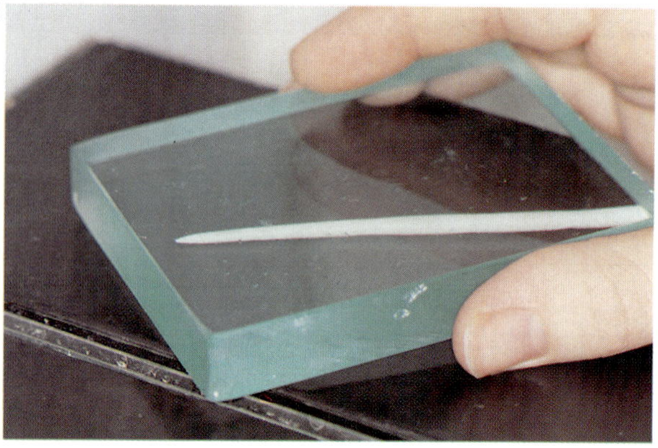

273 Custom-rolling gutta percha — Case 9e. The quality and consistency of the gutta percha needs to be chosen carefully. Most 'stick' materials are too brittle, and the melting point of the commercial points is often too high. Some practice is required before uniformly tapered points can be rolled between warm glass mixing slabs or tiles once the material has been softened in hot water.

274

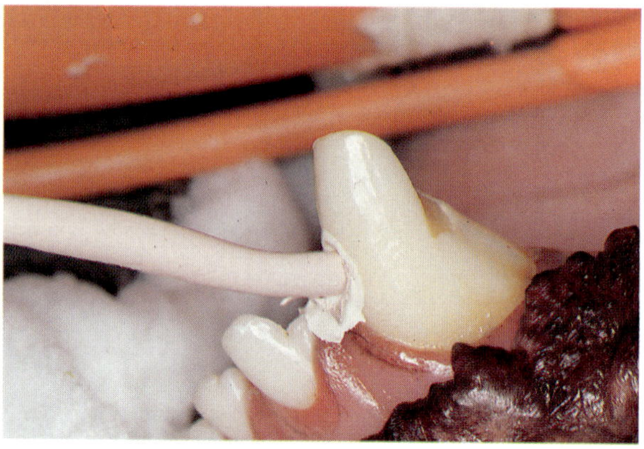

274 Placing a root filling — Case 9f. Obturating a canal with a custom-rolled gutta percha point and sealer.

275 Radiograph of a completed root filling — Case 9g. A well-condensed custom-rolled gutta percha illustrates that this technique is not unique to the treatment of captive wild animals. No apical surgery was performed on this young animal as the relatively short history of apical infection should resolve through the healing potential of the animal and the well-obturated root canal.

275

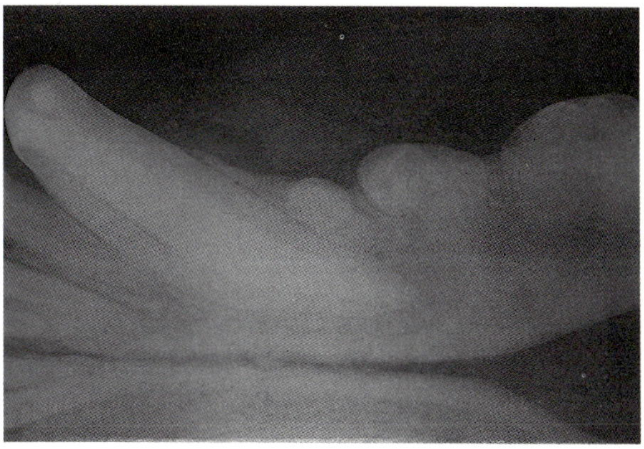

Posterior teeth

It is important in cases of facial trauma to thoroughly examine the posterior and anterior teeth. Road traffic accidents or kicks received from horses that result in fractures of the canine teeth of dogs can also cause fractures of one of the carnassial teeth, either in the same, opposing or contralateral quadrant.

276

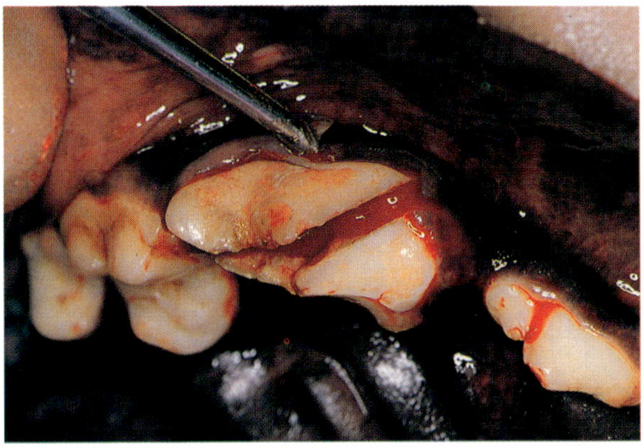

277

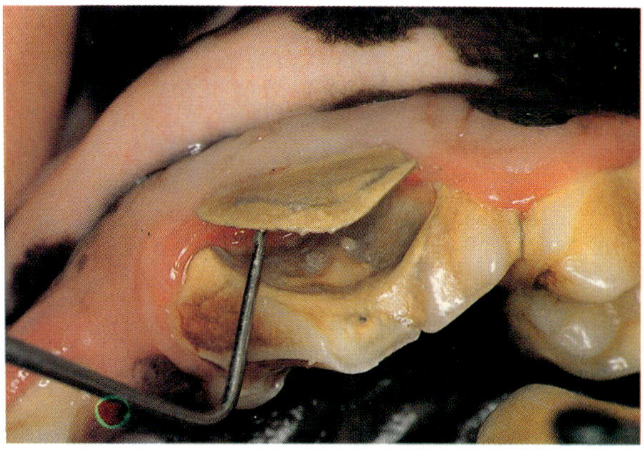

278

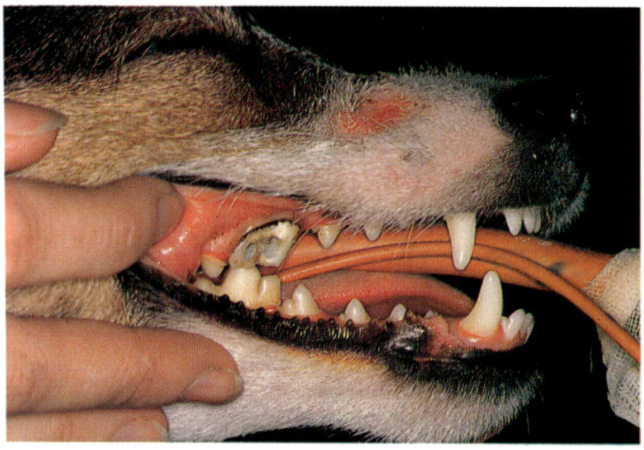

276 Fractured upper premolar. Often the fracture of the posterior teeth demands extraction, but some can be saved through endodontic treatment.

277 Slab fracture. Oblique or 'slab' fractures of the buccal wall of premolars are not uncommon in bone and rock chewers. These usually involve the pulp chamber and a purulent discharge is visible through the small exposure.

278 Nose irritation. In the differential diagnosis of oronasal lesions, dental diseases should be borne in mind as a possible aetiology. The nasal ulceration of this dog was thought to be of dermatological origin; however, the scratching stopped and the ulceration healed once the infected upper fourth premolar had been root-filled.

279

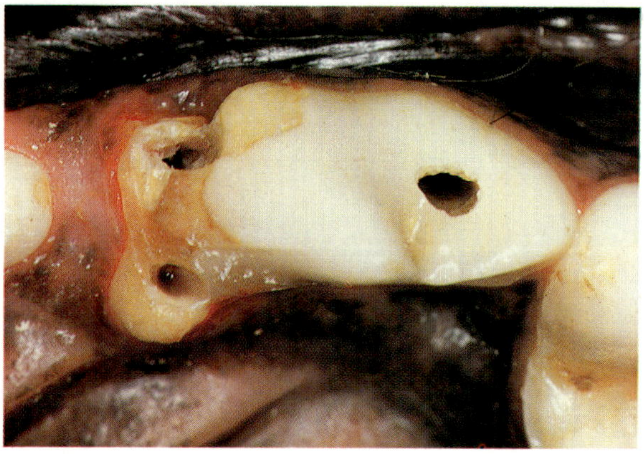

280

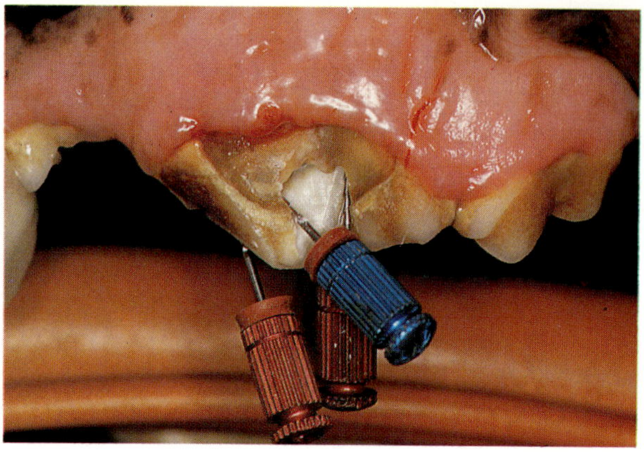

279 Access cavities. The endodontic treatment of these multi-rooted teeth must be considered as if the canals were separate teeth. It is desirable to keep the access cavities as separate as possible, depending on the trauma already present, so as not to weaken the crown.

280 Files in canals — Case 10a. The endodontic files in the canals of this upper fourth premolar demonstrate the severe divergence of the roots that is usually present. The position of the palatal root requires operators to study specimens before they can be confident of finding it consistently. The approach is from a more buccal angulation than expected. In small breeds and old animals it sometimes proves impossible to find the palatal canal in the time restraints general anaesthetics impose. It is permissible in these instances to amputate and extract the palatal root, while the other two canals are filled as normal.

281

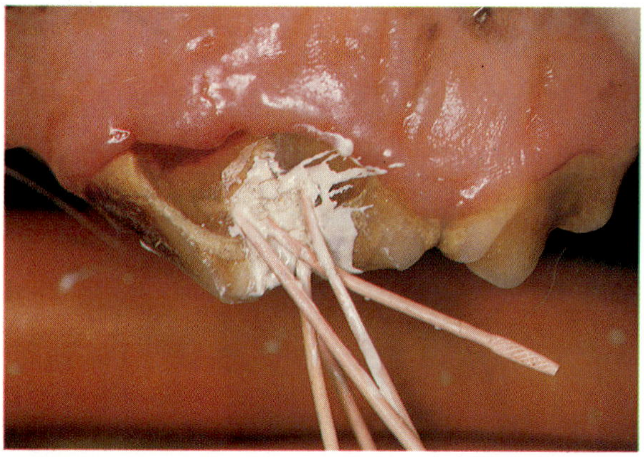

282

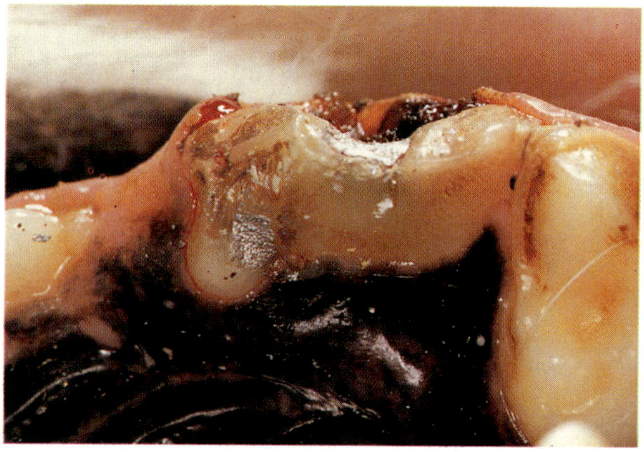

281 Gutta percha in the canals — Case 10b. The canals are obturated in the same way as single-rooted teeth.

282 Final restorations — Case 10c. Amalgam was used to seal the access cavities.

Surgical endodontics

This modality entails the curettage of the apical granuloma, abscess or cyst, and resecting the apical 10% of the tooth through a mucoperiosteal or extra-oral flap, usually in conjunction with a conventional root-filling technique.

The criteria for apicectomies are quite specific and should not be used as an alternative to poor orthograde endodontic technique. Radiolucent periapical areas or abscesses are not an automatic indication for apicectomies. Animals, especially when young, possess great healing potential, and if root fillings are carried out to a high standard, most periapical lesions will resolve.

Apicectomies should be reserved for:

- Draining chronic periapical infections in older animals, where retention of the tooth may be indicated.
- When active apical infection is present, but an orthograde approach is not possible as the root canal is blocked and cannot be passed.
- When conventional root canal treatment has failed, but the extraction of the tooth is contraindicated because of clinical reasons.

Retrograde root fillings

Gutta percha points and zinc oxide eugenol-based cement are an excellent sealing combination; there is no advantage in using a separate apical seal unless the gutta percha point is unable to form a perfect apical seal.

If a canal is blocked or conservative root canal treatment has failed, or the gutta percha cannot be condensed due to mechanical aspects of the root canal, a retrograde seal has to be created surgically at the apical end of the root canal. Amalgam is the material of choice for these restorations.

There are disadvantages to retrograde amalgam fillings:

- Amalgam is considered more of an irritant to the periapical tissues than gutta percha or zinc oxide eugenol cement.
- Apical resorption during the healing phase may cause the retrograde restoration to be displaced if its retention is unsatisfactory.
- If a retrograde filling is used on its own, without following the basic principles of orthograde endodontics, the treatment may fail as a result of the necrotic contents of the canal percolating into the periapical tissues through lateral canals.

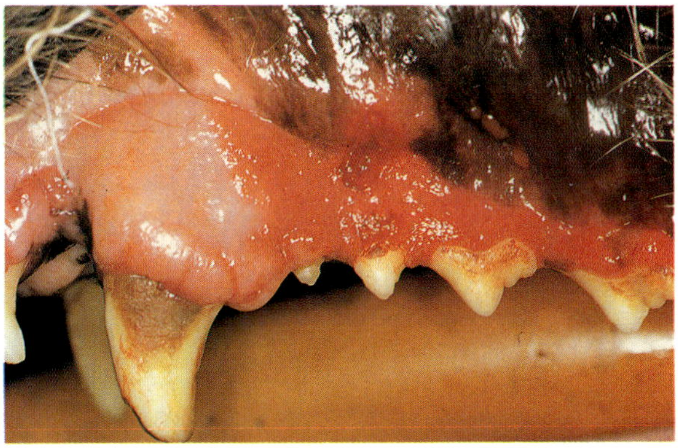

283

283 Purulent discharge in the buccal sulcus — Case 11a. This chronic gingival infection was erroneously treated as periodontal disease. The upper permanent canine was fractured and infected. Probing of the sinus tract indicated a draining periapical abscess.

284 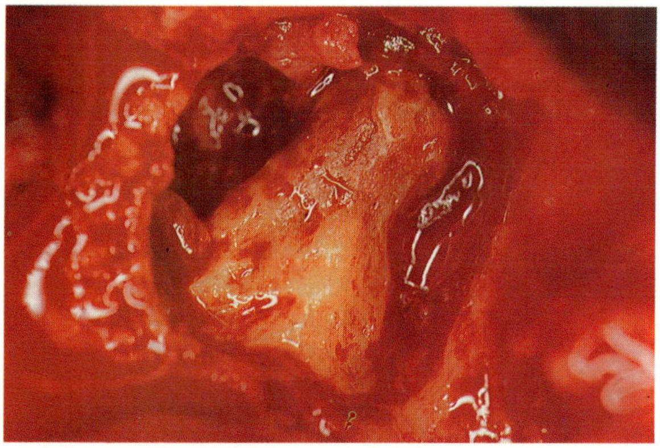

284 Flap reflected — Case 11b. Apical surgery was the treatment of choice because of the chronic sinus tract and the limited healing potential of this middle-aged animal. The reflected labial flap confirmed the presence of apical osteolysis. The site of the incision should be chosen with care as the lateral nasal artery lies within the mucoperiosteum, in close proximity to the root of the upper canine.

285 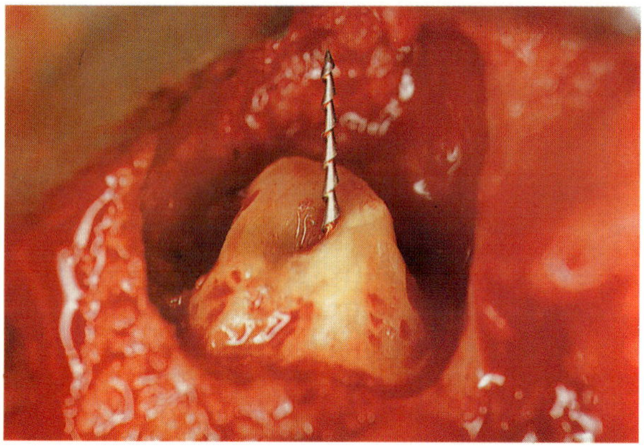

285 Resected tip and file in a canal — Case 11c. The root tip was resected with a fissure burr at an angle bevelled towards the operator to improve access to the apex. Orthograde endodontics was performed to clean and fill the canal. The periapical granulation tissue was curetted to healthy, bleeding bone.

286 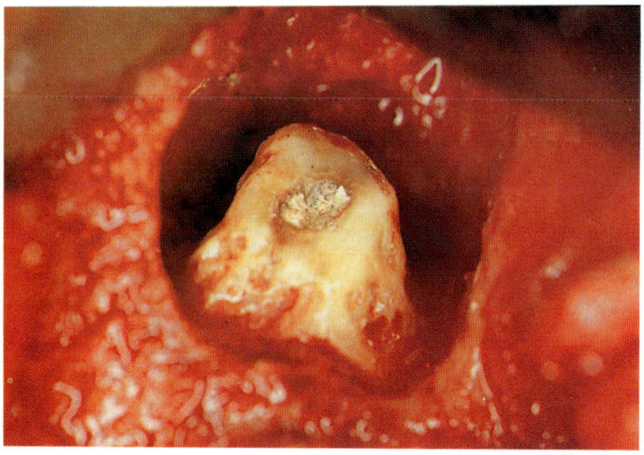

286 Completed root filling — Case 11d. Orthograde root filling (gutta percha and zinc oxide eugenol sealer) was placed. The condensation of the material was not judged to be sufficiently dense.

287 Cutting retrograde cavity — Case 11e. A retrograde cavity was cut with an inverted cone for the amalgam filling.

287

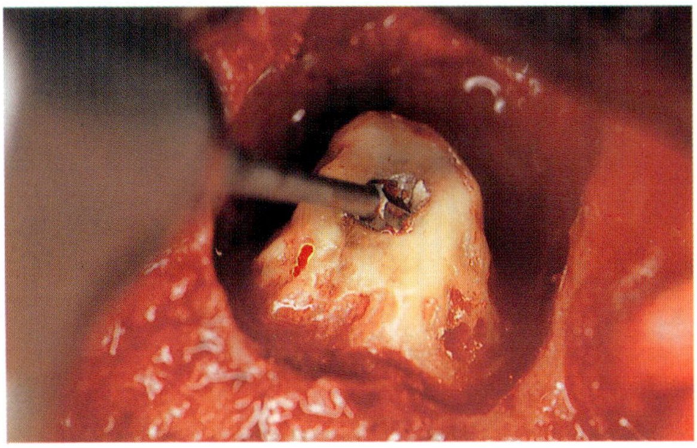

288 Amalgam in place — Case 11f. Retrograde amalgam root filling in place.

288

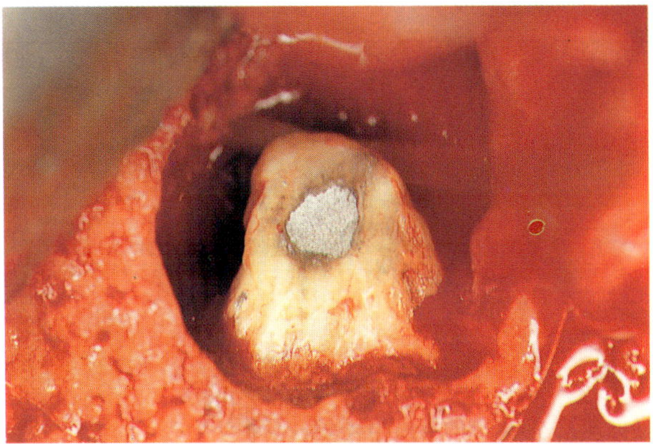

289 Postoperative follow-up — Case 11g. Six months postoperatively. No recurrence of apical infection, sinus tract or gingival inflammation was evident.

289

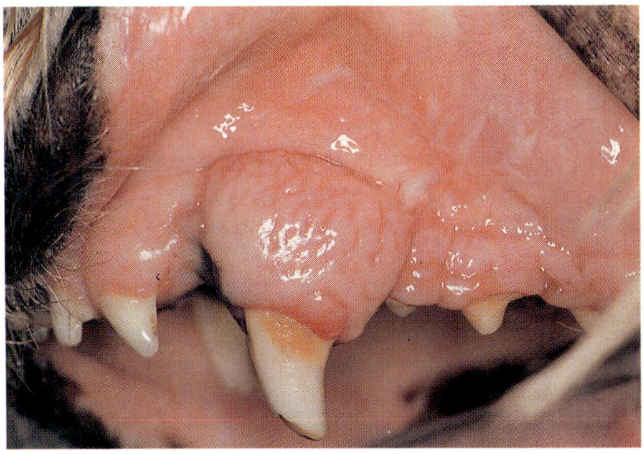

Prophylactic endodontics

Continuing the principle of utilising the simplest and least-traumatic techniques in veterinary dentistry, endodontics can occasionally be used in situations where surgical intervention may seem the only means of relieving pain and infection that is not caused by pulpal disease.

290
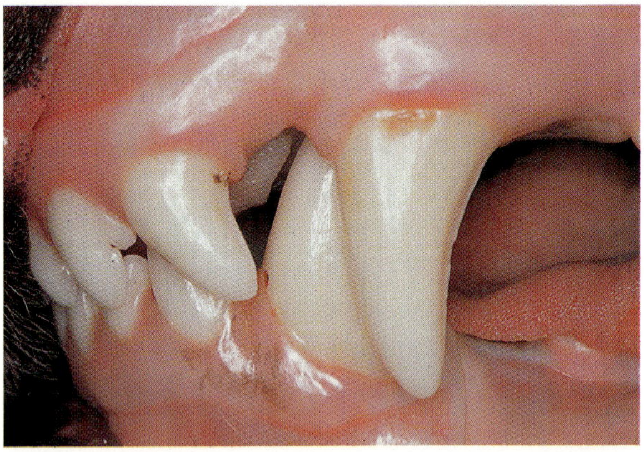

290 Canine traumatising palate — Case 12a. This young dog had a traumatised palatal mucosa through a lingually inclined lower canine. Although orthodontic treatment may be occasionally considered, reduction of the tooth height and treating the exposed pulp of the immature tooth by endodontic treatment is an acceptable procedure. It must be stressed that tooth-height reduction without the appropriate endodontic treatment, in line with the age of the animal, is totally unethical and unacceptable.

291
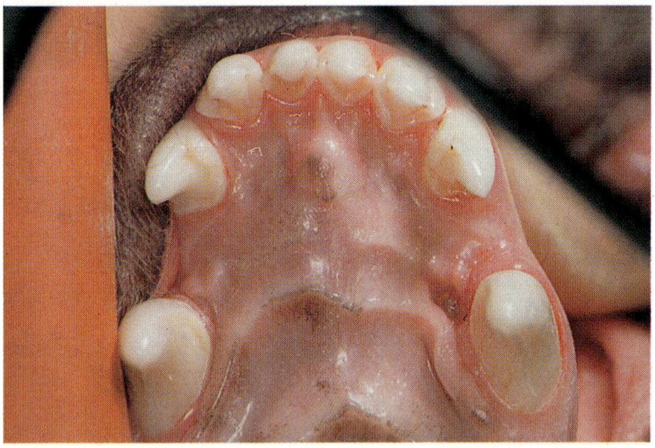

291 Palatal view — Case 12b. Palatal view of gingival damage.

292
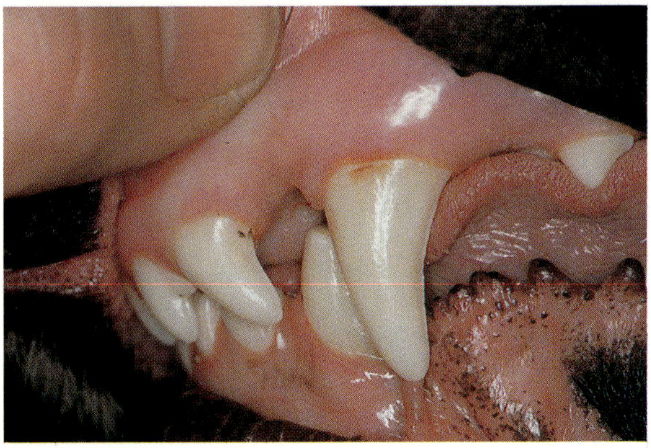

292 End result — Case 12c. The shortened canine after treatment demonstrates the relief of occlusal trauma to the palatal mucosa.

293

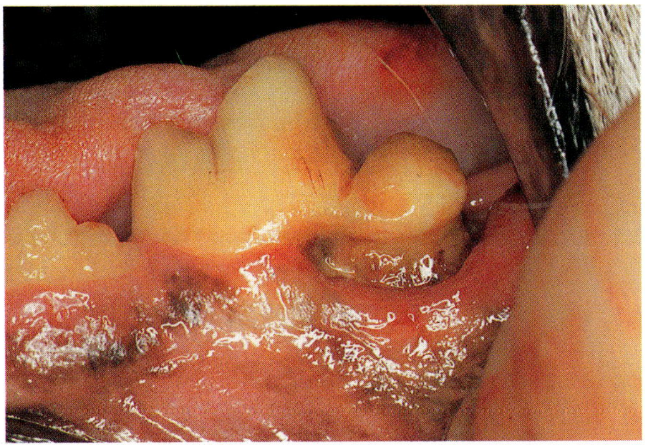

294

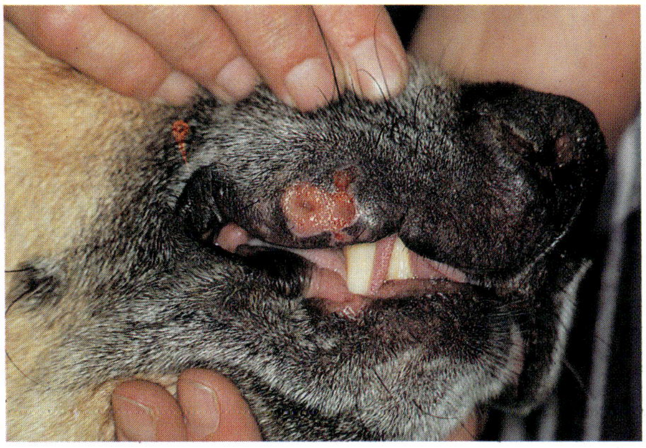

293 Periodontally involved lower molar. If only one of the roots of a vital, multi-rooted tooth has lost its periodontal support it may be permissible to extract the diseased part and leave the well-retained root. This procedure is suitable in old animals, where the extraction of a healthy root from the mandible may involve considerable bone removal. The amputation of the diseased root exposes the pulp tissue, which will in time become necrotic and lead to periapical infection. Endodontic treatment of the retained root affords a predictable and non-surgical alternative in maintaining a comfortable mouth, and prevents iatrogenic fractures in these potentially brittle bones.

294 Traumatised lip. This dog was suffering with idiopathic unilateral facial paralysis, which resulted in continuous trauma to the upper lip from the canine teeth during mastication. Decoronation and root filling the teeth involved was a rapid and atraumatic treatment, preferable to the extraction of these well-retained canines.

295

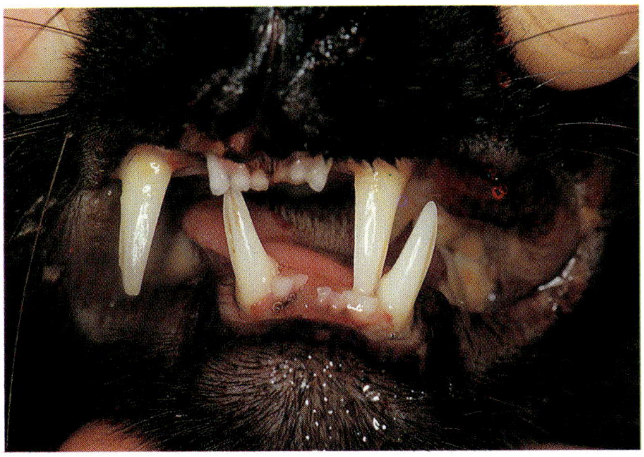

296

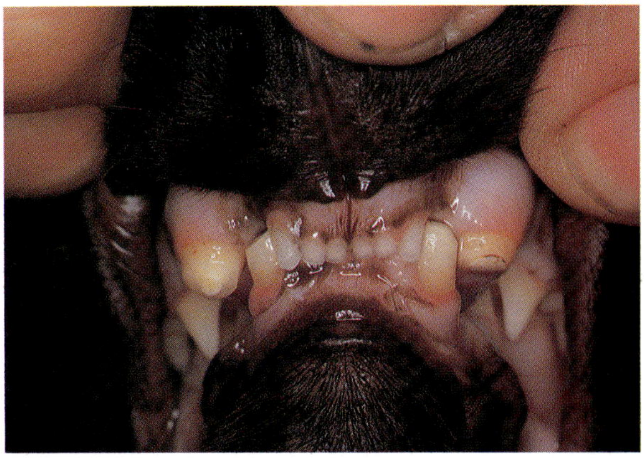

295 Mandibular trauma — Case 13a — cat. This cat suffered symphysial fracture and dislocation of the mandible through a road traffic accident. Reduction of the bilateral temporomandibular dislocations could not be retained and normal dental interdigitation was prevented by the malocclusion of the canine teeth. The animal was anorexic and required intravenous fluid therapy. His general condition was rapidly deteriorating. Radiographic examination did not reveal injuries to the condyles or the base of the skull. Damage to the pterygoid muscles and/or the temporomandibular fossa was suspected. Treatment through bilateral condylectomies and/or extraction of the canine teeth was rejected.

296 Postoperative appearance — Case 12b. Decoronation of all the canines and root fillings were performed. Malocclusion and anorexia ceased immediately and recovery was uneventful. Mastication has remained normal.

Unsaveable endodontic situations

Root canal treatment in veterinary work is not usually performed for aesthetic or functional reasons but to eliminate pain and infection in the least-traumatic way. There are times when teeth cannot be saved or the prognosis is so poor that extractions are positively indicated.

297

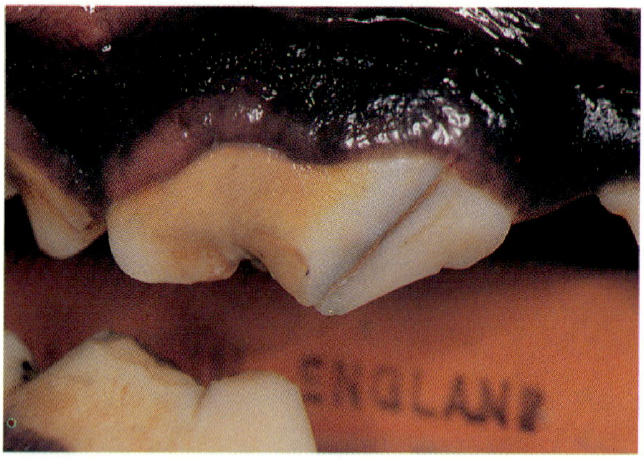

297 Longitudinally fractured upper premolar. Midline fractures of teeth present unsaveable situations.

298

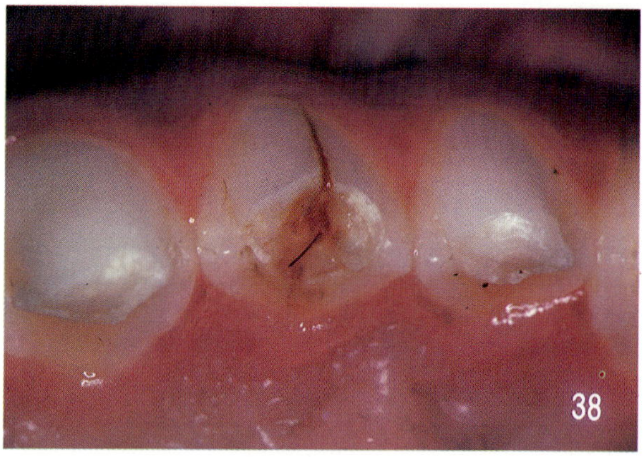

298 Longitudinal fracture of an incisor. Hairline longitudinal fractures invariably extend to an infrabony point of the root and will eventually contribute to the formation of an abscess.

299

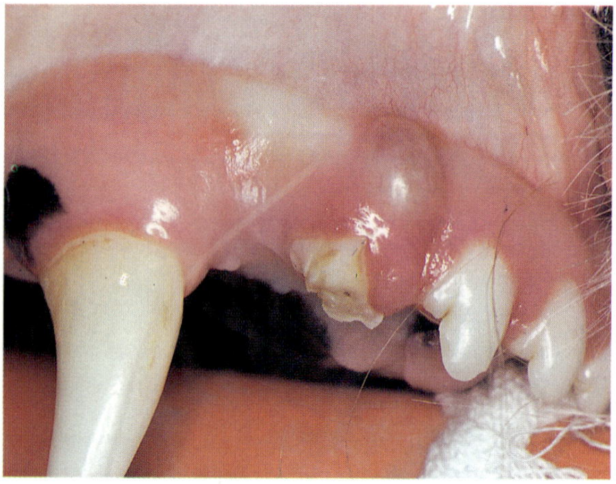

299 Lateral abscess associated with a longitudinal fracture.

300

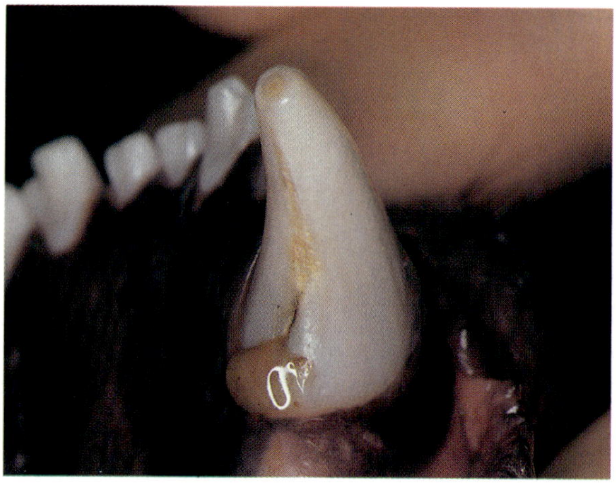

300 Longitudinal fracture of lower canine. Longitudinal fracture of the crown extends into the root of the tooth with a purulent exudate discharging through the crack. The extraction of such teeth is mandatory.

9 Restorative Prosthodontics

The popular press often sensationalises the restoration of dogs' teeth with crowns, as many people like to see the anthropomorphic treatment of animals. The most common tooth in carnivores to fracture and have its restoration attempted is the canine tooth. Dog owners, on finding their pet sustaining such an injury, frequently request restoration to its original form. They believe that the animal will be unable to eat with a tooth of reduced height, failing to appreciate that domestic animals rarely utilise these teeth in the process of mastication. It is the duty of the attending professional to explain to the client that endodontic treatment on animals is performed so as to provide the least traumatic treatment in establishing oral health and not necessarily to maintain or restore function. Restorations performed to satisfy the desires of clients without taking into consideration the clinical needs of the animals are unethical. Before discussing the techniques of restorative prosthodontics for animals, it is important to examine the necessity of such treatment, the mechanics and the associated problems.

An animal's tooth may be fractured as a result of its activities as a working dog, through destructive behaviour, such as chewing rocks, fences or bones, or through accidental trauma.

The primary functions of the canine teeth in carnivores are gripping and killing prey as well as defence; a secondary function of the lower canines may be to keep the tongue from drooping on the side, where it could be damaged by the premolars on closure of the mouth.

Domestic dogs certainly do not suffer from having teeth of a reduced height, and it is highly debatable that a working dog is at a disadvantage and not able to fulfil its function when a canine tooth is shorter than normal. Many dog handlers believe that a better grip results from the use of the posterior teeth rather than the canines, and most working dogs are trained accordingly. There is little doubt that a 1.5 cm long fractured canine can be almost as efficient as a fully restored 3 cm crown. It must also be appreciated that it is impossible to reverse behavioural activities that may have brought about the original injury, and that failures of dental prostheses are high.

The natural crowns of dogs' canines are conical in shape, so that retentive, parallel crown preparations on human lines are not possible. If only minimal crown length has been lost, much tooth substance needs to be sacrificed to gain retention for a prosthesis, and the size of the opposing teeth may also need to be reduced to obtain clearance. If a moderate amount of crown height has been lost, there may be insufficient supragingival tooth material remaining to retain a crown prosthesis; additional anchorage in the form of prefabricated, or custom cast metal posts must then be cemented into a modified root canal space for retention purposes. Carnivores have long roots in relation to their body sizes, especially of their canine teeth, but the natural canine crown length is almost as long as the root support, which places great leverage forces on these teeth. This fact is demonstrated by the frequent fractures of these elongated structures. The natural curve of the dog's canine does not lend itself to post-restorations: usually, only half the root length can be utilised for retention purposes and the mechanical forces would be high on a post that is much shorter than the ideal post/crown ratio (i.e. where the post length is twice the coronal restoration height). Failure of the restoration or fracture of the root itself may result.

Because of the dental anatomy, the occlusal and mechanical forces that are specific to the animal, crown restorations for dogs do not necessarily offer protection to the remaining tooth substance, as in human dentistry. In fact, they may contribute to the loss of a perfectly functional tooth, with root fractures occurring through the increased stress a post creates on the remaining root.

Dog owners in the 'show world' often request the replacement of missing teeth with a fixed bridge prosthesis. The restoration of such defects on animals is totally unethical, irrespective of whether they are genetically, periodontally or traumatically precipitated. Considerable damage would be created to the perfectly healthy adjacent teeth through such unnecessary procedures.

There will be exceptional circumstances when dental surgeons are asked to undertake the restoration of animals teeth with crown prosthesis. This chapter puts forward guidelines on how to avoid elementary errors and on how dentists can adapt their knowledge and skills when such treatment is genuinely indicated.

301

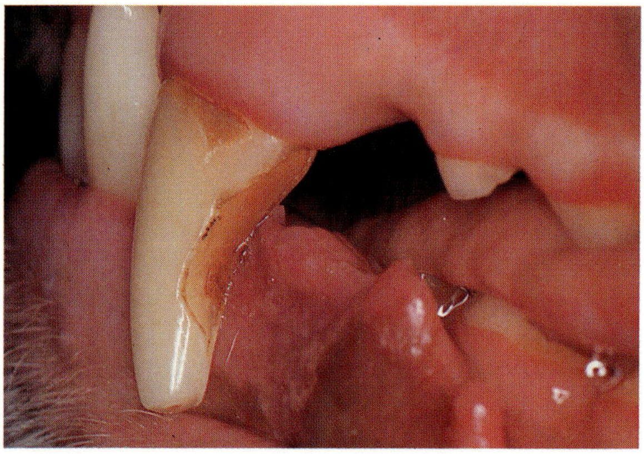

301 Canine tooth of fence chewer. A young dog, demonstrating the amount of tooth loss that can take place through such destructive behaviour. Restoration of these abrasion lesions is positively contraindicated. The behaviour will continue and rapid failure of the treatment, be it with filling material or full-coverage prosthesis, will occur.

302

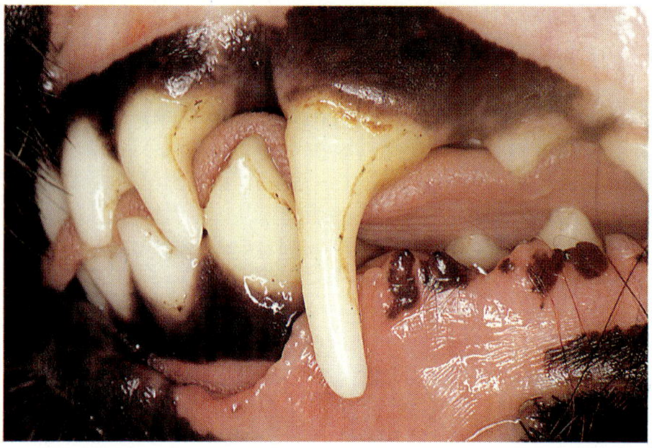

302 Rock chewer — Case 1a. Middle-aged dog with moderate wear of the canine and third incisors.

303

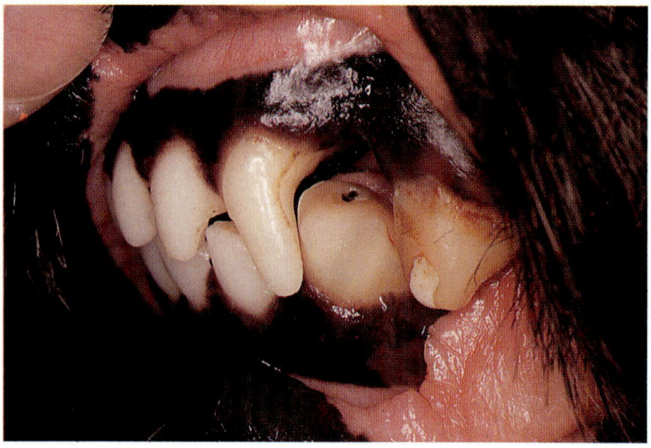

303 One year later — Case 1b. The teeth have been fractured through continued destructive behaviour. Full-coverage restorations would have stood no chance of long-term retention.

Examples of crown restorations in dogs

The cases below were performed at a time when the author, like so many professionals crossing the species barrier, presumed that human techniques could and should be directly transposed onto animals. His criteria have changed considerably over the years with the experience and clear understanding gained into the dental needs of animals. The author's prerequisite for restorative prosthodontics for animals are now quite specific: it must be proven that a reduced crown height presents a functional handicap before cases are restored. No treatment is performed for aesthetic reasons. The cases below do not fulfill the current criteria but are used to illustrate the principles of full coverage restorations in veterinary dentistry.

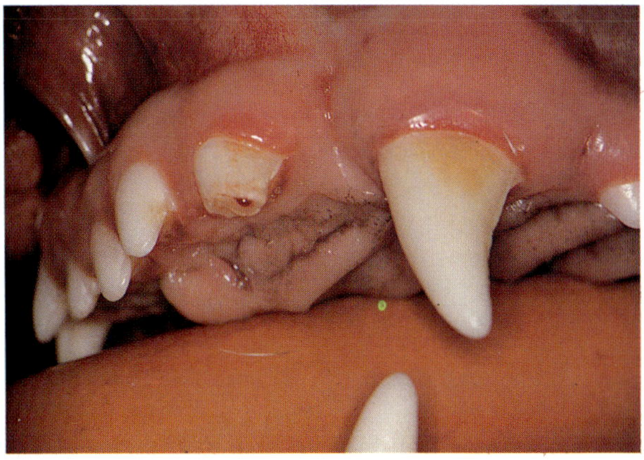

304

304 Fractured third incisor — Case 2a. Fractured upper third incisor of dog through trauma. Vital pulp exposure is evident.

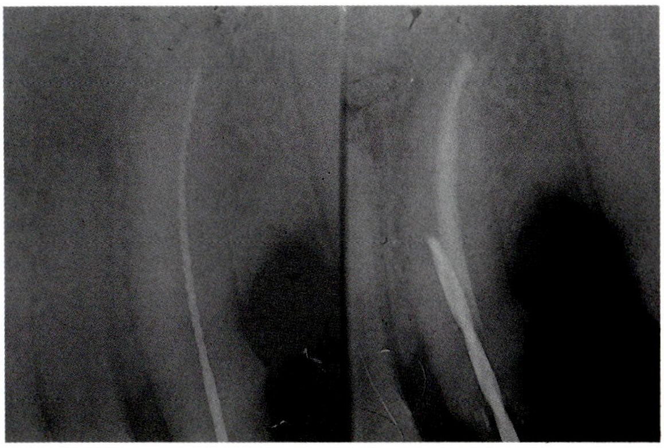

305

305 Radiographs of third incisor — Case 2b. The curvature of the root canal can be instumented with moderately fine endodontic files. The post preparation can only be achieved to a certain length before the curved root is perforated.

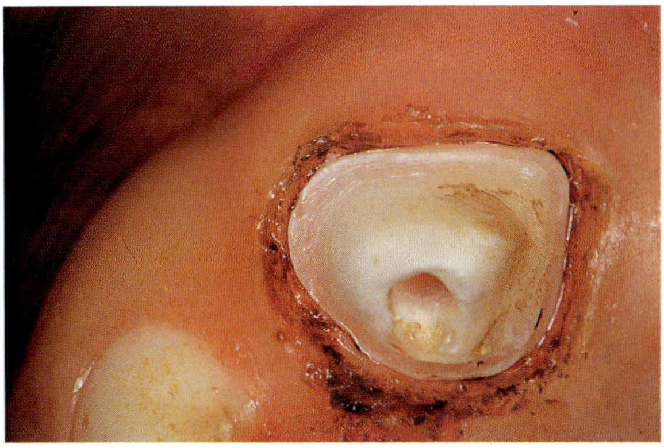

306

306 Close-up of coronal preparation — Case 2c. Coronal preparation is made in such a way as to give maximum retention.

307

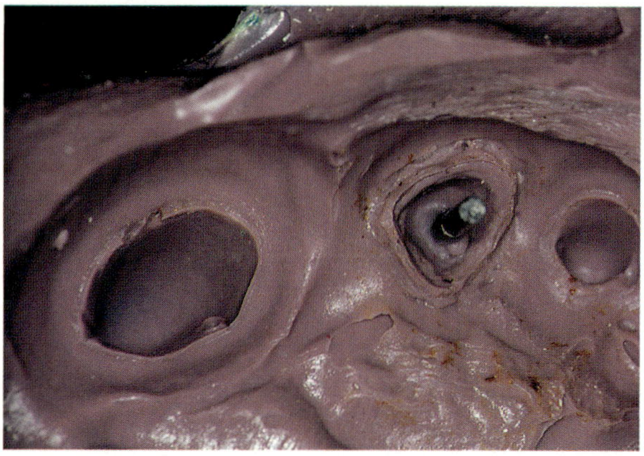

308

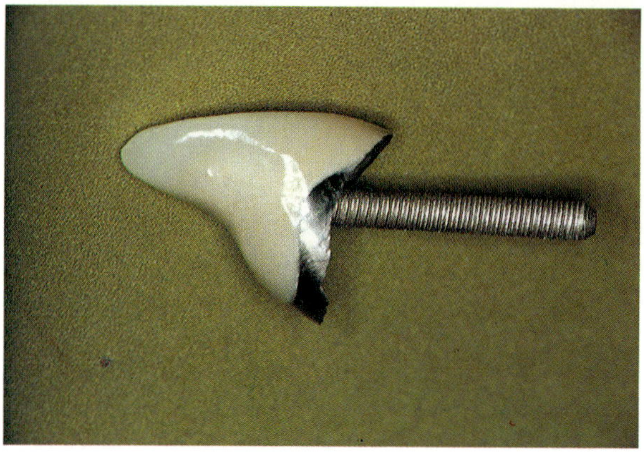

307 Impression — Case 2d. Impression of the preparation and the dental arch is made in an elastic material using a special tray.

308 Close-up of single casting — Case 2e. Maximum retention is obtained if the post and coronal casting are made as a single unit as this eliminates the weakness of a cement interface between the post and crown.

309

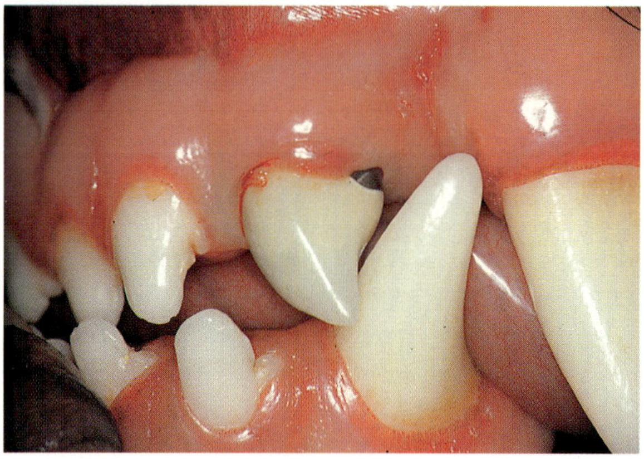

310

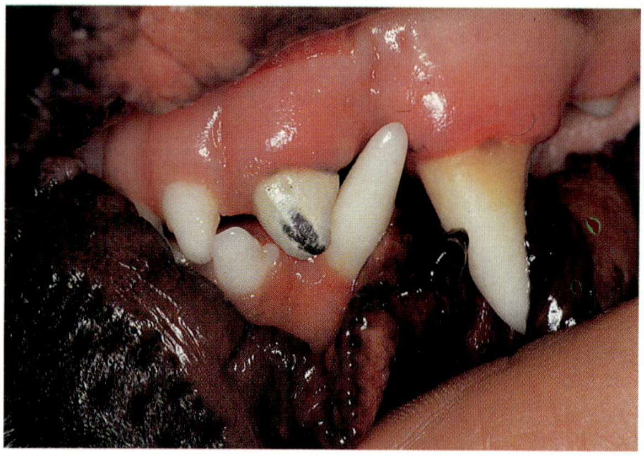

309 Cemented crown — Case 2f. The restoration is cemented in place.

310 Fractured porcelain — Case 2g. The restoration was not lost over a follow-up period of three years, although the porcelain fractured in the testing environment of the mouth of a 60 kg dog. within a few weeks

311

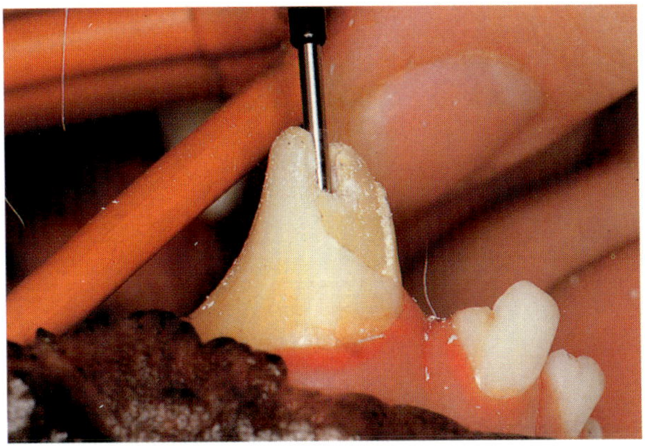

312

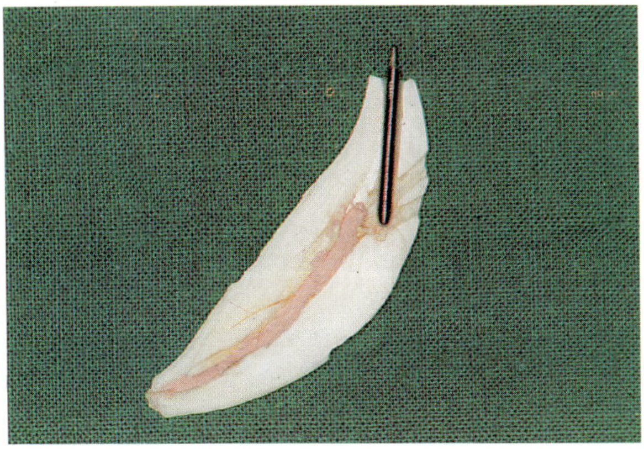

311 Fractured tip of working dog's canine — Case 3a. The infected root canal was treated endodontically. A post reamer in the root canal illustrates how the path of the post cannot follow the natural curvature of the root without further tooth preparation, which in turn would reduce the retentive element of the remaining supragingival natural crown.

312 Curved root and post length — Case 3b. Cross-section of a root-filled canine tooth illustrates the limiting factor the curved root canal has on the post length that can be utilised, and the maximum internal retention that can be obtained.

313

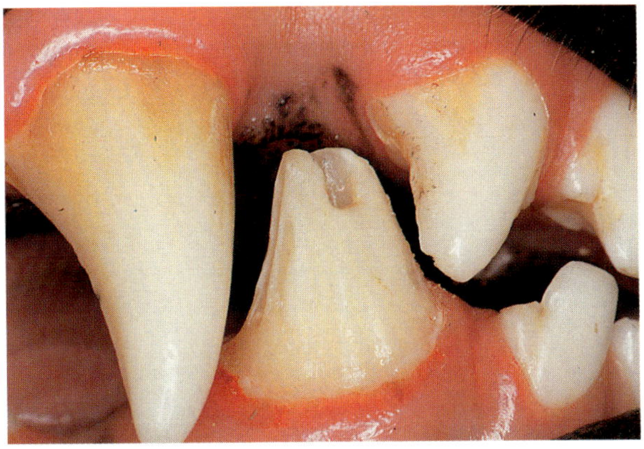

314

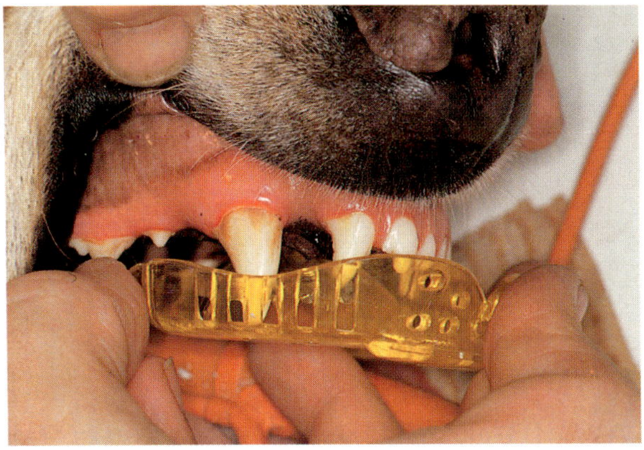

313 Preparation of remaining crown — Case 3c. The areas of occlusal contact of the mandibular canine tooth are at its mesial and distal surfaces. Clearance needs to be created at these points for the casting, having the maximum conservation of tooth substance in mind for retention and strength.

314 Try in of human impression tray — Case 3d. Human stock trays fit poorly to the differently shaped dental arches of dogs.

315

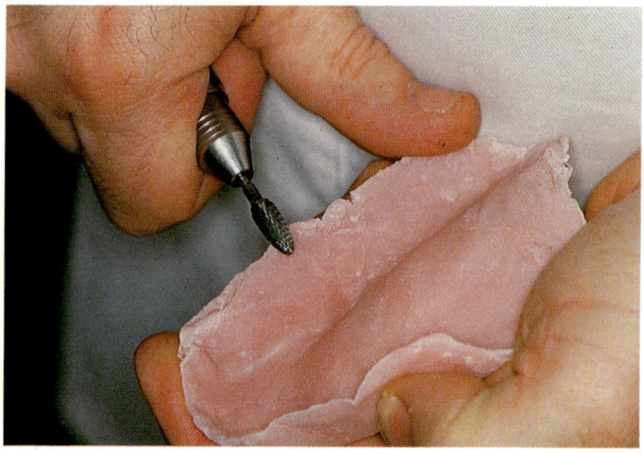

31

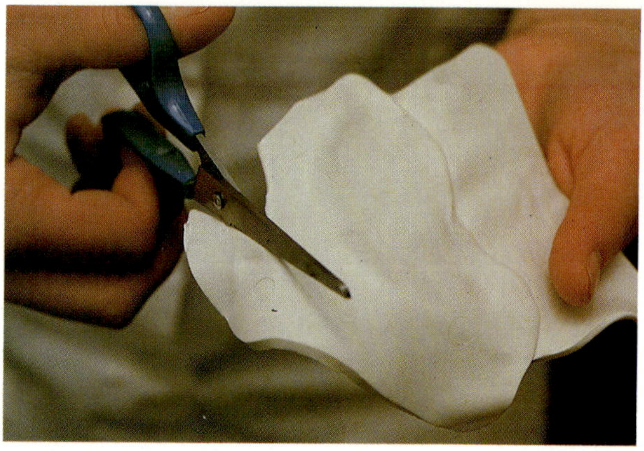

315 Special tray — Case 3e. A custom-made tray is the only way of making an accurate impression of an animal`s jaw. The trays may be fabricated out of 'cold cured' acrylic. This is a time-consuming procedure if performed during the same anaesthetic period as the endodontic treatment and preparation of the tooth. If prefabricated from acrylic on a similar-sized model or skull, adjustments of dimensions are usually difficult or impossible.

316 Handling tray material — Case 3f. The ideal tray material is thermoplastic, which may be prefabricated prior to treatment. It can be rapidly adapted as necessary to the correct shape and size of the jaws during anaesthetic.

317

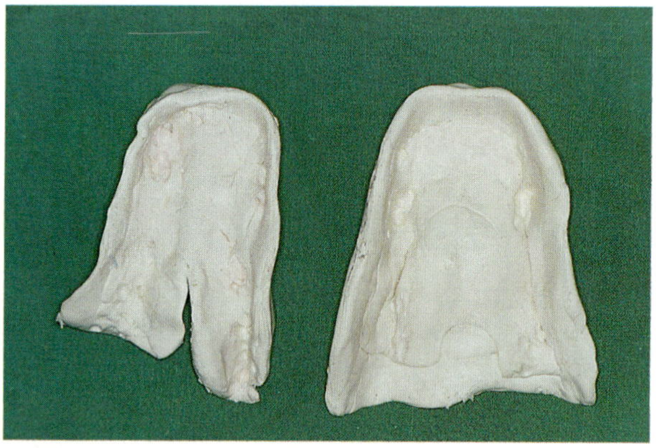

31

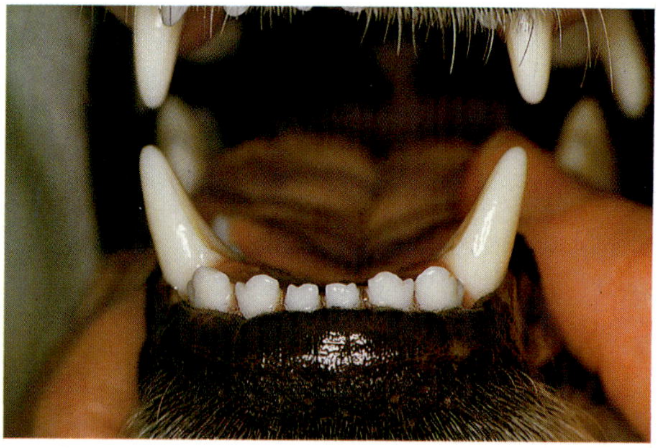

317 Trays made up — Case 3g. The trays can be made to any dimension and can be easily added to.

318 Divergent lower canines — Case 3h. Because of the natural divergence of the lower canines' crowns and the undercuts these create, any full arch impression can be easily distorted at important areas when the tray is removed from the teeth.

319

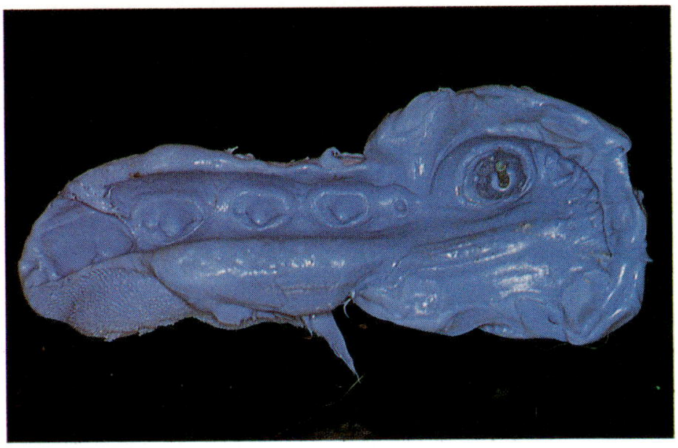

319 Partial tray — Case 3i. It is advisable to take the working impression in a partial tray, so that the line of withdrawal of the impression is within the normal limits of elasticity of the impression material and the internal tray space available.

320

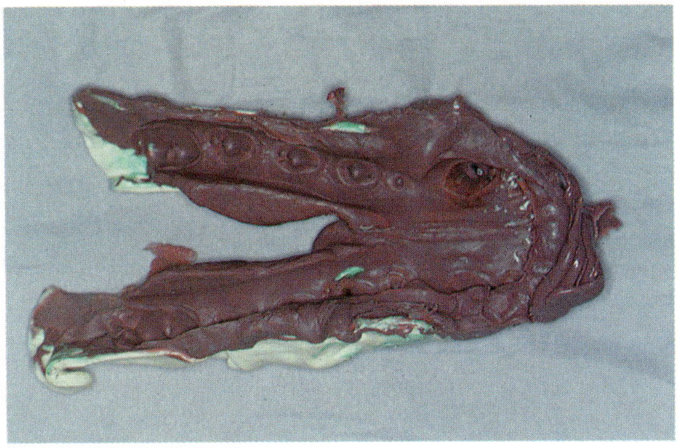

320 Full arch impression — Case 3j. An overall, full-arch impression is also advisable, so that the laboratory can analyse the occlusion before casting the restoration.

321

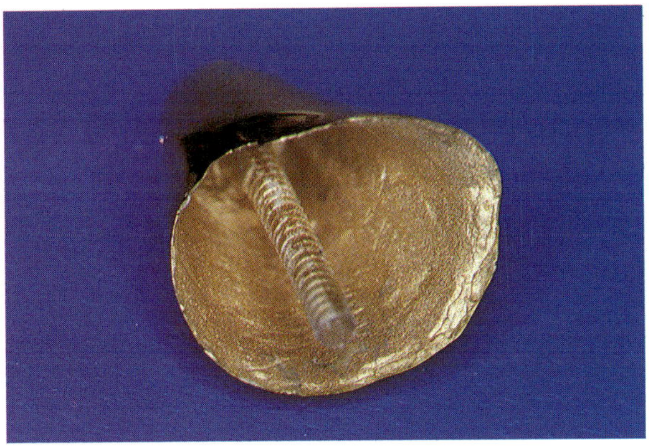

321 Close-up of one-piece casting — Case 3k. For maximum retention, a one-piece casting was made, with the post an integral part of the restoration. The crown is shorter in height than a natural tooth to minimise mechanical stress factors.

322

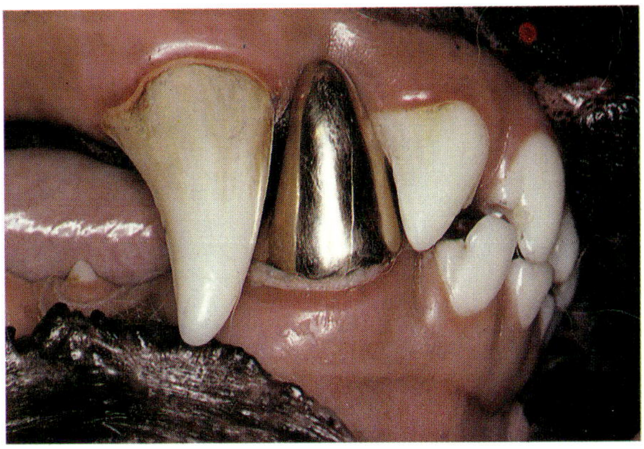

322 Crown cemented — Case 3l. The crown was cemented with a composite cement for maximum compression strength.

10 Oral Surgery: I. Extractions

Dental extractions are one of the most frequently performed operations in veterinary surgery. Operators must be familiar with the limitations of conservative dentistry in a veterinary environment, as it is unkind to subject animals to such treatment if a high degree of success cannot be predicted. Atraumatic, planned extractions are often the most realistic and therapeutic form of care when considering the dental needs of animals. Utilising the correct techniques with ideal instrumentation can help provide a stress-free procedure for the operator.

The extraction of teeth should not be treated lightly as in orthopaedic terms they are open fractures. Oral structures are often abused and the healing potential of the mouth is taken for granted. Careless extraction techniques can create chronic problems and may jeopardise the life of the veterinary patient. The removal of teeth should be carefully planned and thought-out, with the full range of instruments and equipment available to perform the operation. It is important that the operator understands the mechanics by which teeth are retained in the alveolar bone, because only by appreciating the fundamental principles can the operations be performed systematically and with the minimum of trauma to the patient.

Anatomical considerations

Teeth are supported in the mandible and the maxilla by the alveolar bone. In carnivores the periodontal ligament, which attaches the roots to the lamina dura of the sockets, is narrower in width than in herbivores or omnivores, so little movement of the teeth is allowed to take place. In the wild, carnivores' teeth are primarily used for catching, killing and tearing prey and it is imperative that they are locked in their sockets: tooth mobility is usually only present at the advanced stages of periodontal disease. The teeth of older animals are more brittle and the roots may be ankylosed to the bone. Carnivores' roots are long when compared with their body sizes; but other retentional factors are more relevant in the extraction process.

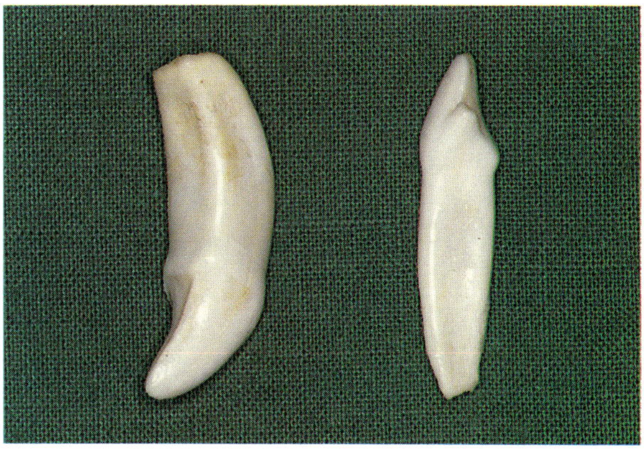

323

323 Incisors. The primary function of the carnivores' incisors is the tearing of meat, and great stresses are created by such forces. As the bone support around the incisor teeth in both the mandible and maxilla is limited, these teeth often have the highest root support to crown dimension ratio. The incisor roots are often curved and flat in cross-section, with concave lateral root surfaces; they produce an anti-rotational, retentive mechanism, which must be considered in the extraction process.

324

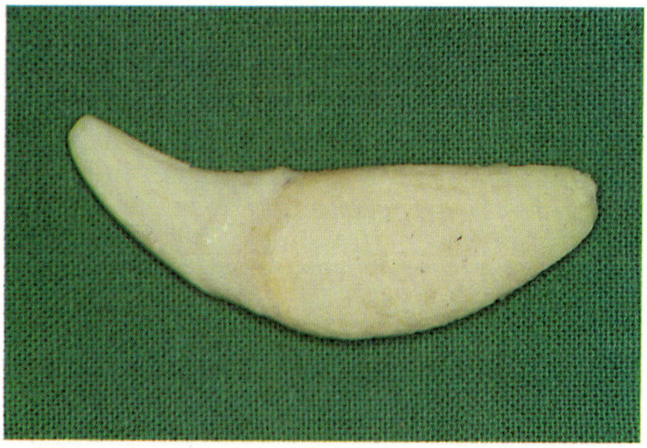

324 Canine — dog. The canine teeth of most carnivores have crown lengths which are slightly shorter than their roots. This leverage can create extreme stress on the retention of the roots in the alveolar bone. The canine tooth of the dog has a curved root with an oval cross-section. Its maximum bulbosity is not at the cemento-enamel junction or the alveolar crest, but some distance apical to it. Through this feature, alveolar bone locks the root into the jaw.

325

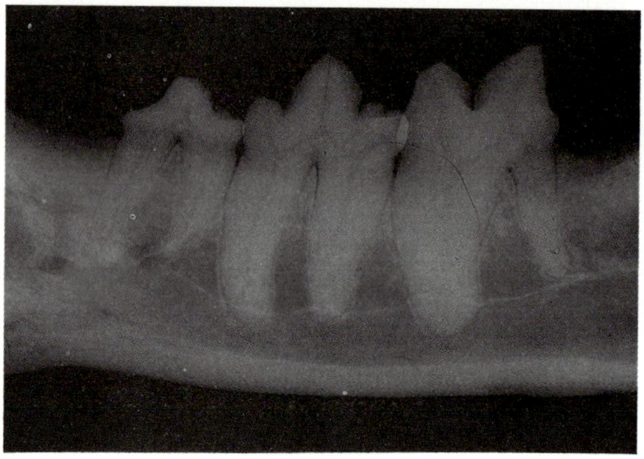

325 Radiograph of posterior teeth — cat. In most of the posterior teeth, the mechanics employed for tooth retention are multiple roots. The furcation of the roots extends to the cemento-enamel junction of the premolars/molars to maximise the root lengths. Divergence of the roots, which locks the teeth in the alveolar bone, is another important retentive aid. The posterior teeth of felids often have curved, bulbous apices, which increases the retention.

Basic principles

The basic principles of dental extractions are to reduce or eliminate the retentive factors of the roots and not to apply forces on the teeth with forceps until such a level of mobility has been obtained that the instrument can be used solely for the delivery of the teeth or roots. This systematic approach is especially true in the veterinary field, working with small animals, where the leverage one can exert with dental forceps is such that either the roots or the jaws can be easily fractured.

326

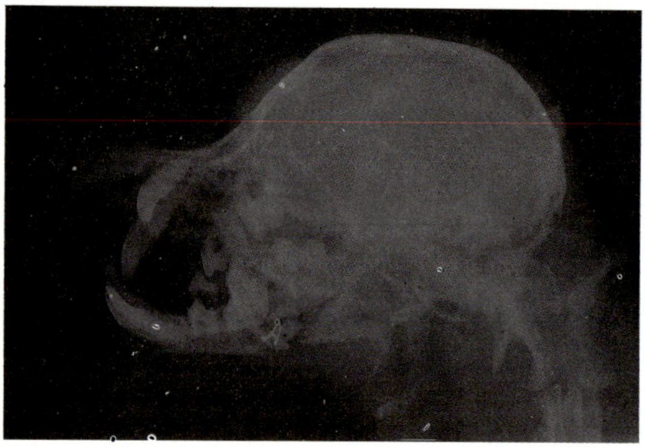

326 Radiograph of fractured mandible. Careless extraction technique, ignoring basic principles and using excessive force, can lead to life-threatening injuries. This referred dog suffered a fractured mandible through an extraction of the lower first molar. The immobilisation of the fragments was poor. Three weeks postoperatively, a severe osteomyelitis resulted and required further surgery.

327

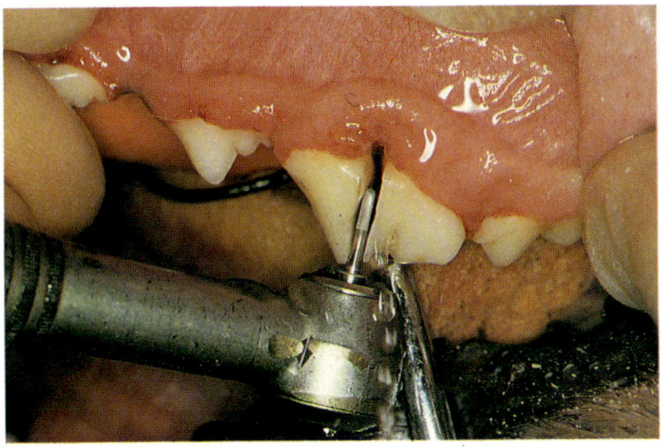

328

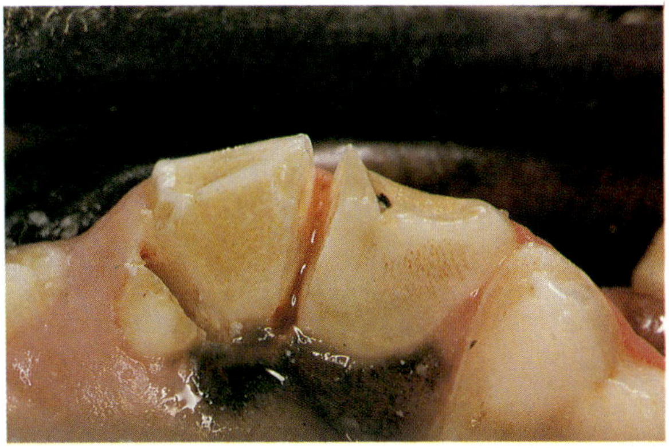

327 Sectioning of crowns. Little benefit is achieved by working against the mechanical factors that retain the teeth. By analysing which elements need to be overcome, extractions are performed more quickly and with less trauma to both the patient and the operator. Sectioning a multirooted tooth at the furcations often increases the mobility of each root considerably. The tungsten burr used in the air rotor is constantly irrigated with water to prevent the alveolar bone and the burr from overheating.

328 Occlusal view. An upper fourth premolar is sectioned into three segments according to the position of the roots. If the small palatal root is not separated from the mesiobuccal root it can considerably increase the difficulty encountered in their extraction.

329

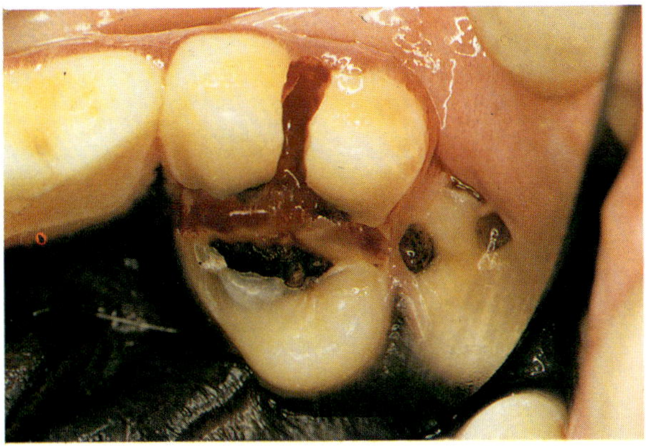

330

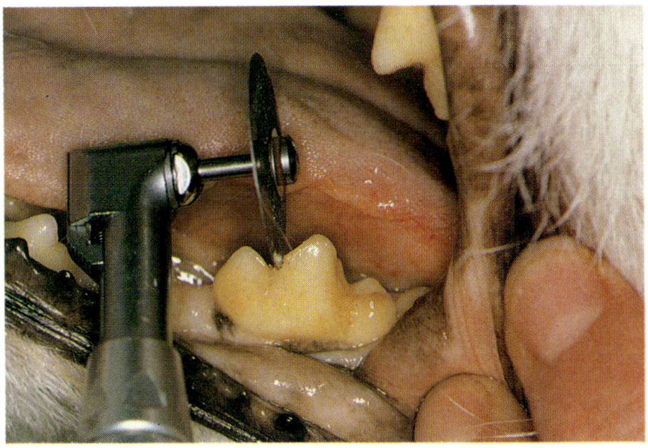

329 Upper first molar. The sectioning of the upper molar into a palatal and two buccal segments eliminates much of the elevation and socket dilation that needs to be performed to extract these tri-rooted teeth.

330 Diamond disc. Veterinary practitioners must be warned against the use of a diamond disk for sectioning teeth. This idea will come as a horrifying suggestion to dental surgeons, but the technique has been put forward in the veterinary field. Wheels are dangerous, especially in the confined space of the mouth of an unconscious small animal. The torque of such a large-diameter rotary instrument can easily become uncontrollable, resulting in lacerations to the tongue, cheek, lips and palatal artery of the patient, or the fingers of the operator. The use of the correct burrs in a low or high-speed handpiece can achieve tooth sectioning with far greater accuracy and safety.

331
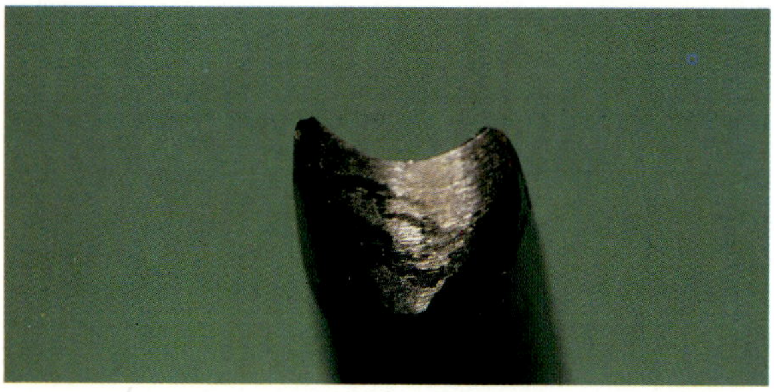

331 Tip design of a Coupland chisel. The most useful hand instrument in the extraction of teeth is the Coupland chisel. The design of the blade is of utmost importance. Some versions have little similarity to the original design and are less efficient in their action. The blades should have a straight edge to their working tips, which affords a positive and safe rest and resists slipping — unlike designs with pointed or rounded tips. The blade should be razor sharp, which aids in the cutting of the epithelial attachment, the periodontal ligament and the penetration of the instrument into the narrow periodontal space.

332
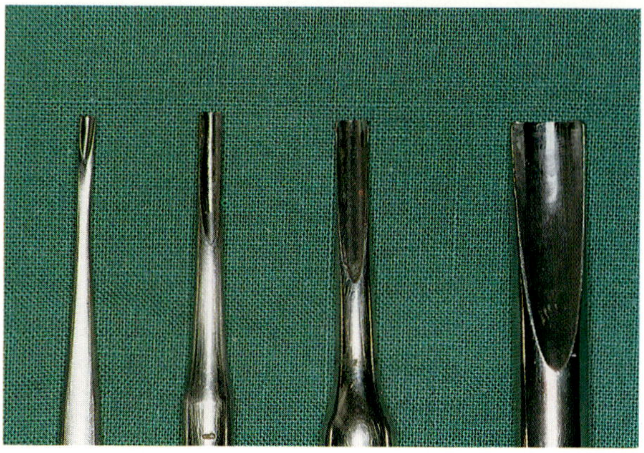

332 Coupland chisels. The size of the instrument should closely reflect the size of the root being elevated. Coupland chisels are available in different widths, from 1.5 mm to 9.5 mm.

333
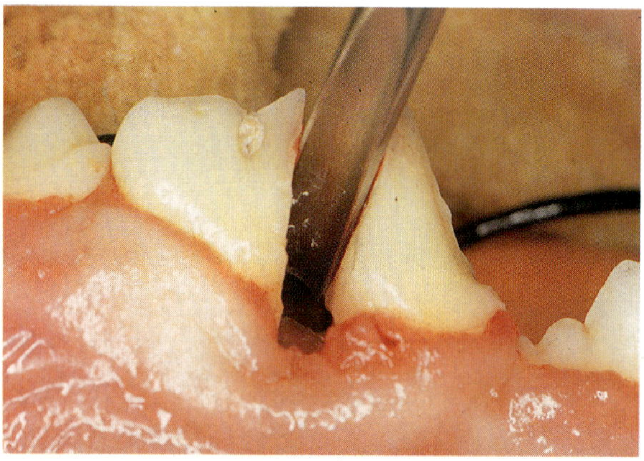

333 Separating segments. Once the crown of a posterior tooth has been sectioned to alveolar bone, the elevator can be used to separate the segments by gently rotating the instrument with the tip in the coronal cut. This will give the operator an indication of whether delivery of the roots can be achieved with the use of elevators only, or whether a full surgical procedure is necessary.

334
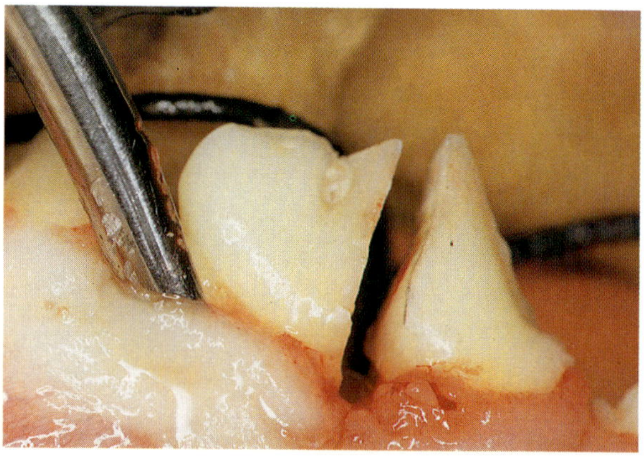

334 Use of an elevator. Elevators should never be used to lever teeth out of the sockets as the forces created by such an action are enormous and may fracture the root or the mandible. The Coupland chisel is first used to sever the gingival attachment from the tooth to be extracted. The blades of chisels should then be worked between the roots and the alveolar bone of the socket to tear the periodontal ligament, starting with narrow instruments and changing to wider elevators as appropriate. The elevator is also used to force the tooth out of the socket through the line of least resistance. A fulcrum point on the alveolar bone and not the adjacent teeth must be used. The force employed in elevation must be applied extremely carefully, taking into consideration the strength and anatomy of the jaws and the tooth being extracted. The principle of elevation is to use the tip of the elevator in a well-controlled rotating motion on its long axis between the root and the fulcrum point.

An important factor in the extraction of teeth is their location. The bone of the maxilla is less cortical than the mandible; it is softer in consistency and easier to dilate the sockets to help the extraction process, but when examining the bulbous, divergent and hooked roots usually little benefit will be gained.

Surgical extraction techniques

If any difficulty is encountered in the extraction process, and the tooth resists elevation because of root anatomy, or if the operator is unable to retrieve fractured roots through the socket, it is futile, time-consuming and damaging to the surrounding tissues to continue the extraction process blindly. Applying increased force or using forceps will only damage the root or the jaw. Time is saved and the procedure will be less traumatic if a deliberate open technique is employed, through the reflection of a full-thickness mucoperiosteal flap, to complete the extraction.

335

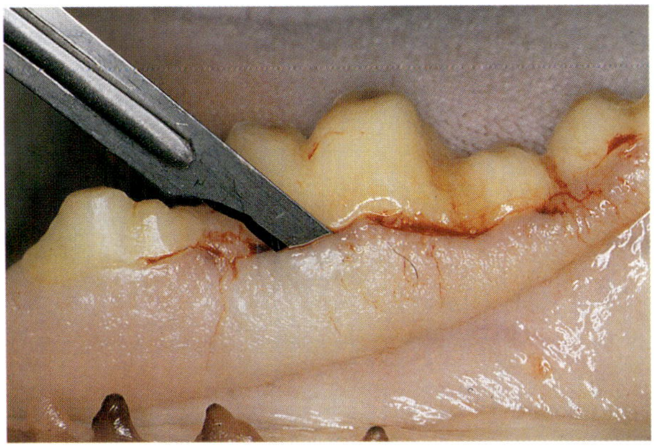

336

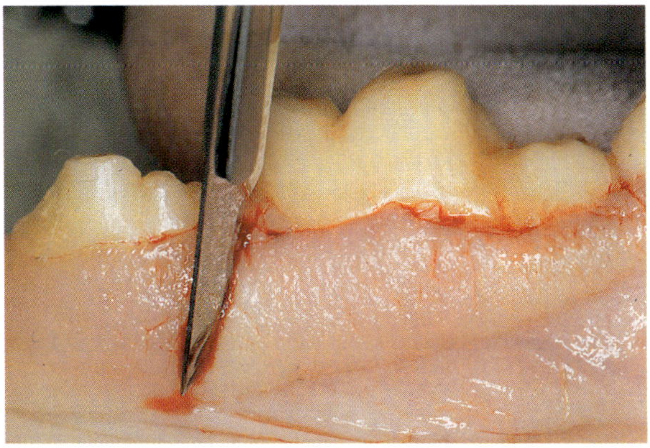

335 Gingival sulcus incision — cadaver. A horizontal incision is made in the gingival sulcus. The incision should extend beyond the width of the tooth to be removed, the extension depending on a number of factors:

- The maximum mesiodistal dimension expected as a result of divergent roots.
- The position from where alveolar bone is to be removed so as to aid postoperative gingival approximation and primary healing. Vertical suture lines should lie over a healthy table of bone for predictable healing to take place. If relieving incisions are made over an area where bone is to be removed to facilitate extraction, the chances of flap dehiscence are greatly increased. In extraction sites where oronasal/oro-antral fistulas may be created during surgery, predictable flap approximation is of vital importance.
- The desirability of avoiding vertical relieving incisions because of anatomical structures in the region.

336 Relieving incision — cadaver. A relieving incision is important for gaining access to the apical region of the alveolar bone through adequate flap reflection. A single, vertical incision is usually adequate to raise a sufficient sized mucoperiosteal flap. The incision is slanted away from the tooth to be extracted, so that the base of the flap is longer than the coronal aspect. This feature allows for a broad-based flap, with an excellent blood supply, that heals through primary intention. In certain locations, such as the premaxilla or the mental foramen, extended vertical incisions may encounter vessels and nerves that should be avoided during extraction procedures. Surgical access can be greatly facilitated in these areas by increasing the rostrocaudal length of the flap and making the relieving incision in a safe area. There are no disadvantages in extending the flap in the rostrocaudal dimension and they heal just as rapidly as a short wound.

337

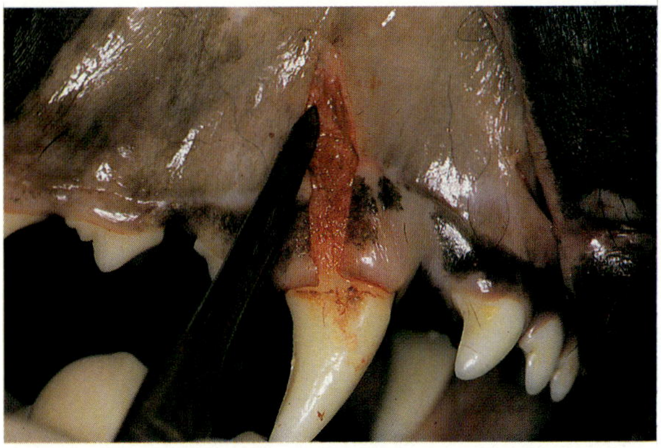

337 Incorrect flap design — cadaver. Incisions made over areas where alveolar bone is to be removed are contrary to all principles of oral surgery. The suture line will lie over an osseous defect and healing will be unpredictable due to the increased danger of flap dehiscence.

338

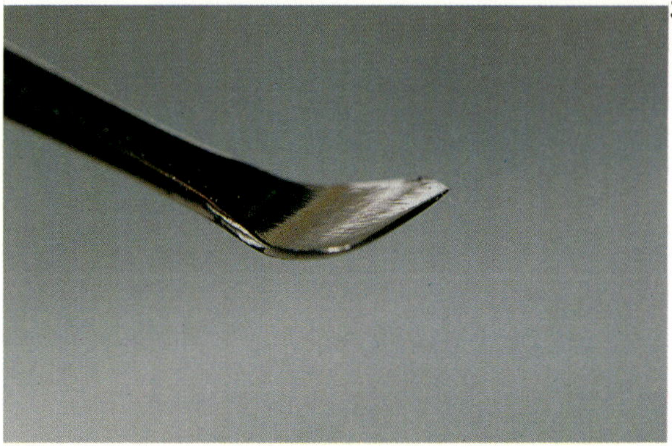

338 Periosteal elevator. A periosteal elevator is usually a flat, sharp instrument that should only be used for the separation of the mucoperiosteal flap from the alveolar bone.

339

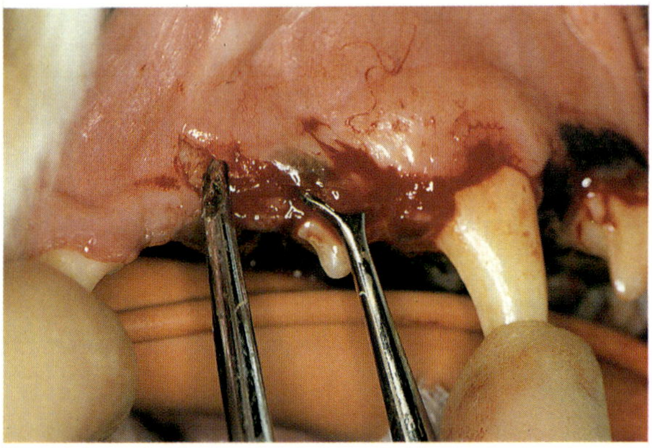

339 Canine flap — Case 1a. The mucoperiosteum must be fully sectioned through to bone before its elevation is attempted, otherwise separation between the gingiva/alveolar mucosa and the periosteum is created. This causes difficulty in flap elevation and unnecessary trauma to the soft tissues. Flap reflection is started by applying pressure at the gingival margin towards the flap that is to be reflected in a peeling fashion. The sharp end of the instrument is used at the coronal aspect of the relieving incision, although in the case of some carnivores the gingivae is extremely well bound to the bone and it is easier to start elevation of the flap slightly apical to the mucogingival junction.

340

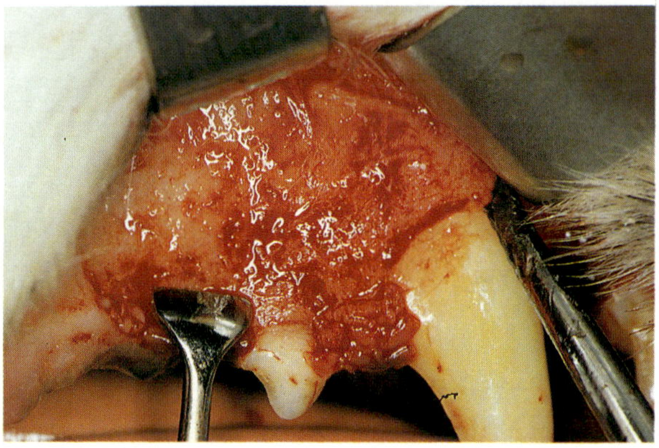

340 Flap reflected and retracted — Case 1b. A mucoperiosteal flap that is generous in the rostrocaudal dimension has many advantages over a short flap. The size of a flap determines the visibility to the operation site and facilitates instrumentation. Less stretching and trauma is created to the soft tissues through a well-designed flap, which is conducive to healing. The flap is retracted during osseous surgery to:

- Afford good access and visibility to the surgical site.
- Protect the flap from inadvertent trauma from rotary instruments during bone removal.

341 Burr selection. For rapid removal of vertical bone, round tungsten or steel burrs are used. The use of air rotors appears to be an attractive technique in the removal of alveolar bone but their use is to be avoided once a mucoperiosteal flap has been reflected for a number of reasons:

- The burrs used in air rotors are usually shorter in their working length than normal surgical burrs, so that access to deeper cuts is limited.
- The shanks of these instruments are thin and can fracture in use, especially when being used for drilling at their maximum depth. Fractured air rotor burrs can be lost in the soft tissues.
- Air rotors do not give the operator the tactile feedback that is so important in oral surgery.
- Most air rotors use air mixed with water for irrigation. This may give rise to emphysemas if the air is blown below the mucoperiosteal flap into the soft tissues.

Straight handpieces driven by electric or air micromotors give the tactile and speed control, as well as the torque and power, that is required to remove alveolar bone efficiently and safely.

342 Surgical burrs. For guttering, tungsten carbide, tapered-fissure, bone-cutting surgical burrs with coarse self-clearing channels are most useful. These burrs maintain their cutting efficiency for a long time and do not get clogged with bone chips during surgery.

343 Bone removal — Case 1c. The maximum bulbosity of the canine root is covered with alveolar bone, which resists attempts at extraction and needs to be judiciously reduced before elevation is attempted. The principle of alveolar bone removal in the extraction of teeth is to remove the minimum amount of vertical height necessary from the alveolus to gain mobility of the roots for delivery. Usually, buccal or labial bone is removed; only in exceptional circumstances is lingual bone removed in the lower jaw. Under no circumstances should both areas be reduced, as this may seriously weaken the mandible. Oral surgery demands continuous irrigation during bone removal with rotary instruments to:

- Cool the alveolar bone and, therefore, prevent overheating and bone necrosis.
- Cool the burr to prevent its overheating and the loss of cutting efficiency.
- Wash away bone chips that would clog the burrs.
- Maintain good visibility of the surgical site.

One of the greatest obstacles in oral surgery is the poor visibility due to the quantity of blood and water present. Irrigation in the required volume of water demands surgical aspiration to ensure proper visibility.

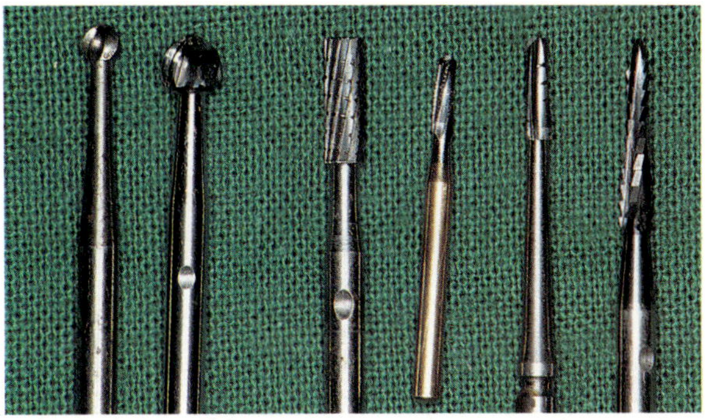
341

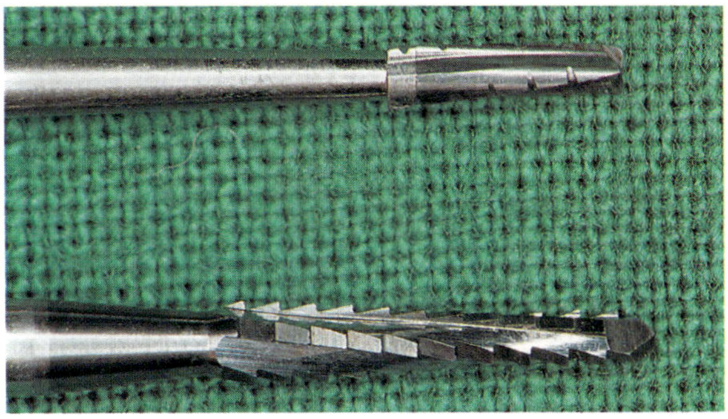
342

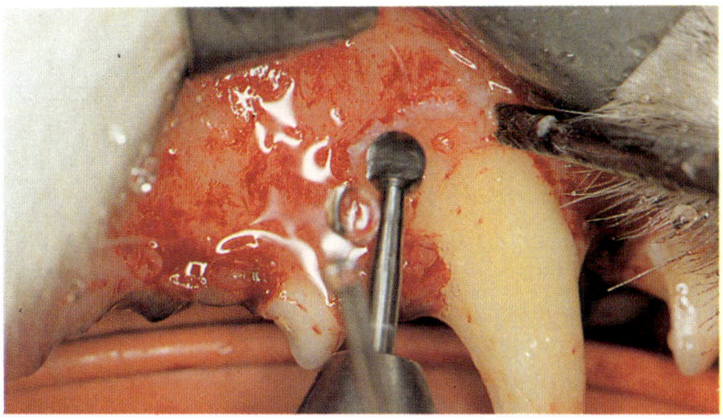
343

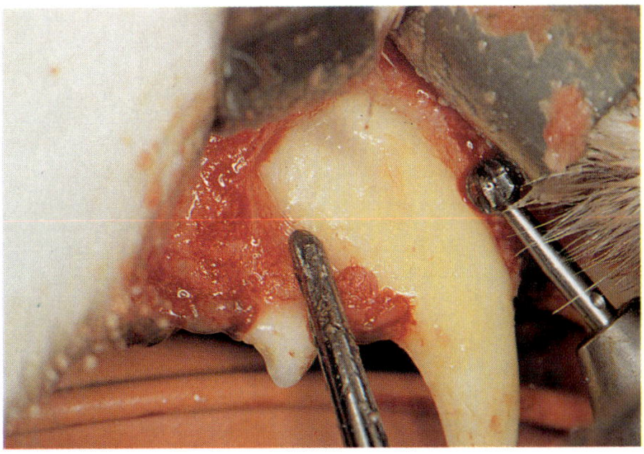
344

344 Exposure of root bulbosity — Case 1d. Once adequate vertical bone has been removed to expose the maximum dimension of the canine tooth, elevation may be attempted, but further bone can be removed through 'guttering' to facilitate disimpaction.

345 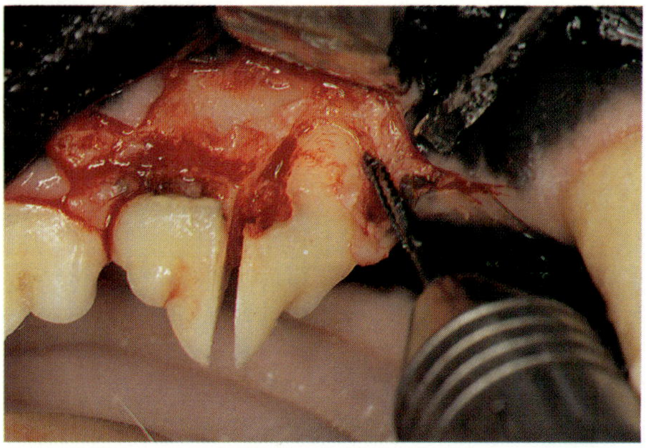

34[illegible] 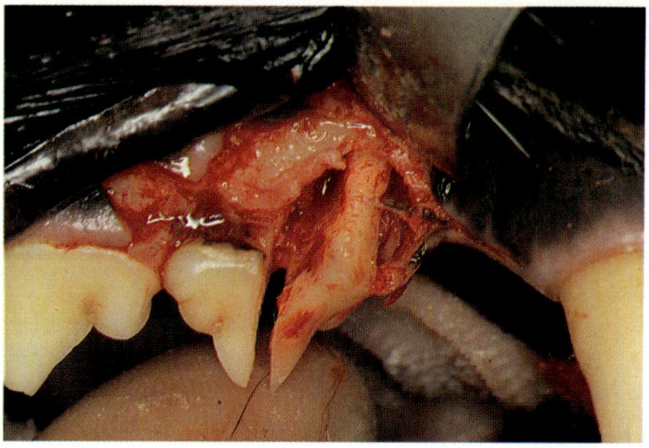

345 Guttering with fissure burr — upper premolar — Case 2a — feline. Guttering increases the internal dimensions of the socket without excessively reducing the vertical height and weakening the jaw, and it creates fulcrum points to aid elevation. The tooth was sectioned at the bifurcation with an air rotor before flap reflection.

346 Buccal bone removed — Case 2b. It is helpful to remove some of the interalveolar septum to facilitate an easier path of elevation; fulcrum points are created through guttering around the root.

347 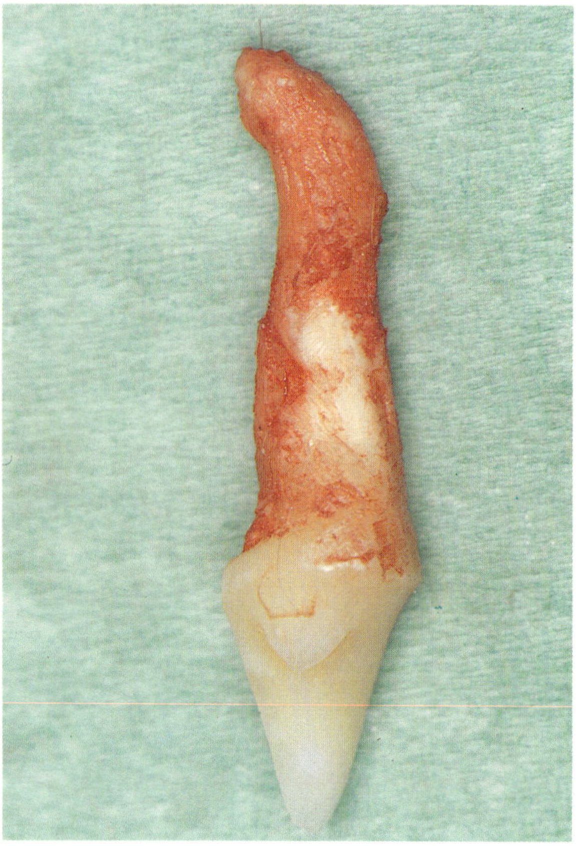

347 Elevated root — Case 2c. Careful elevation is required as the roots are long, fine, curved and brittle, often with bulbous apices.

348 Extraction completed — Case 2d. Careful examination of the surgical site is necessary after the delivery of the roots. Irrespective of whether the extraction was simple or an open surgical procedure, loose fragments of bone and granulation tissue should be debrided to aid healing. Any sharp spicules of alveolar bone that are attached may also be rounded off with the aid of a round burr or rongeours. The socket is irrigated with water only. Air or air/water spray must not be blown into an extraction socket as it may create an emphysema. In this case, a small perforation into the nasal cavity is visible. The importance of a well thought-out flap design, impeccable reflection and closure assures uneventful healing of a potentially serious condition.

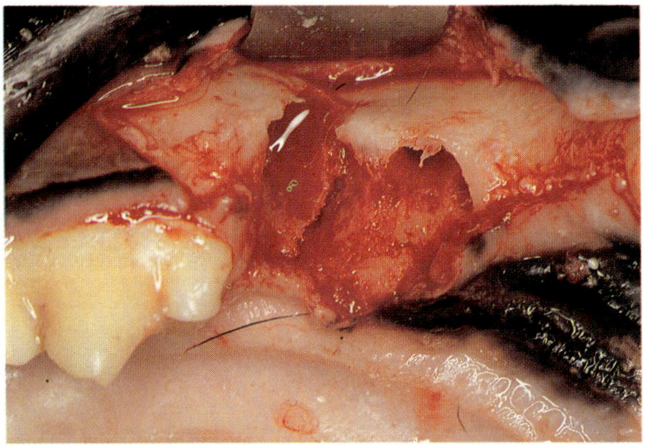
348

349 Incising the periosteum — Case 2e. Basic principles of oral surgery must be followed for a predictable fistula repair. Mucoperiosteal flaps do not stretch, and suture lines under tension are likely to break down. To increase the vertical dimension of the flaps and close the defect without tension, two or three relieving incisions are made in the periosteum in an rostrocaudal direction at its full length. Care must be exercised not to perforate the gingiva or the alveolar mucosa with the relieving incisions. To facilitate fistula repair, other steps need to be performed:

- The gingival margins of the flaps should be freshened up.
- The buccal margin of the alveolar bone often needs to be rounded off to facilitate that the flap lies in a better position for approximation.
- Reflection of the palatal mucosa and, if necessary, rounding off and reducing the height of the palatal margin of the alveolus can also improve closure.

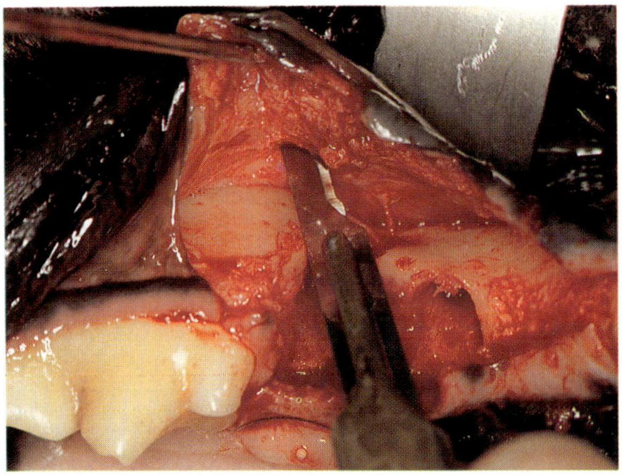
349

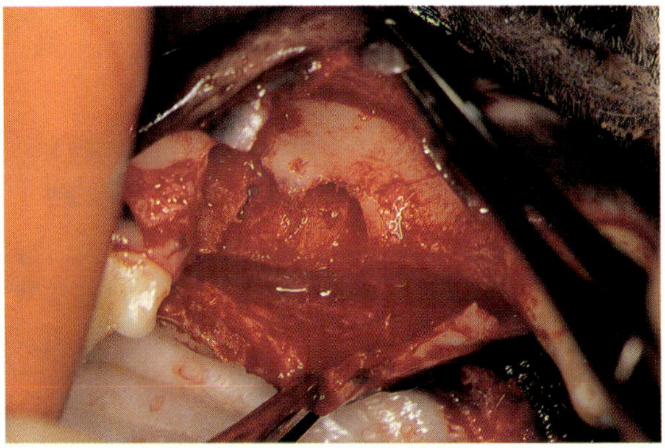
350

350 Buccal and palatal flaps mobilised — Case 2f. Both buccal and palatal flaps have been elevated and only the periosteum has been incised.

351 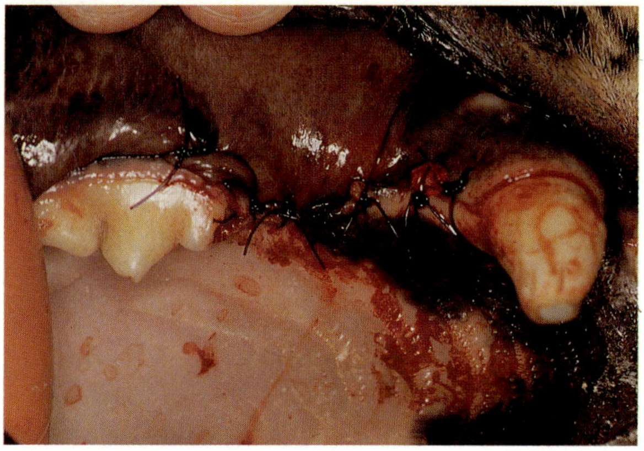

351 Flap sutured — Case 2g. Excellent approximation of the flap margins has been created which allows for predictable primary healing. The flap is carefully closed, free of tension, with resorbable sutures. The use of an intra-alveolar pack is contraindicated unless an abnormal haemorrhage needs to be controlled.

Guidelines for the treatment of retained and fractured roots

Certain practical guidelines must be given to the general practitioner on how to deal with retained roots and those fractured during extraction.

Buried roots are occasionally found during routine radiographic examination of the mouth. If they are totally buried subgingivally, with no communication into the oral cavity, and there are no signs of active infection, no treatment should be embarked upon. Often, the pulp of these roots has remained vital and the roots will stay symptomless for life.

If a tooth being extracted has an infected root canal, every part of the root should be removed; otherwise, any periapical infection will not resolve.

If the pulp of the tooth being extracted is alive and the fractured apex is well below bone level, there is a good possibility that the pulp will remain alive, especially if the gingival flap is carefully sutured over it. In this way the pulp has a double blood supply — through its apical foramen and the covering periosteum — which allows it to remain vital and symptomless.

A reasonable effort must be made to retrieve fractured roots, but the increased anaesthetic risks caused by prolonged surgery and the risk of removing a considerable height of alveolar bone, especially in a weak mandible, must be weighed against the potential danger posed by a retained root apex.

The practice of blindly 'atomising' fine feline roots or retained apices using high-speed drills is contrary to all principles of oral surgery and must be strongly frowned upon. This illogical and amateurish technique in no way benefits the patient and can create considerable iatrogenic trauma. Either roots need to be removed in total, or allowed to remain buried if judged to be harmless.

Haemostasis

In the great majority of veterinary dental extractions, haemostasis does not present a problem. Firm digital pressure employing a gauze pack invariably stops the gingival and alveolar bleeding that is normal after oral surgery.

Mucoperiosteal flaps, if raised, should always be sutured. In cases of excessive alveolar haemorrhages the use of electrocautery, or tying off the bleeding vessels, is usually not practical or possible. Other means must be utilised to create the predictable clot. Bone wax has not proved to be a satisfactory means of controlling alveolar haemmorhages. Resorbable cellulose or collagen, plain or preferably saturated in a thrombin solution are excellent agents in haemostasis. The gingiva is sutured over the packs without tension. In the case of gingival haemorrhages it is often helpful to create a level of ischaemia in the margins of the sockets through the use of tension sutures which assist haemostasis.

Retained primary teeth

352 Permanent canine erupting — upper primary retained — Case 3a. Retained primary canines often cause their permanent successors to erupt in a traumatic lingual position (see also **96–98**, Chapter 5.) Early planned intervention can prevent and, in some cases, correct a traumatic occlusion which at a later age can cause pain and demands more invasive treatment. If the condition is treated early, before the lower canines have fully erupted, the alveolar bone may be flexible enough to allow for drifting to take place and an atraumatic occlusion to develop.

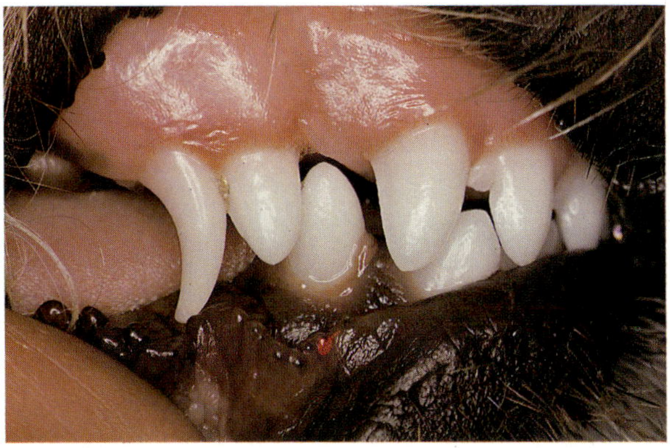
352

353 Elevating primary canine — Case 3b. The aetiology of retained canines is unclear. Possibly, pressure from the erupting permanent tooth has not been at the right position to encourage root resorption of the primary tooth. A hereditary element to the aetiology is highly likely. Usually, the primary teeth are firm and their roots still fully formed. Attempting to elevate the tooth or extract it with forceps will frequently result in root fracture, as the roots are extremely long, thin and brittle. An even more dangerous consequence of blind elevation of the primary tooth is the accidental elevation of the permanent canine tooth. As it is still in the development stage, the root is not fully formed and it exhibits greater mobility than the primary tooth.

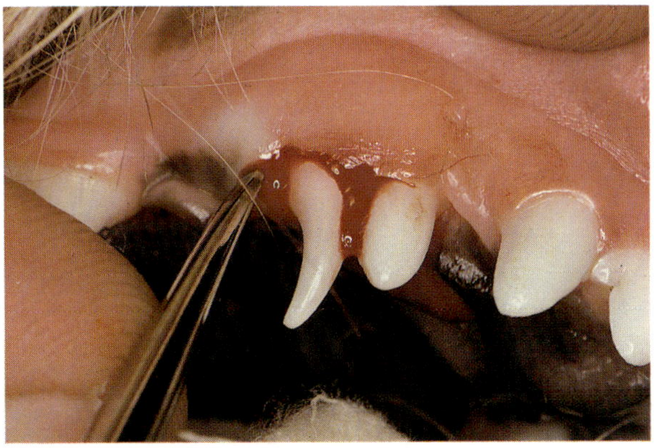
353

354 Flap reflected — retained root visible — Case 3c. The treatment of choice is to reflect a mucoperiosteal flap and work through direct vision.

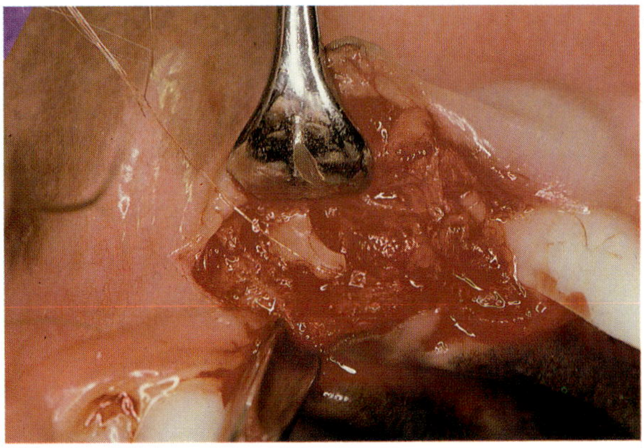
354

355

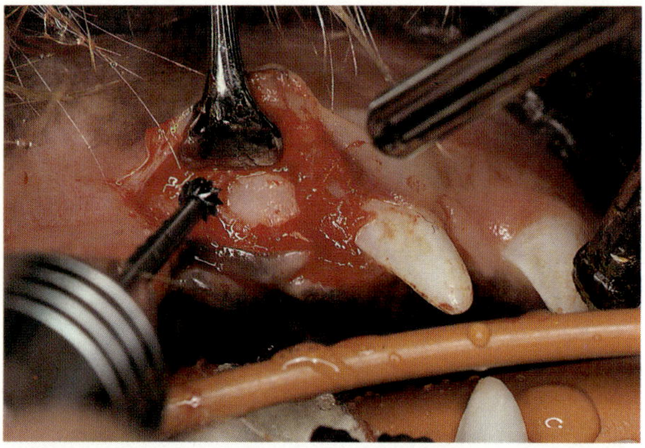

355 Removing bone — Case 3d. The removal of labial bone is usually necessary and is carried out as described above, taking great care not to damage the developing permanent teeth.

356

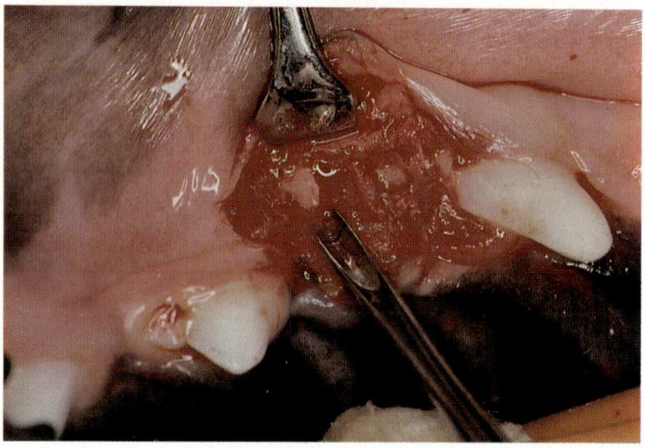

356 Elevating root — Case 3e. Any elevation must be done with extreme care.

357

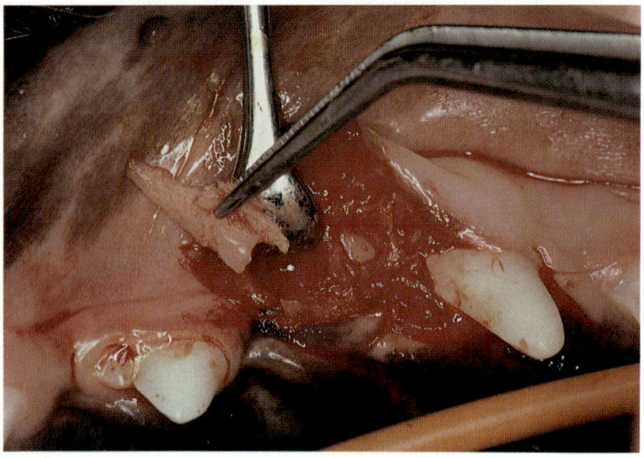

357 Apex retrieved — Case 3f.

358 Primary tooth and comparison with human incisor — Case 3f. When the relatively long primary canine from a wire-haired Dachshund is compared with a permanent human incisor it is easy to appreciate the difficulties encountered in its extraction.

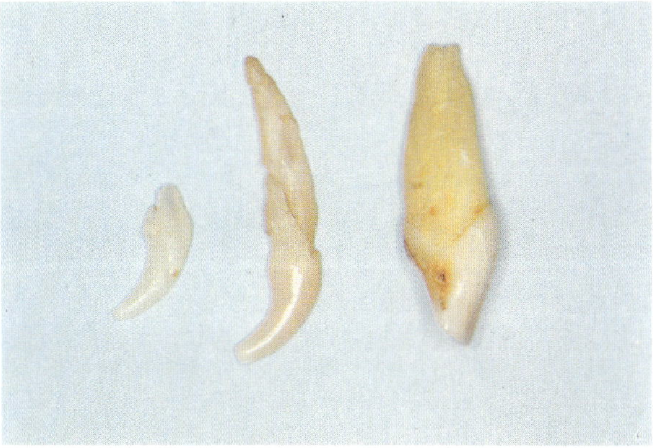

358

359 One-week postoperatively — Case 3g. Sutures removed. The owner of this animal was dedicated enough to apply digital pressure at this stage to the upper canine teeth in a distal (caudal) direction on a daily basis, as directed, to create the necessary space between the upper canine and the third incisor.

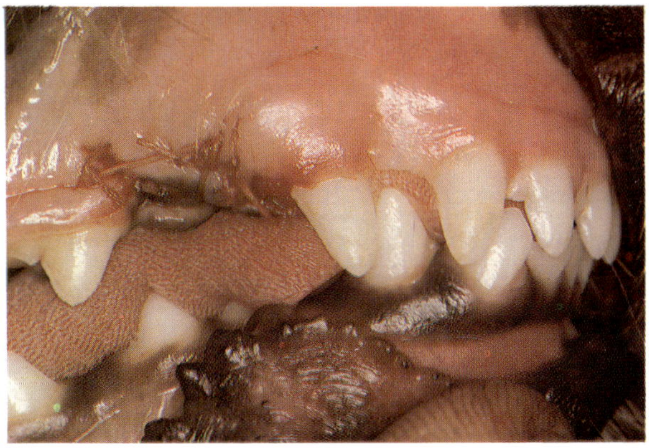

359

360 Final result — Case 3h. Cases must be chosen with care. The owner was successful in retracting the upper canines, and within three weeks a normal-sized diastema was created. This allowed enough room for the lower canines to erupt labially, with minimal assistance through digital pressure, into a non-traumatic occlusion.

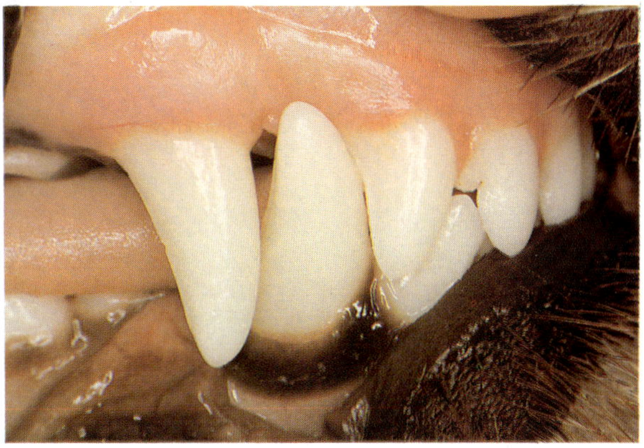

360

Repair of oronasal fistulas

361

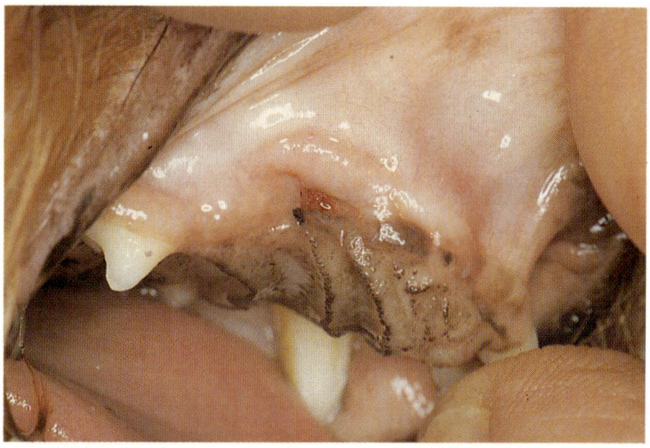

361 Chronic oronasal fistula — Case 4a. This chronic oronasal fistula remained after the extraction of an upper canine tooth. The palatal wall of the socket is also the lateral wall of the nasal cavity. The palatal surface of the canine root is often ankylosed to this thin bone, which is easily damaged during the extraction of the tooth. The mucosal lining of the nose may remain patent, but if a defect is suspected after extraction it is advisable to gently investigate the socket and immediately repair it rather than allow the condition to become a permanent fistula, which in turn can lead to chronic rhinitis. Oronasal fistula repairs often break down as a result of a failure to mobilise the soft tissues sufficiently, so that tension-free flaps may be approximated.

362

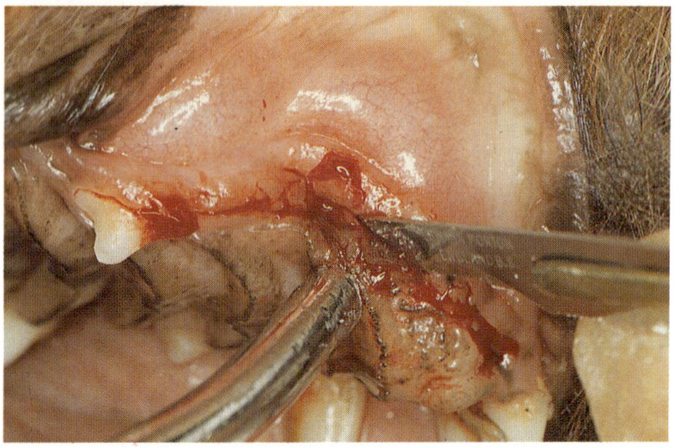

362 Extent of mucoperiosteal flap — Case 4b. By extending the rostrocaudal aspect of the incision a large mucoperiosteal flap can be raised which is easy to mobilise and aids extension in a vertical direction.

363

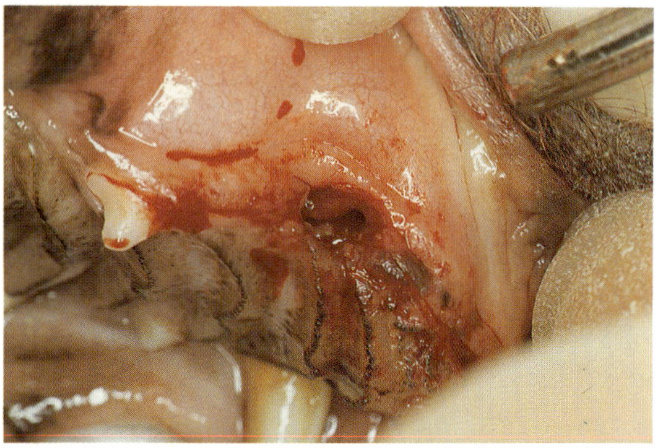

363 Margin of fistula freshened up — Case 4c. The epithelial lining of the fistula must be excised to encourage primary healing to take place.

364 Reflecting flap — Case 4d. Large, full-thickness labial and palatal mucoperiosteal flaps are reflected; if necessary, a relieving incision can be made remote from the osseous defect to aid mobility of the labial flap. Any necrotic material, infected mucosa or nasal conchae are curetted to a healthy base.

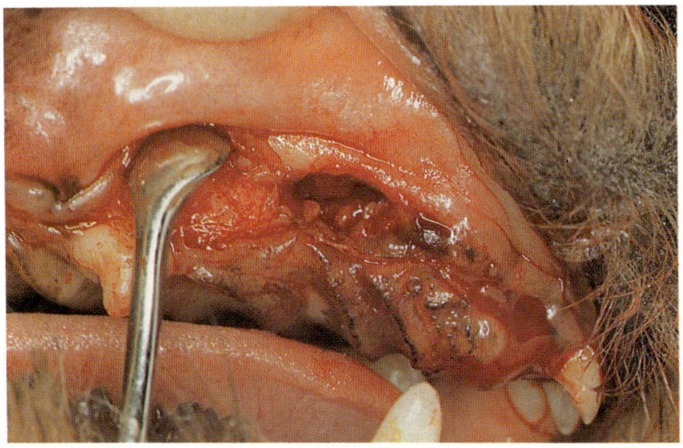

364

365 Rounding off bone — 4e. The labial and palatal margins of the alveolar ridge often need to be reduced in height or rounded off, to allow for the flaps to lie in a better position for approximation.

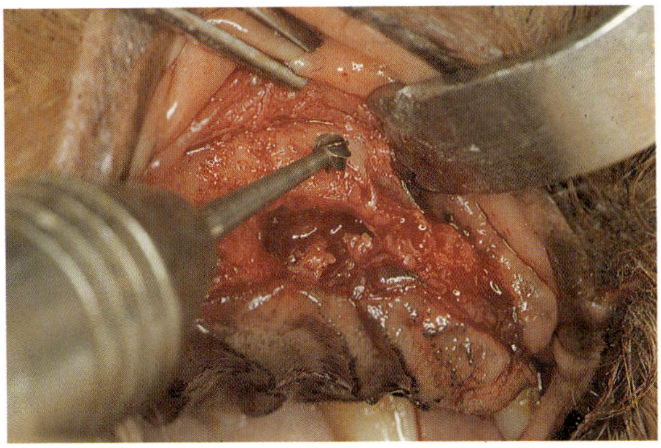

365

366 Incising the periosteum — Case 4f. If necessary the palatal mucoperiosteal flap can also be extended in its gingivopalatal dimension through rostrocaudal relieving incisions. The position of the palatal artery at the caudal aspect of the alveolus should be kept in mind and avoided.

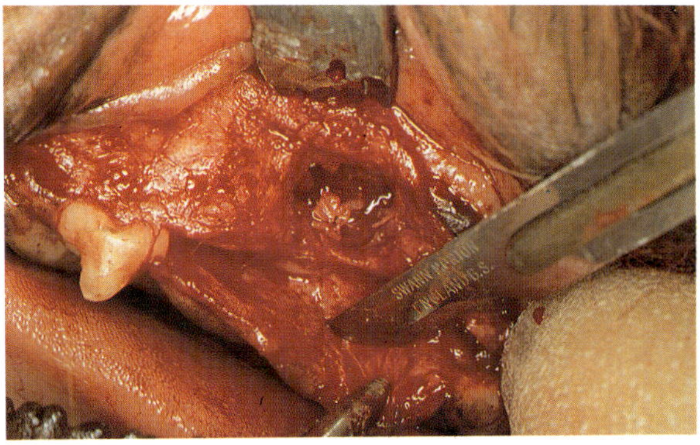

366

367 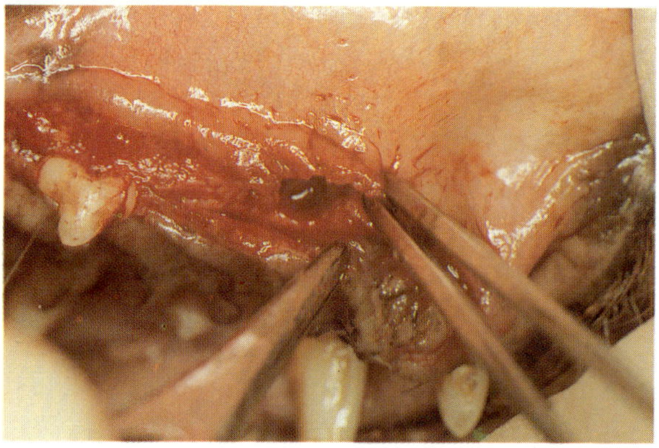

367 Approximating gingival flaps — 4g. Considerable flap mobilisation has been achieved through flap design, relieving incisions and limited alveoplasty.

368 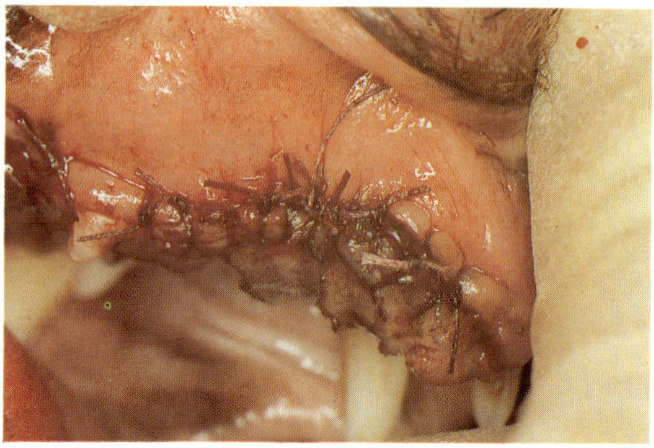

368 Flaps sutured — Case 4h. The flaps are closed with simple interrupted or vertical mattress absorbable sutures that are likely to remain for 14–21 days.

If the size of an oronasal fistula is so large that it is unlikely to be closed by the above technique a large pedicle flap with its base in the buccal sulcus can be utilised and the area from where it is harvested repaired.

In human surgery the flaps are often taken from the palate leaving a denuded area to granulate over, as harvesting the buccal mucosa reduces the sulcular depth. This is significant in denture construction, as the retention of the prosthesis is partly governed by sulcular depth. In veterinary surgery, such considerations do not arise and buccal flaps are recommended.

11 Oral Surgery: II. Orthopaedic Surgery of the Mandible and Maxilla

Fractures of the mandible

Introduction

Fractures of the mandible are characterised by local pain, asymmetry, drooping of the jaw and displacement of the bony fragments. There is generally drooling of blood-stained saliva and malocclusion of the teeth. Road traffic accidents are the usual cause of mandibular fractures in dogs, while cats frequently sustain such fractures as a result of falling from a height. Iatrogenic fractures during dental extraction can be harrowing experiences; they accounted for over 11% of canine mandibular fractures in one series of 157 cases. This complication is particularly likely to occur in the elderly toy breeds of dog with osteopaenic jaws. The commonest sites of mandibular fractures in the dog are the premolar and molar regions. In the cat, symphyseal fractures predominate.

Mandibular fractures may be unilateral or bilateral and are frequently open. They are, therefore, generally contaminated or infected. Most mandibular fractures occur with minimal loss of teeth — the exception being pathological fractures associated with infected tooth sockets. However, although few teeth are removed by the traumatic incident, the fracture frequently involves the roots of the teeth. Tooth loss, and loss of the associated alveolar bone, not only makes reduction of the fracture more difficult but also makes immobilisation less secure. Thus, teeth should be retained wherever possible, even if they have to be removed at a later date.

The diagnosis of mandibular fractures is generally readily made from the physical findings and a history of trauma. It is often necessary to sedate or anaesthetise the animal before a thorough inspection can be performed and it is essential to maintain a patent airway at all times. Any blood clots or debris should be removed from the pharynx before examining the remainder of the mouth (**369**).

Radiography should demonstrate the position and number of fracture lines and confirm the physical findings (**370**). The animal must be positioned carefully to avoid superimposition of bony structures since these can easily obscure the areas of interest. Oblique projections often demonstrate fractures of the mandibular body better than lateral views, and open-mouth views, with non-screen radiographic film placed in the mouth, allow the rostral parts of the mandible to be radiographed without superimposition of the maxilla. Open-mouth views are obtained with the animal in dorsal recumbency and the radiographic beam directed ventrodorsally.

When treating mandibular fractures, the aim is to restore dental occlusion and enable the animal to eat and drink. Occlusion is easiest to check with the jaws closed and the endotracheal tube removed. This can be a nuisance when repairing complicated fractures but can be overcome by introducing the tube through an

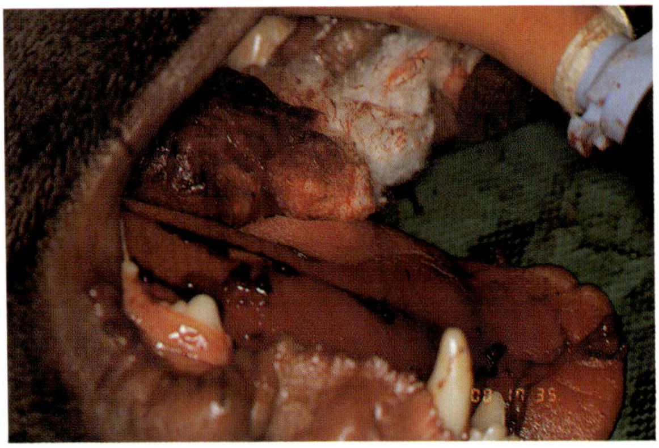

369

369 Acute stage of oral trauma. A caudal mandibular body fracture sustained as a result of being kicked by a horse. The lingual artery was lacerated by a fractured fragment. It is imperative to establish a patent airway and to remove all blood clots from the oropharynx before assessing the extent of any other damage. Blood is most easily removed by suction but, if this is unavailable, swabbing the oropharynx is a satisfactory alternative.

incision made in a similar position to that of a pharyngostomy tube. At the end of surgery the incision can be sutured or the endotracheal tube can be replaced with a pharyngostomy tube (**371**) to facilitate postoperative feeding. Alternatively, the animal can be anaesthetised throughout the surgery with a total intravenous technique using an agent such as propofol. However, it is important to make sure that the airway does not become occluded with blood during the surgery and that the animal remains well oxygenated.

Animals with open fractures should be given perioperative antibiotics. Osteomyelitis is not eliminated following antibiotic therapy but its incidence is reduced with their usage. A broad-spectrum, bactericidal agent with good bone-penetrating properties should be used. To reduce the incidence of infection further, torn gingivae should be sutured where possible. This prevents excessive contamination of the fracture with food and saliva.

370

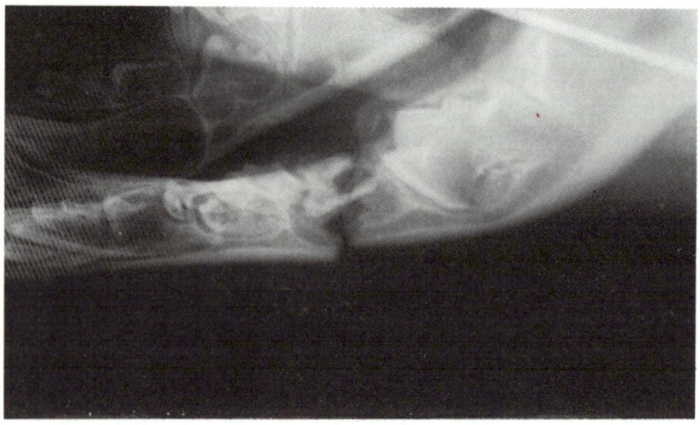

370 Radiograph of a fractured mandible. An oblique projection of the right mandibular body demonstrating a fracture through the alveolus of the fourth premolar tooth. When taking oblique projections, the affected bone should be closest to the radiographic plate so as to minimise magnification and distortion.

371

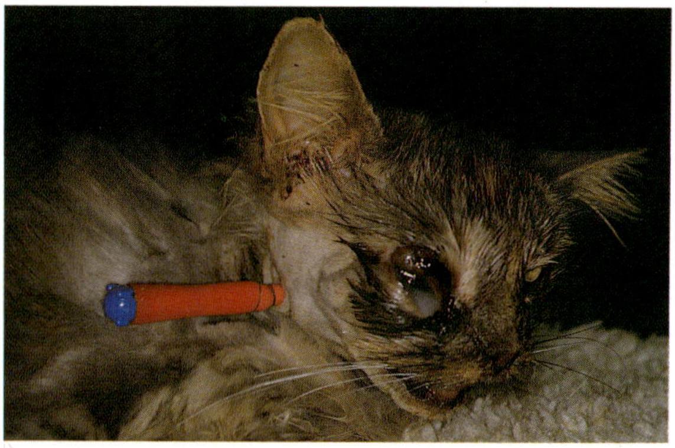

371 Pharyngostomy tube. This cat has a soft, red rubber pharyngostomy tube to make postoperative feeding easier. The tube replaced an endotracheal tube that was used to provide gaseous anaesthesia while the mandibular fractures were reduced. A tape muzzle was used to immobilise the fractures. Liquidised food should be syringed through the pharyngostomy tube at frequent intervals and the tube plugged between times. To prevent it from becoming occluded, the tube should be flushed with water before and after the liquidised food is given.

First aid treatment of mandibular fractures

The rostral portion of the mandible should be supported in a tape muzzle or similar support (**372**). This not only prevents further damage to the weakened area(s) but also makes the animal feel more comfortable. The support should not be so tight as to impair the airway.

Repair of the mandibular symphysis

Most fractures of the mandibular symphysis can be repaired with a simple interrupted stainless steel wire suture placed either between the third incisors and the canine teeth, or immediately behind the canines (**373**). The wire is introduced through the mucosa, passed ventral to the mandibles and brought out in a corresponding position on the opposite side. The ends of the wire are twisted, cut off leaving three or four twists and laid flush with the gingiva.

Alternatively, one end of the wire is introduced through the mucosa, distobuccal to the canine tooth, and pushed out through the skin on the midline ventral to the mandible. The other end of the wire is introduced in a similar manner. The free ends of the wire are then twisted and cut off. The wire can generally be removed after 4–6 weeks with either technique.

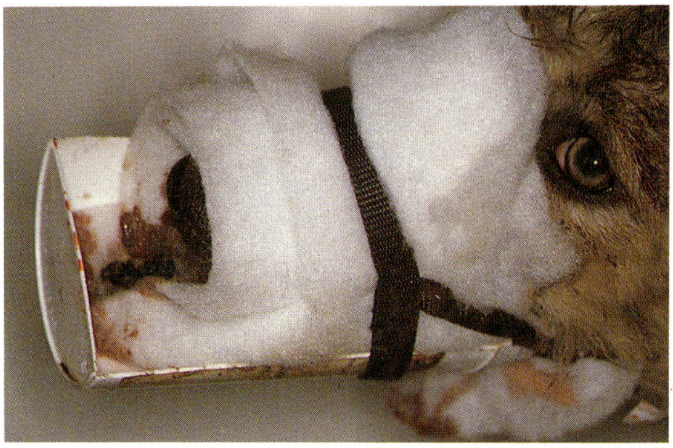

372

372 Emergency support of a mandibular fracture. Comminuted mandibular and maxillary fractures are supported by a cut-out yoghurt pot and a 'Halti'. The dog had been hit by a train, and sustained multiple maxillary fractures and bilateral mandibular fractures.

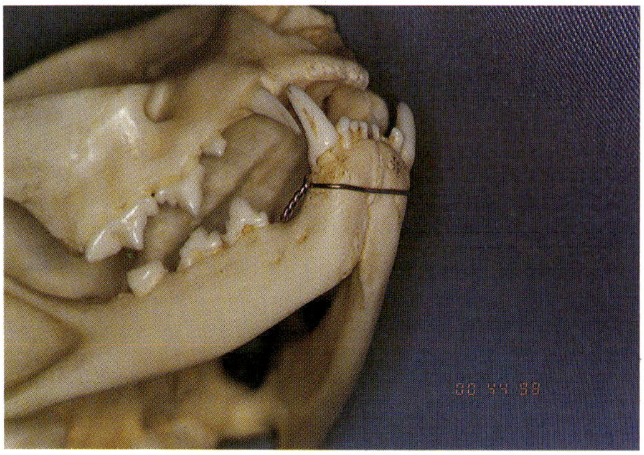

373

373 Symphyseal wiring. The skull of a cat demonstrating a cerclage wire placed around the mandibular symphysis, immediately distal to the canine teeth. The twisted ends of the wire are directed to lie in the space between the canine and the first premolar tooth.

374

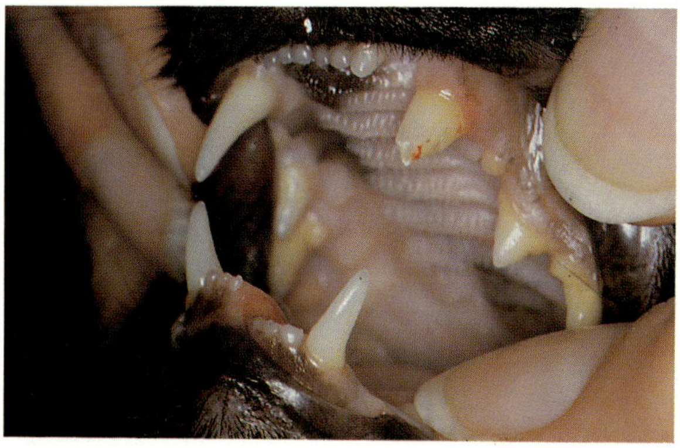

374 Fracture of the mandibular symphysis — Case 1a. Occlusal discrepancy seen in a two-year-old cat that had been hit by a car three days previously. The mandibles could be moved independently of each other, but there was little other damage, except for a fracture of the upper left canine tooth. The symphyseal fracture was immobilised with a cerclage wire.

375

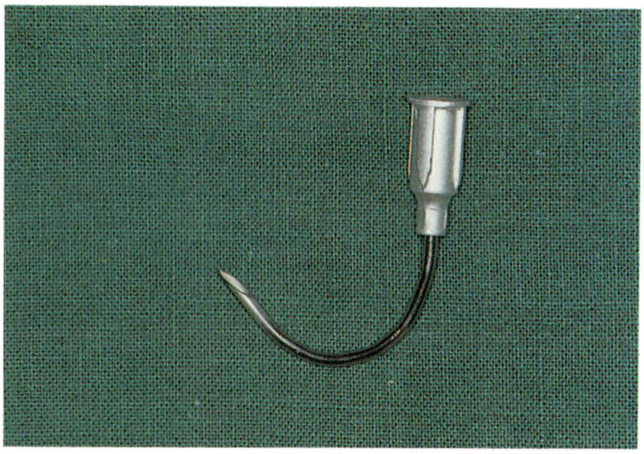

375 Passing cerclage wire — Case 1b. To facilitate passing the wire around the mandibles, a simple wire passer can be fashioned from a hypodermic needle.

37

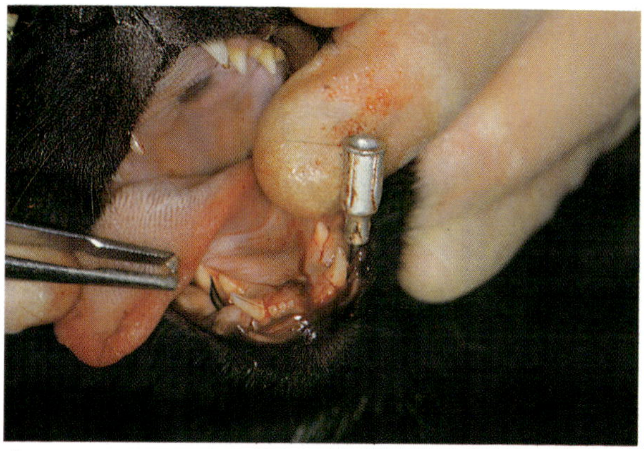

376 Directing the needle subcutaneously under the symphysis and threading the wire through it. If the fracture is oblique and the mandibles slide on each other as the wire is tightened, a lag screw or small pin should be used to counteract the shearing forces.

377 Screw immobilisation of symphysis. A lag screw can be used to immobilise an oblique fracture of the mandibular symphysis. The screw is placed distal to the canine teeth but mesial to the mental foramen. Since the symphysis is a synarthrosis, it may repair with fibrous tissue rather than by osseus union. This does not appear to affect the outcome, and fibrous healing may actually stabilise the symphysis more rapidly.

377

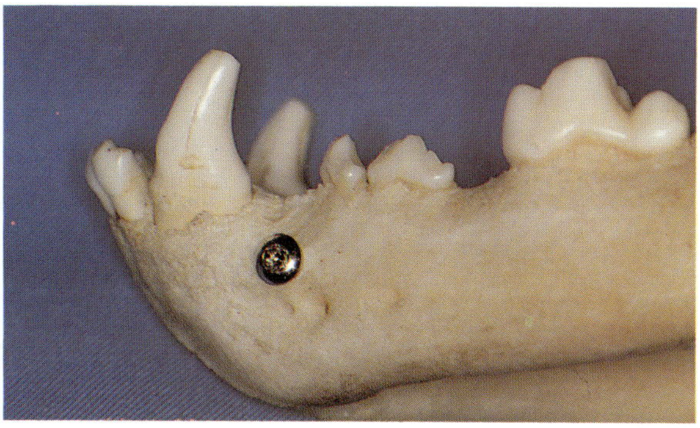

Repair of mandibular body fractures

The tension band side of the mandibular body is the alveolar border. Thus, provided the ventral border of the ramus is intact, interdental wiring or interfragmentary wiring between the tooth roots is often adequate. This is fortunate since the rostral portion of the mandible has only a small area of bone for attaching implants such as plates.

If the fracture is distal to the second premolar tooth it can be immobilised either by a tape muzzle or by plate fixation. Fractures rostral to the molar region tend to heal more rapidly than those situated more caudally, and as a general rule tape muzzles are effective. However, the likelihood of dental malocclusion is greater with a tape muzzle and plate fixation will provide a more secure repair. Plates are easiest to apply in the molar region since there is greatest space and the mandibular bone is thickest.

The application of an external fixation splint using polymethyl methacrylate (acrylic resin) as the connecting bar is an alternative repair technique. Numerous configurations can be used and the method is both cheap and versatile.

Interdental wiring

Interdental wiring can be performed in one of two ways: simple interdental wiring (**378**) and transfurcational interdental wiring (**379**). Transfurcational interdental wire can be left *in situ* unless its removal is indicated because of osteomyelitis, implant loosening or associated soft-tissue problems.

Interfragmentary wiring

Interfragmentary wiring can be used to repair oblique and certain multiple fractures. A longitudinal skin incision along the ventral

378

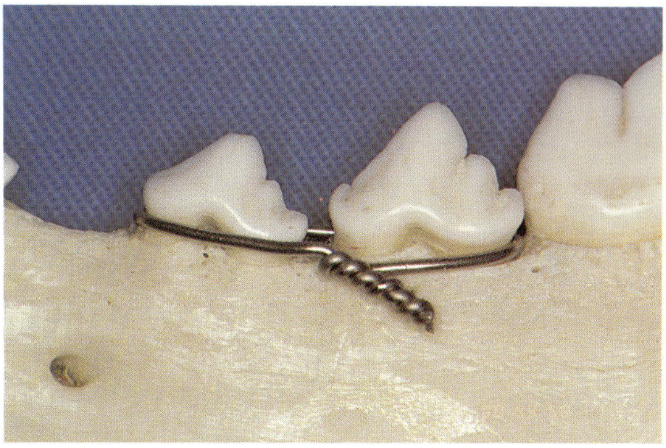

378 Simple interdental wiring. A length of stainless steel wire is taken around the bases of the teeth on either side of the fracture line. The teeth should be firm within their sockets for this method to succeed.

379

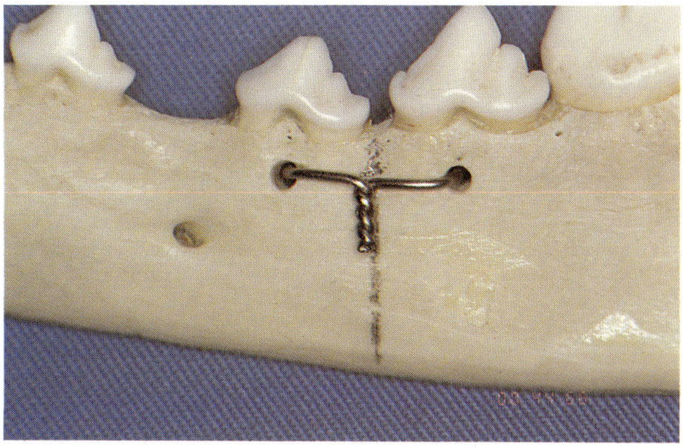

379 Transfurcational interdental wiring. Alternatively, the wire can be taken between the roots of the adjacent teeth. The drill holes are best made with a small Kirschner wire, drilled from the buccal aspect. The wire should be threaded through both drill holes from the lingual aspect before the fracture is reduced.

380

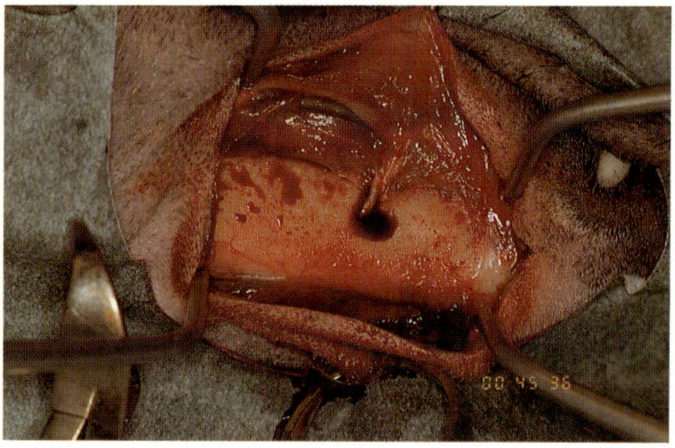

380 Exposure of the mandibular body. Surgical access to the mandibular body is readily achieved by subperiosteal elevation of the digastricus muscle. The mental neurovascular bundle is seen distal to the root of the canine tooth.

381

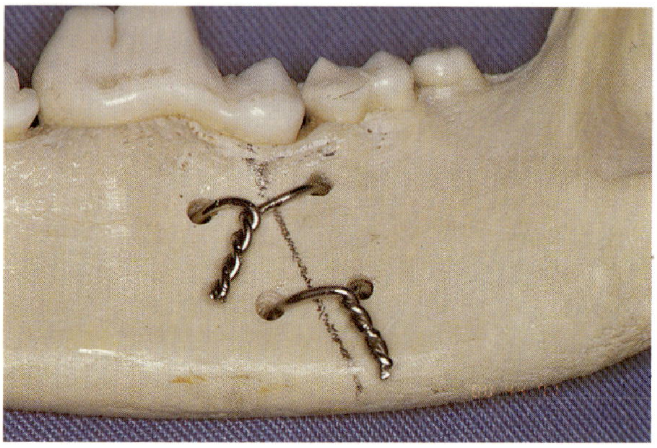

381 Interfragmentary wiring. The wire, or wires, are placed at right angles to the fracture line. The implants may be left in situ, unless there are associated problems.

border of the mandibular body exposes the digastricus muscle caudally and the platysma muscle rostrally. Subperiosteal elevation and retraction of these muscles provides good access to the mandibular body (**380**, **381**).

Tape muzzles

Tape muzzles should only be used where the fracture is stable and dental occlusion can be maintained by the canine teeth. Muzzles for dogs are usually made of tape. They consist of an encircling band around the maxilla and mandible, with a second band that goes behind the ears and connects to both sides of the first band.

Tape muzzles for cats (**382**) are best fashioned from zinc oxide tape. They may need to be sutured to prevent them from slipping.

Muzzles can be used as the sole method of immobilisation or they can be used as additional support following internal fixation of fractures. When used as the sole method of support,

382

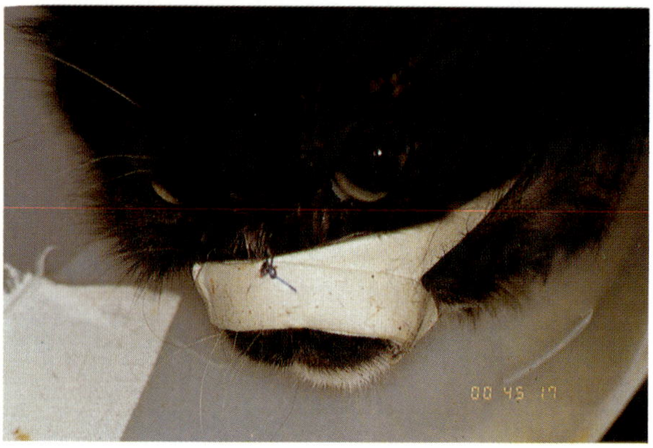

382 Tape muzzle. This kitten sustained a fracture of the right mandibular body. Following reduction, the fracture was immobilised with a tape muzzle sutured to the animal's nose and to the skin beneath the chin. An Elizabethan collar prevented the kitten from removing the muzzle.

regular checks must be made to ensure the canine teeth are maintaining jaw alignment if malocclusion is to be avoided.

Bone plates

Bone plates provide good rigidity but must be contoured accurately if occlusion is to be achieved. The plate is placed laterally, near the ventral border of the mandibular body, so that the screws avoid the tooth roots (**383**).

Ideally, the screws should not enter the mandibular canal, but it is not always possible to achieve this. In any case, the mandibular artery within the canal has often been damaged by the original insult so that its function is already impaired.

A variety of bone plates may be used to immobilise fractures of the mandibular body. The most useful plates are manufactured by the ASIF/AO group and include reconstruction plates, veterinary cuttable plates and small dynamic compression plates.

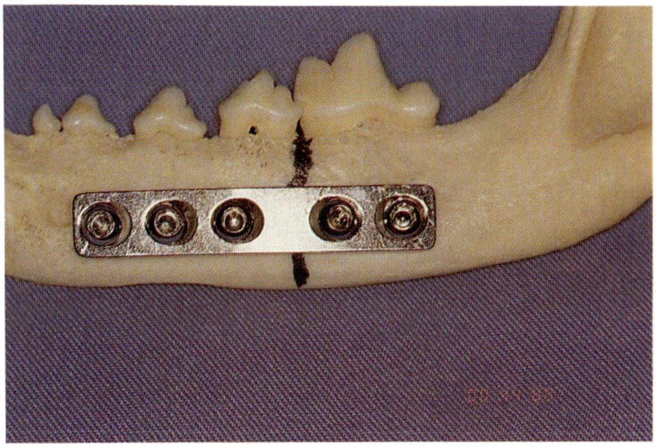

383

383 Compression plate on a mandibular body. A five-hole 2.7 mm dynamic compression plate is applied to the mandibular body. The screws either side of the fracture line are placed eccentrically within the screw holes of the plate so as to compress the fracture line and achieve high interfragmentary forces.

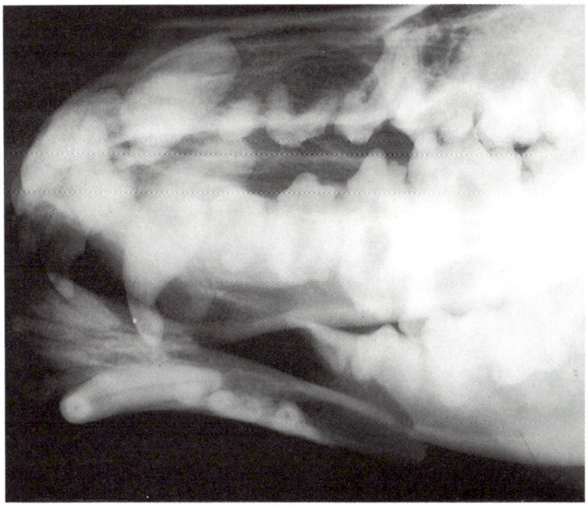

384

384 Pre-operative radiograph — Case 3a. A lateral oblique projection of the mandibular body and symphysis demonstrating an oblique fracture between the second and third premolar teeth and a symphyseal separation.

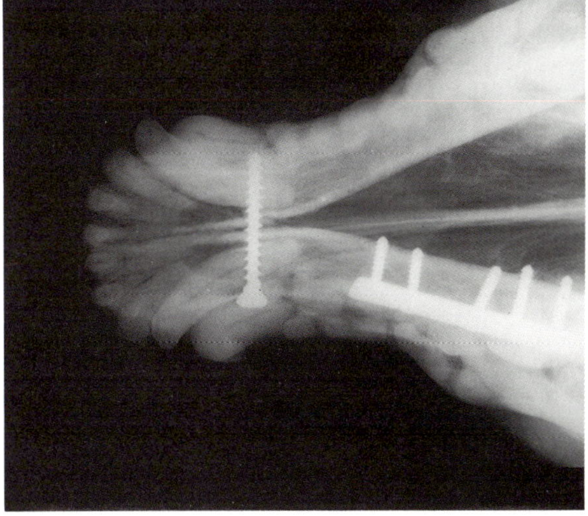

385

385 Postoperative radiograph — Case 3b. A post-operative radiograph demonstrating repair of the mandibular fracture with a bone plate. The symphyseal separation was repaired with a lag screw. Nose facing to the left of the page.

386

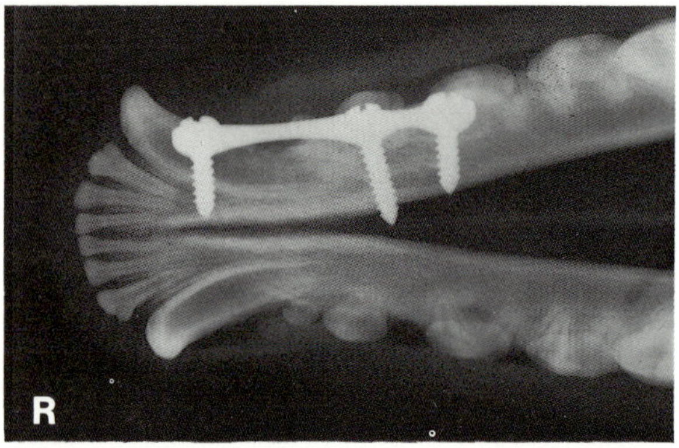

386 Immediate postoperative radiograph — Case 4a. Radiograph of a dog aged approximately seven months. The dog was involved in a road traffic accident and sustained a fracture of the mandibular body, which was repaired with a bone plate and screws. Unfortunately, dental anatomy was ignored by the operator and both canine teeth were perforated with the rostral bone screw. Nose facing to the left of the page.

387

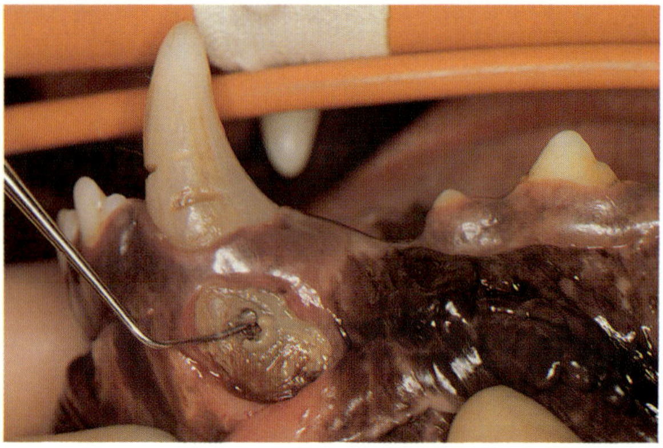

387 Two years later — Case 4b. The damaged tooth became infected and caused an abscess. The mucous membranes around the sinus tract had been repeatedly sutured over the defect, but failed to heal for obvious reasons. At referral, chronic osteomyelitis was present with severe halitosis and hypersalivation. The animal was in pain and resented its mouth being touched or examined.

388

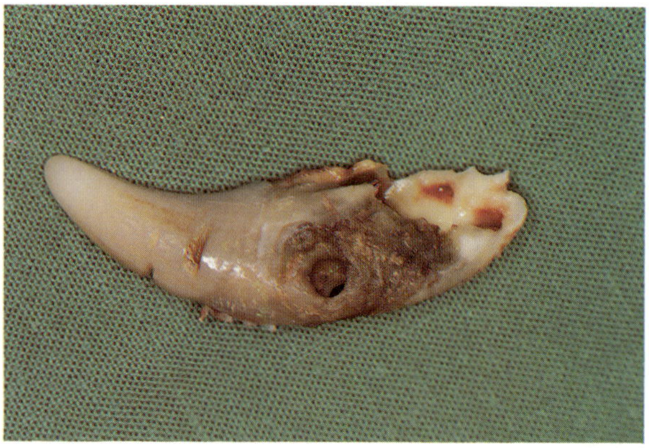

388 Extracted canine — Case 4c. Due to the severely weakened mandible, and the risk of further fractures, the canines were extracted at two separate sessions, with a period of six months between surgery to allow for osseous healing. To minimise the force exerted on the weakened mandible, an open procedure was used. Alveolar bone was carefully removed with rotatory instruments; no forceps were used, as these could easily exert an excessive force. Healing was uneventful and within weeks the animal allowed its mouth to be examined.

External fixation splint

This device is useful for repairing multiple fractures, bilateral fractures or fractures where stability is difficult to maintain because of missing or highly comminuted fragments. Ideally, two pins should be placed in each fragment; the pins are then joined by either a connecting bar and clamps (Kirschner type of fixator) or with 'cold cured' acrylic. In some rostral fractures a single pin is sufficient, provided it is drilled transversely through both halves of the mandible.

The acrylic fixator has a number of advantages over the more conventional Kirschner type of fixator: it is quicker to apply and the pins need not be all in the same plane before they are joined to the bar. As a result, pin placement, particularly when using many small pins, is easier.

The fixator is applied with the jaws closed and the teeth occluded. The pins are inserted through small stab incisions in the skin and drilled through the soft tissues and bone. High-speed drills should be avoided, since they encourage thermal necrosis and subsequent pin loosening. There should be little or no soft-tissue tension on the pins to reduce the likelihood of pin tract infection.

Small Steinmann pins or Kirschner wires should be used. When using a 'sausage' of acrylic, the ends of the pins may be bent over to provide better purchase in the moulded material. Alternatively, the pins can be pushed through plastic tubing, which is then filled with acrylic. Self-curing acrylic generally takes 6–10 minutes to harden, after which excess pin length can be cut off with pin cutters.

389

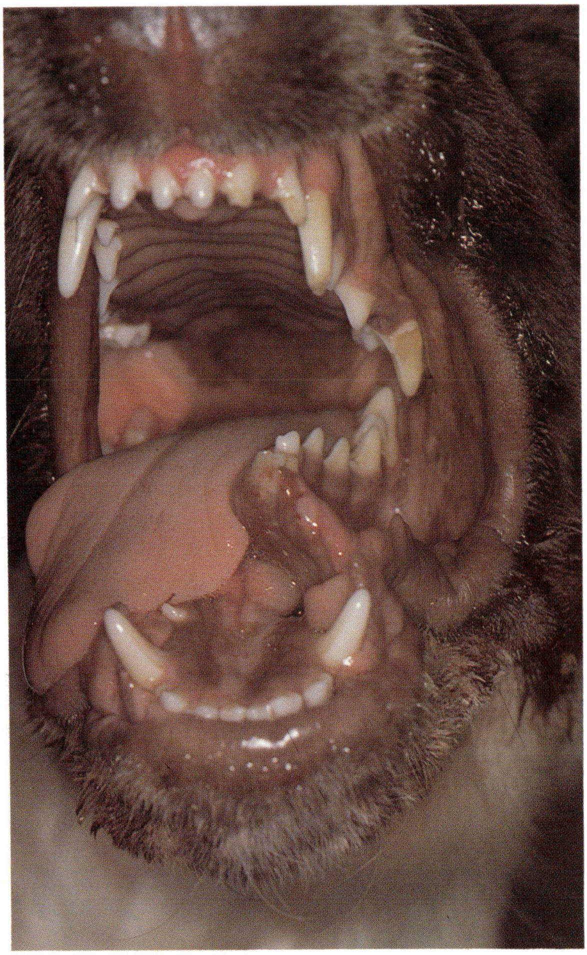

389 Bilateral mandibular body fractures caused by a kick from a horse — Case 5a.

390

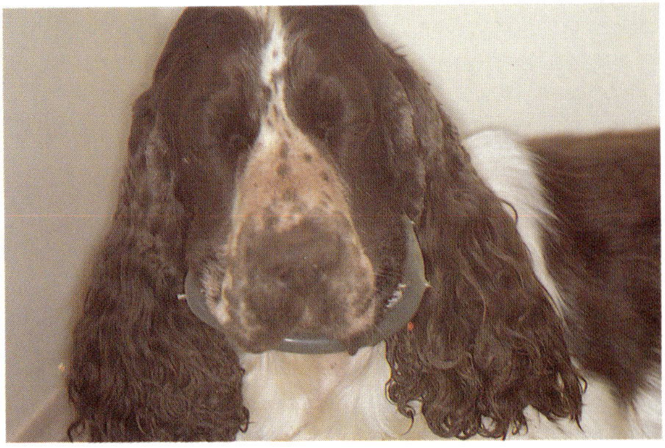

390 Immediate postoperative appearance — Case 5b. Five minutes after recovery from general anaesthesia, using an intravenous 'propofol' infusion. The fractures were reduced and immobilised with an external fixator. The connecting bar was constructed of methyl methacrylate injected into polythene tubing with a 60 ml catheter syringe.

391 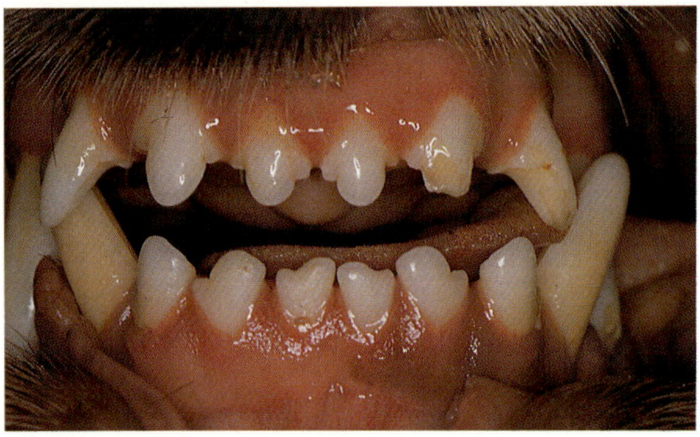

391 Six weeks postoperatively — Case 5c. The fractures have healed and there is good occlusion.

Repair of the ramus

Many fractures of the ramus can be treated conservatively since they possess considerable inherent stability due to the large masticatory muscles surrounding the area. Moreover, the thinness of the bone of the ramus limits the use of internal implants. Small bone plates and Kirschner wires are the most suitable forms of internal fixation.

Bone plates

A ventrolateral approach is used to expose the ramus. The platysma muscle is divided to expose the digastricus muscle. The masseter muscle is subperiosteally elevated to expose the masseteric fossa and the angular region of the mandible. If further exposure is required, a second incision can be made along the ventral border of the zygomatic arch and the temporomandibular joint. The underlying soft tissues are divided along the same plane and reflected ventrally. The muscle between the two incisions is then elevated to expose the remainder of the ramus.

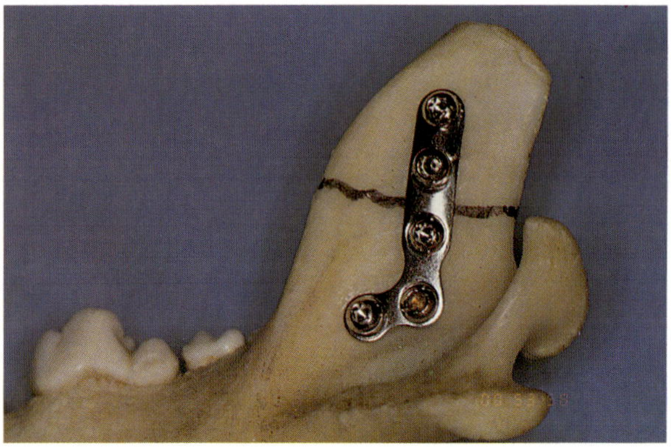 39

392 Plated ramus. A small bone plate can be used to repair fractures of the ramus. The plate shown is a mini L-plate produced by the ASIF/AO group.

393 Primary incision to ramus — Case 6a. A ventral skin incision followed by division of the digastricus muscle exposes the masseter muscle. This is subperiosteally elevated to expose the angular region of the mandible. Further retraction of the masseter muscle permits access to the masseteric fossa.

393

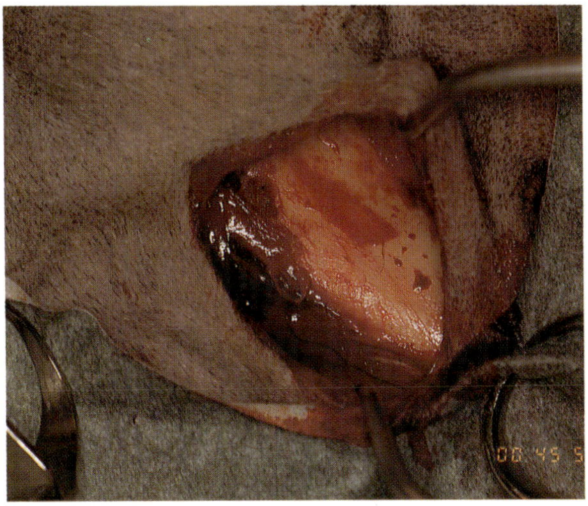

394 Accessory incision — Case 6b. To increase the exposure of the ramus, a second incision is made along the ventral border of the zygomatic arch, taking care not to enter the temporomandibular joint capsule. The soft tissues between this and the first incision are elevated with a periosteal elevator.

394

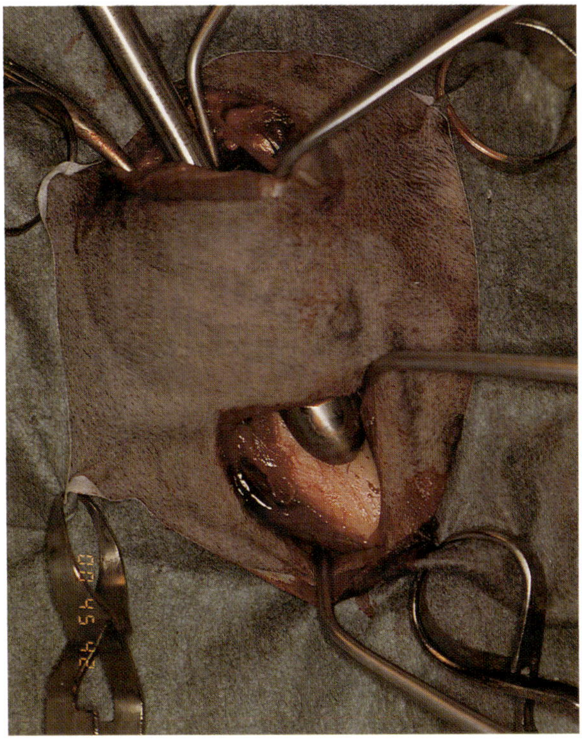

Kirschner wires

Kirschner wires can be used to maintain temporary reduction of the fracture while some other form of internal fixation is used, but generally they do not provide sufficient immobilisation on their own. Additional support can sometimes be provided with a tape muzzle.

395 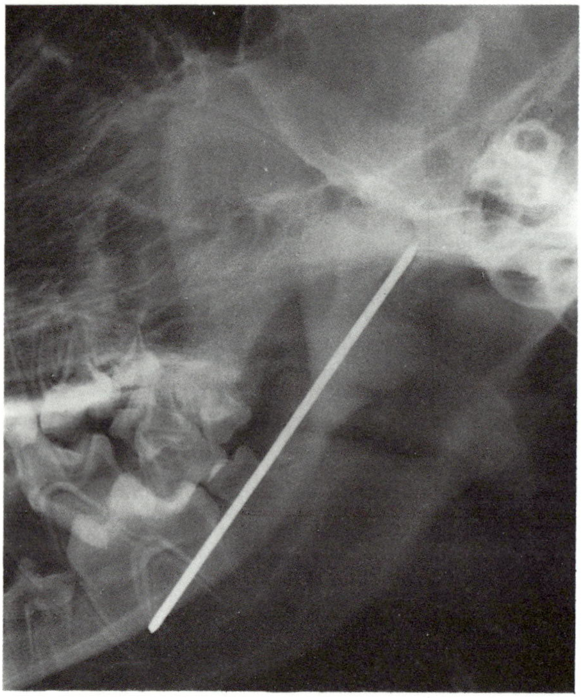

395 Postoperative radiograph — Case 7a. Fracture of the ramus of a six-month-old dog. The fracture has been immobilised with a Kirschner wire.

396 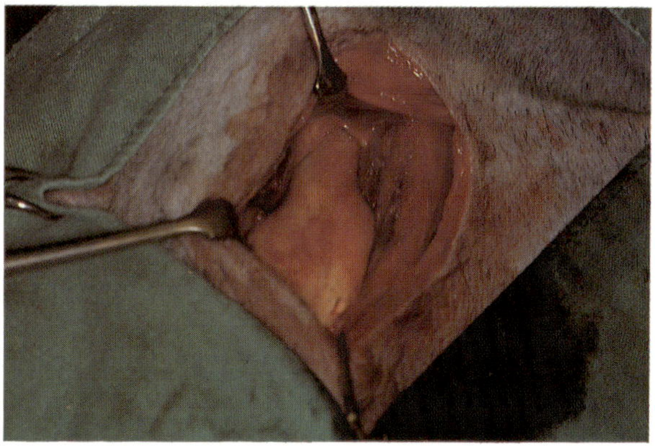

396 Intraoperative view — Case 7b. The fracture can be seen below the top Langenbeck retractor. The Kirschner wire can be seen exiting the ventral border of the ramus prior to being cut flush with the surface of the bone. Additional support was provided by a tape muzzle applied for two weeks postoperatively.

Fractures of the maxilla

Fractures of the maxilla involve either the nasal and/or maxillary bones. The aims of treatment are similar to fractures of the mandible, namely the restoration of dental occlusion and the ability to eat and drink.

Most maxillary fractures are multiple. The fragments may remain in alignment or they may be depressed. Epistaxis, swelling of the region and asymmetry are the usual physical findings, with or without crepitus and subcutaneous emphysema. Radiography is often disappointing because of the confusing appearance of the multiple fracture lines.

Fixation of simple maxillary fractures is not often required. Severely depressed fractures may be elevated and wired in position but, generally, open reduction is avoided.

Fractures that result in malocclusion may be immobilised with a tape muzzle as described previously. Alternatively, interdental wiring can be employed, possibly with further support provided by acrylic. Primary teeth are not ideal candidates for interdental wiring as the teeth lack the bulbosities and the necessary undercuts. It is permissible to use a rotatory instrument to score the enamel of the primary teeth to gain retention.

Multiple or grossly unstable fractures of the maxilla are best repaired using external fixation and acrylic connectors.

397 Alveolar maxillary fracture. The maxilla was immobilised with an external fixator, similar to that seen in **390**.

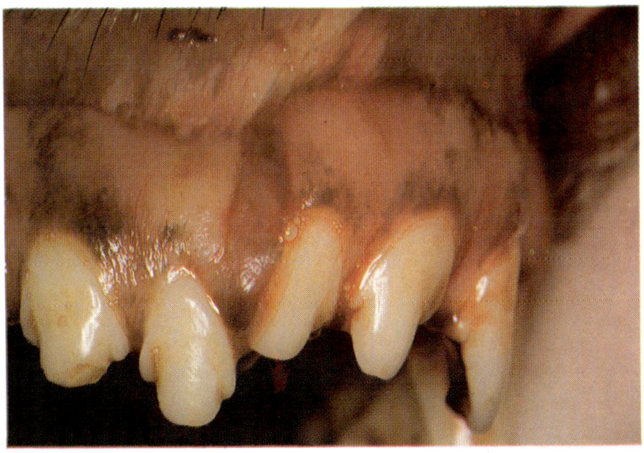

397

398 Multiple maxillary and mandibular fractures — Case 8a. A comminuted, open fracture of the mandible of the same animal as seen in **372**. In addition, the puppy had bilateral mandibular body fractures and multiple maxillary fractures.

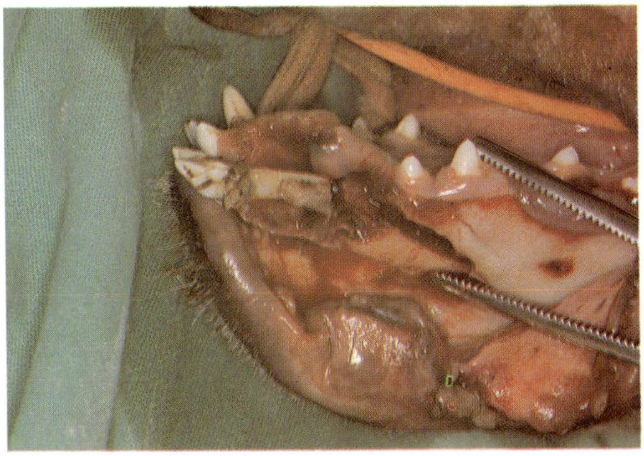

398

399 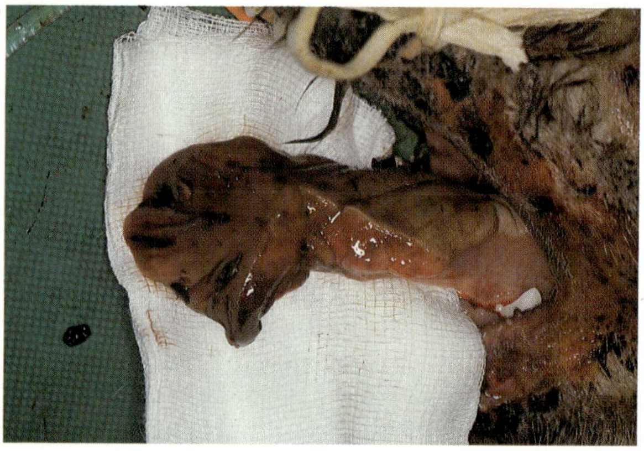

399 Pre-operative appearance — Case 8b. The severely lacerated tongue prior to cleansing and debridement. The tongue was cleaned, debrided and sutured with a continuous simple suture of polyglactin 910 (Vicryl®).

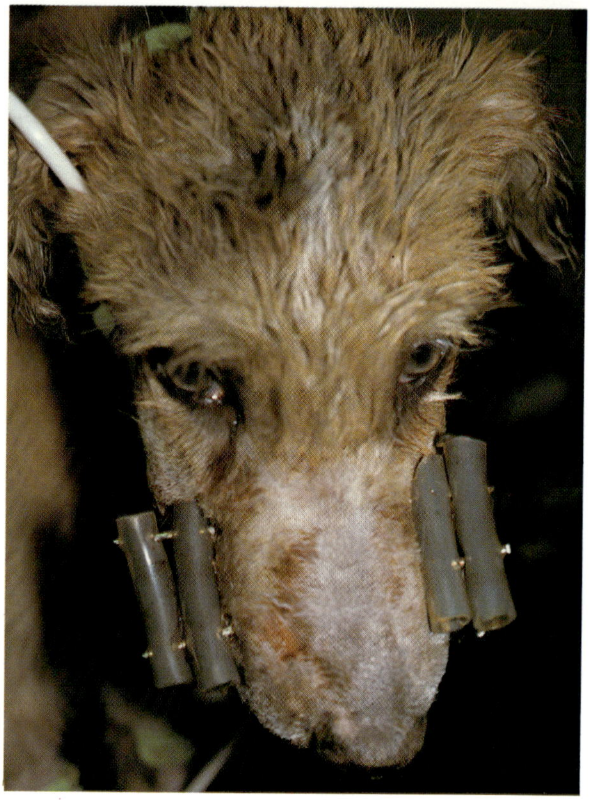 40

400 Five days postoperative — Case 8c. The maxillary fractures have been immobilised with an external fixator.

401 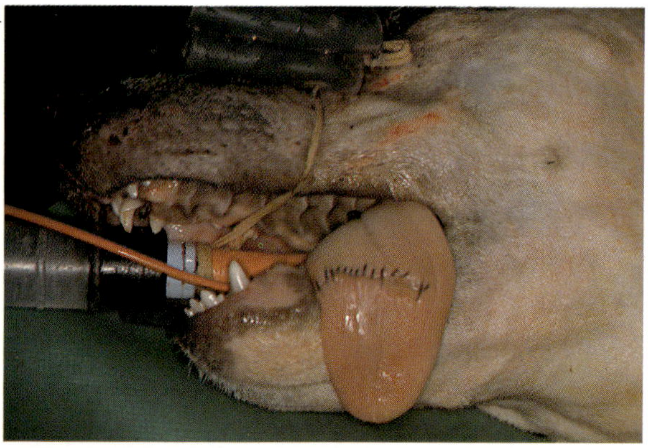

401 Five days postoperatively — Case 8d. The bilateral fractures of the mandibular body were grossly overridden, causing marked malocclusion. At this stage the mandibular fractures were immobilised with compression plates, interfragmentary wires and Kirschner wires. The tongue is healing satisfactorily.

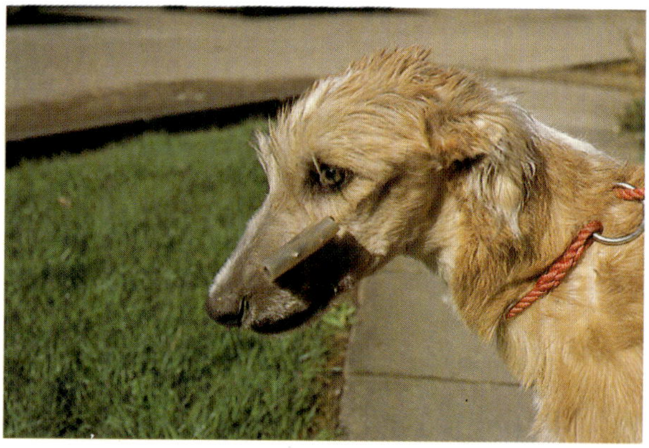 4

402 Five weeks postoperative appearance — Case 8e. The puppy was fed via a gastrostomy tube for the first 10 days after the mandibular fractures were repaired. It was then fed a soft diet per os. Atrophy of the muscles of mastication is evident but the range of temporomandibular joint movement was good, as was dental occlusion. The external fixator was removed at this stage.

403 Alveolar fracture in a six-month-old puppy — Case 9a. The animal was bitten by a much larger dog and sustained bilateral mandibular body fractures and a unilateral fracture of the caudal maxillary alveolar process. Simple interdental wiring was insufficient. The maxillary alveolar process could not be immobilised and the buccal segment was displaced through occlusal forces.

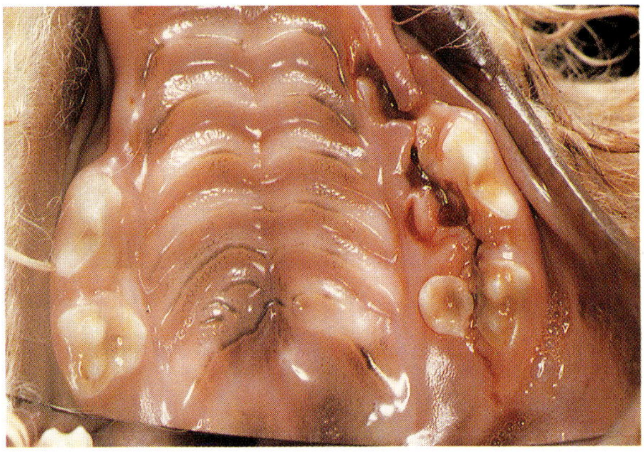

403

404 Intra-oral splint *in situ* — Case 9b. An intra-oral splint was made from a self-curing acrylic (for handling material, see **715–717**). The material was not allowed to set in contact with the oral mucosa, because of the heat that the material generates, but was repeatedly inserted and removed to maintain the desired shape. Once the initial set had taken place, the material was placed in warm water, which not only speeded up the procedure but also leached out free monomer that may be an irritant to the oral mucosa once the splint has been wired in. Holes were drilled in the splint at the appropriate places and stainless steel wire was used to wire the appliance to the dentition.

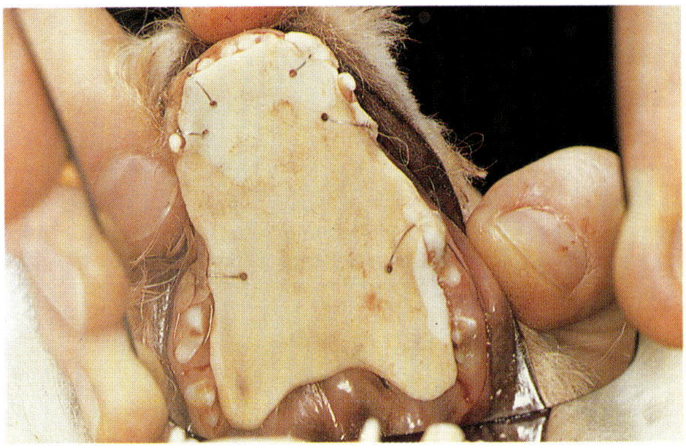

404

405 Two-weeks postoperatively — Case 9c. The intra-oral splint was removed, as healing was expected to be rapid at this age. The palatal mucosa was in good condition and minimal food packing was present under the appliance. The buccal cortical plate was stable. Two weeks later the fourth permanent premolar was being exfoliated with a purulent discharge from its gingival sulcus. It was found that the tooth was infected, having been devitalised through the original trauma. Only a thin shell of enamel had been formed.

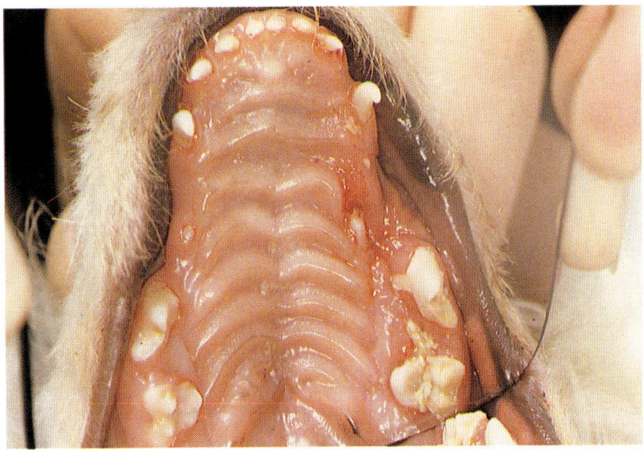

405

406

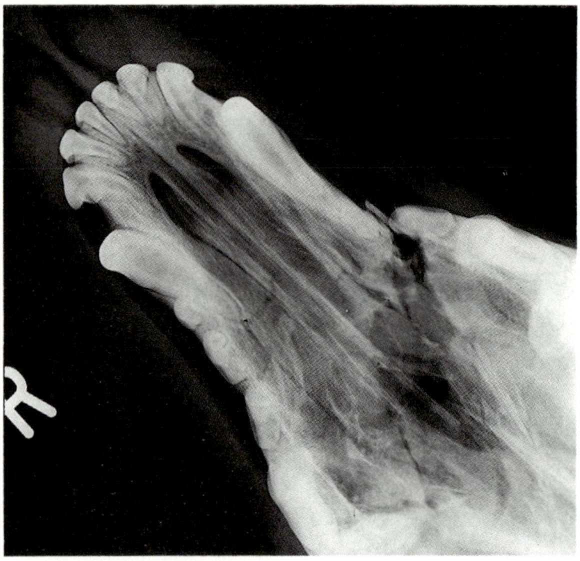

406 Multiple maxillary fractures — Case 10a. An intra-oral radiograph of a 10-month-old puppy which ran into a car shows multiple maxillary fractures, with gross displacement of the rostral aspects of the upper jaw.

407

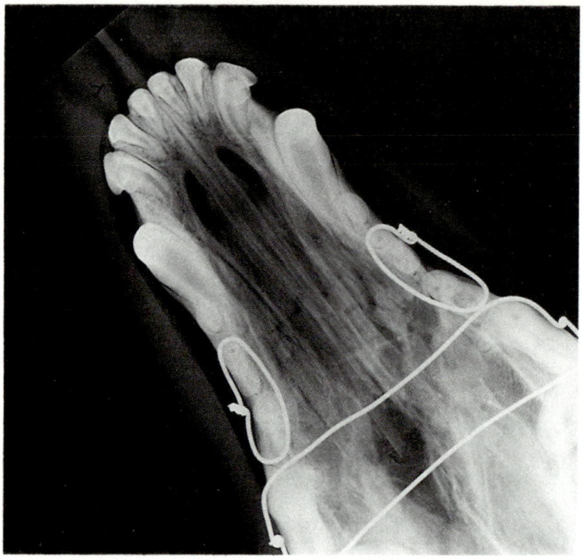

407 Postoperative radiograph — Case 10b. The fractures have been immobilised by wires around the base of the teeth on each side of the fracture line. The hard palate has been repaired with a wire suture inserted submucosally.

Temporomandibular luxation

Traumatic luxations

Luxations of the temporomandibular joint may occur with or without fractures of the mandible. The luxation is generally rostrodorsal in the dog (**408**). Cats more frequently sustain additional fractures of the adjacent osseous structures, since the joint is relatively well protected by the large zygomatic arch found in this species. Additional fractures include fractures of the condyloid process, the articular process or the zygomatic process of the temporal bone.

40

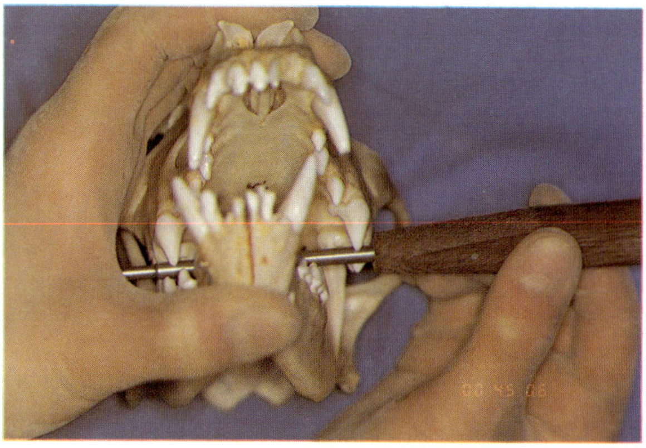

408 Temporomandibular luxation. Luxations of the temporomandibular joint in the dog are usually rostrodorsal. The mandible is deviated away from the side of the luxation. Reduction involves using a wooden dowel or metal pin placed between the molar teeth as a fulcrum, and pushing up on the chin. This disengages the mandibular condyle and pushes it into the temporomandibular joint.

Congenital luxations
Temporomandibular dysplasia may cause instability of the joint, resulting in the coronoid process catching under the zygomatic arch. The condition is most frequently seen in basset-hounds (**409**) and occurs when the mouth is opened wide, such as when the dog yawns. The coronoid process can be palpated lateral to the zygomatic arch and the dog is unable to close its mouth. The subluxation can be reduced by opening the mouth a little wider to disengage the coronoid process and manipulating the mandible into a normal alignment. The subluxation may occur sporadically at first, but it generally becomes more frequent. Surgical correction of recurring cases is possible by removing that part of the zygomatic arch that interferes with the coronoid process (**410, 411**).

409

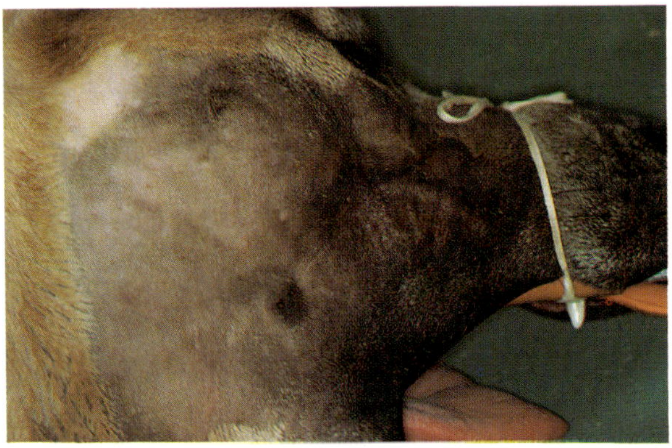

409 Temporomandibular dysplasia in a basset-hound — Case 10a. Subluxation of the temporomandibular joint is evident. The coronoid process can be seen distorting the facial contour.

410

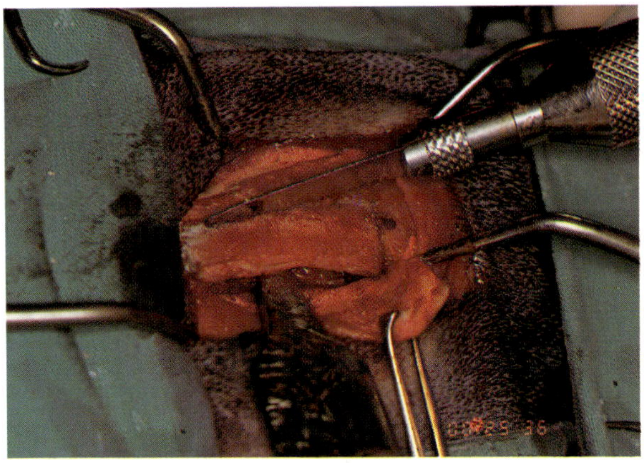

410 Resection of the zygoma — Case 10b. The ventral portion of the zygomatic arch that interferes with the coronoid process is removed with a reciprocating saw. Retention of the dorsal part of the arch preserves the facial outline.

411

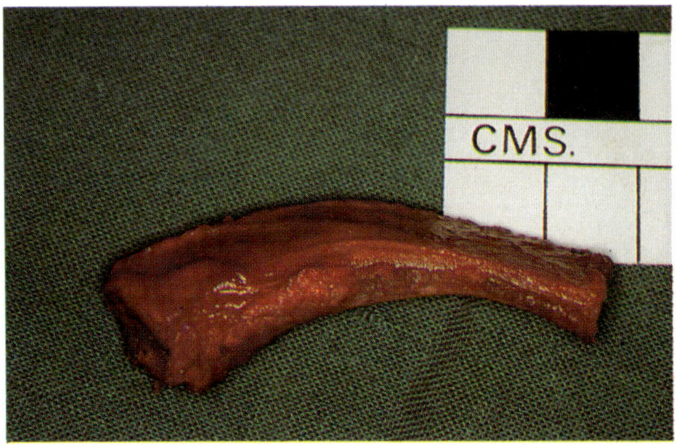

411 Resected portion of the zygoma — Case 10c.

12 Oral Surgery: III. Tumours

Signs and symptoms

Oral tumours are common presentations in both the dog and the cat. Early clinical signs include tooth loss, halitosis and facial deformity, although many lesions can reach an advanced stage before they are noticed and presented for treatment. Pain and dysphagia are rare clinical signs, except in tumours that involve the tonsil or tongue. Nodal metastasis may cause enlargement of the regional lymph nodes in the cervical region.

Aetiology

The aetiology of most oral tumours is unknown, although environmental carcinogens have been implicated in the development of the now uncommon tonsillar carcinoma in dogs. The feline leukaemia virus may be involved in the aetiology of some oral lymphoid tumours in the cat.

Assessment of the tumour

Many oral tumours have a similar appearance, irrespective of their histological type, and a standard protocol for examination of both the primary and potential secondary sites is essential:

The primary tumour (T). The site and extent of the primary mass should be inspected and accurately recorded for later comparison. Tumours adjacent to bony structures (i.e. mandible, incisive or maxillary bone) should be radiographed using intra-oral studies, supplemented by oblique views of the oral cavity where appropriate, to confirm the presence of any *bone involvement*.

Regional lymph nodes (N). Regional lymph nodes (mandibular and retropharyngeal) should be palpated to assess their size and mobility in order to detect *nodal metastatic deposits*.

Distant sites (M). Right and left lateral views of the thorax should be taken to detect any distant *metastatic deposits*.

The anatomical stage of the tumour should be recorded using the World Health Organization TNM staging system:

Stage I. Primary tumour less than 2 cm diameter — no bone involvement or metastatic disease.
Stage II. Primary tumour less than 4 cm diameter — no bone involvement or metastatic disease.
Stage III. Primary tumour greater than 4 cm diameter — no bone involvement or metastatic disease; or any primary tumour with bone involvement; or any tumour with ipsilateral lymph node involvement.
Stage IV. Any tumour with bilateral lymph node involvement; or any tumour with distant metastatic disease.

Histological identification

The histological tumour type should be identified as accurately as possible in all cases *prior* to the instigation of any treatment.

Biopsy techniques

Samples are best removed from the oral cavity under general anaesthesia with the airway intubated, using a cuffed endotracheal tube, and the pharynx packed with gauze swabs to prevent aspiration of any debris. Occasionally, samples can be removed from the sedated patient after infiltration of local anaesthetic around the biopsy site.

Superficial samples may be collected using alligator forceps or, for deeper and often more representative samples, incisional wedge or punch biopsy techniques should be used. Needle aspirate and core techniques are inappropriate for biopsy of oral tumours and rarely recover representative samples.

Samples should be transferred to 10% formol saline solution or 'Susa' fixative for fixation.

In cases where the regional lymph nodes are thought to be involved, needle aspirate biopsy should be performed to detect metastatic deposits.

Tumour classification

A wide variety of tumours is found in the oral cavity and accurate identification of tumour type is crucial to the selection of the most suitable treatment. The most frequent types include:

Benign or locally-invasive oral tumours
- Peripheral odontogenic fibroma (previously termed fibromatous or ossifying epulis).
- Basal cell carcinoma (previously termed acanthomatous epulis).
- Ameloblastoma.

Malignant oral tumours
- Squamous cell carcinoma.
- Fibrosarcoma.
- Malignant melanoma.
- Other less common tumours include osteosarcoma, chondrosarcoma, salivary gland adenocarcinoma.

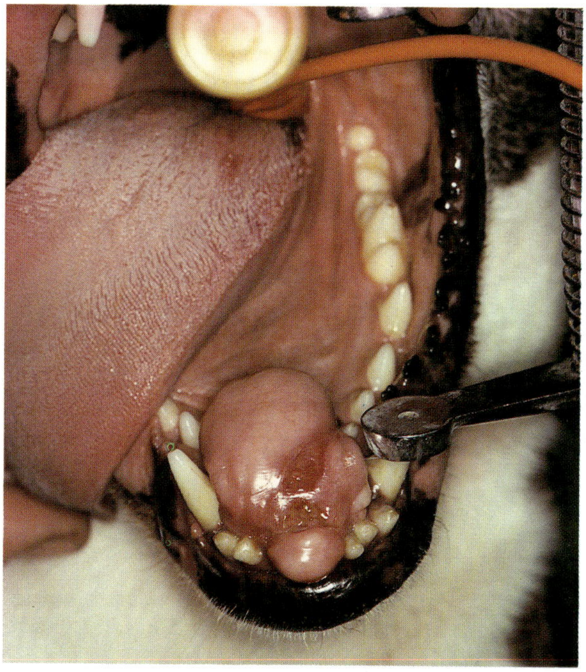

412

412 Peripheral odontogenic fibroma. Previously classified as fibromatous or ossifying epulides, peripheral odontogenic fibromas often have a shiny, non-ulcerated surface and are firmly attached to the gum. Radiographically, these tumours demonstrate varying degrees of mineralisation. They develop slowly and although they may disrupt the dentition through their sheer physical size they never invade or damage the underlying alveolar bone.

Treatment. Peripheral odontogenic fibromas can be very successfully managed by surgical excision. Surgical margins should, however, be extended into the underlying bone since local excision will inevitably result in recurrence.

413 Gingival hyperplasia. This degenerative condition is commonly encountered in dogs with poor dental hygiene and seems to be particularly common in the boxer. Because of its appearance it is often confused with the peripheral odontogenic fibroma and mistakenly regarded as having a neoplastic aetiology. Lesions are frequently mineralised and very firmly attached to the gingivae. Untreated lesions can reach spectacular proportions, as in the case illustrated, and give rise to dysphagia and halitosis.

Treatment. Lesions should be removed surgically with rongeurs or by diathermy. Any associated periodontal disease should be dealt with to reduce the risk of recurrence of the condition.

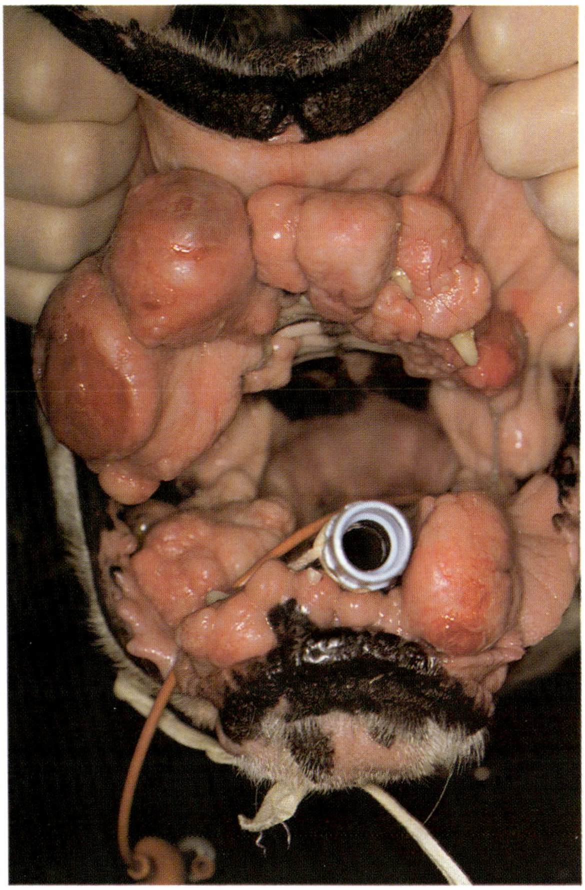
413

414 Basal cell carcinoma. Previously termed the acanthomatous epulis this benign tumour behaves in a locally aggressive fashion. It invariably invades adjacent alveolar bone and may exhibit rapid growth. Additionally, its ulcerated appearance often gives rise to suspicions of malignancy although there is no risk of metastatic spread.

Treatment. Basal cell carcinomas can be consistently cured by surgical removal, using wide local excision with margins of approximately 1 cm on all aspects. Radiation therapy is equally successful in curing this tumour although the lack of available radiation facilities combined with a significant risk of malignancy developing subsequently at the irradiated site compromise this alternative approach. Partial mandibulectomy or maxillectomy is, therefore, the treatment of choice.

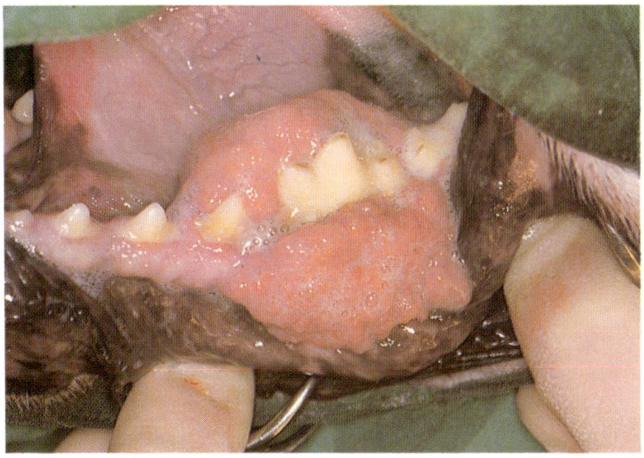
414

415 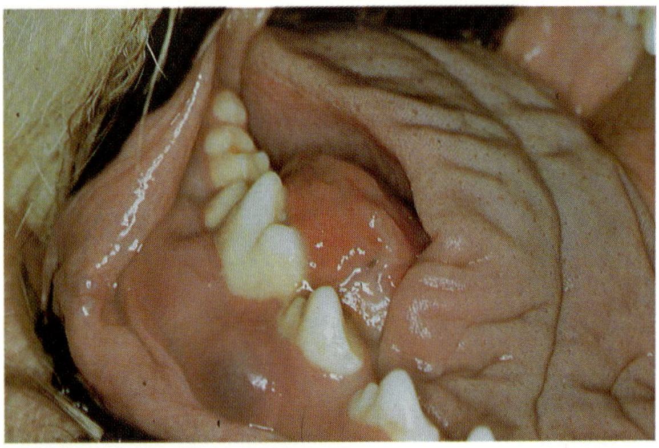

415 Ameloblastoma. This is an unusual benign tumour and almost always involves the mandible. It has a characteristic cystic, expansile appearance which is seen to be multilocular on radiography.

Treatment. Local excision, employing minimal surgical margins or even vigorous curettage of the internal aspects of the cystic structures, invariably achieves a cure.

416 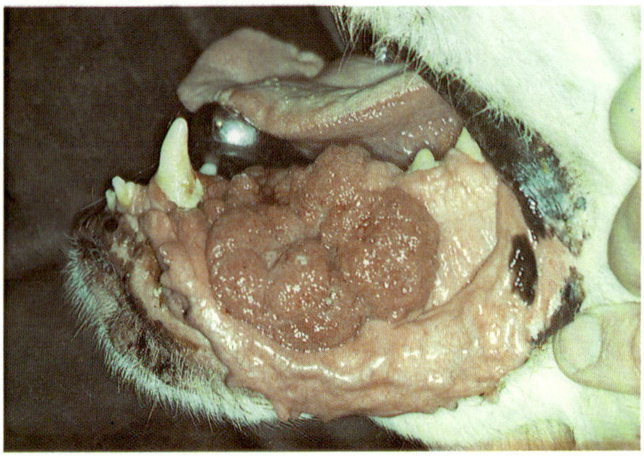

416 Squamous cell carcinoma (gingival). This is the most common type of malignant tumour found in the oral cavity of both the dog and the cat. The lesion is often ulcerated, dental disruption is common and bone invasion is found in approximately three-quarters of cases. Metastasis is slow to occur but may be detected in the regional (usually mandibular) nodes in 10% of cases.

Treatment. Wide local excision (margins of not less than 1 cm on all aspects), dictating mandibulectomy or maxillectomy, is frequently successful, with one-year survival rates of over 85% reported. Radiation therapy is a useful alternative to surgery, particularly where combined with hyperthermia, achieving one-year cure rates of 70%.

417 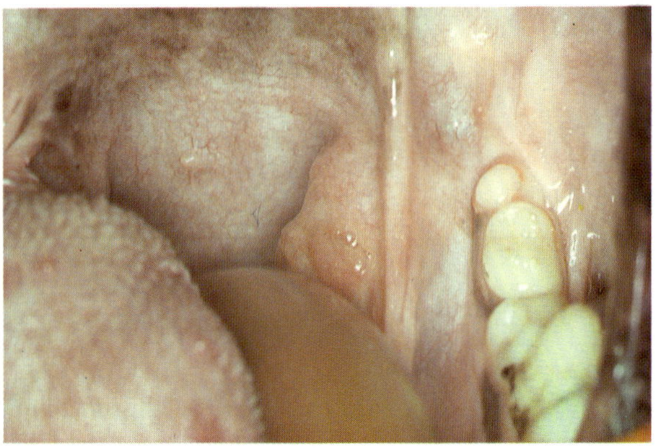

417 Squamous cell carcinoma (soft tissue). The tonsil (see illustration) and tongue are the most important non-gingival sites for squamous cell carcinoma in both the dog and the cat. Dysphagia is, consequently, often encountered. Tonsillar lesions are highly metastatic and eventually involve the regional (retropharyngeal) nodes in almost all cases.

Treatment. Surgical excision with adequate margins is rarely possible and local recurrence is a consistent outcome. Radiation therapy may be useful in palliating the disease in some cases but the primary problem of dysphagia often persists and survival exceeding a few months is rare.

418 **Fibrosarcoma.** These tumours are often large and occupy a relatively caudal position within the oral cavity, especially in the maxillary region. Bone invasion is almost invariably found and metastasis will eventually develop in 20% of cases.

Treatment. The difficulty of achieving compartmental resections in the oral cavity means that surgery alone cannot be relied upon to achieve a more consistent cure for fibrosarcoma. One-year survival rates of 45% have, however, been reported. Similarly, radiation therapy does not achieve guaranteed results although survival rates of up to 50% have been reported where radiation has been combined with hyperthermia. A combined modality approach (i.e. surgery plus radiation) may be a more rational means of dealing with this type of sarcoma.

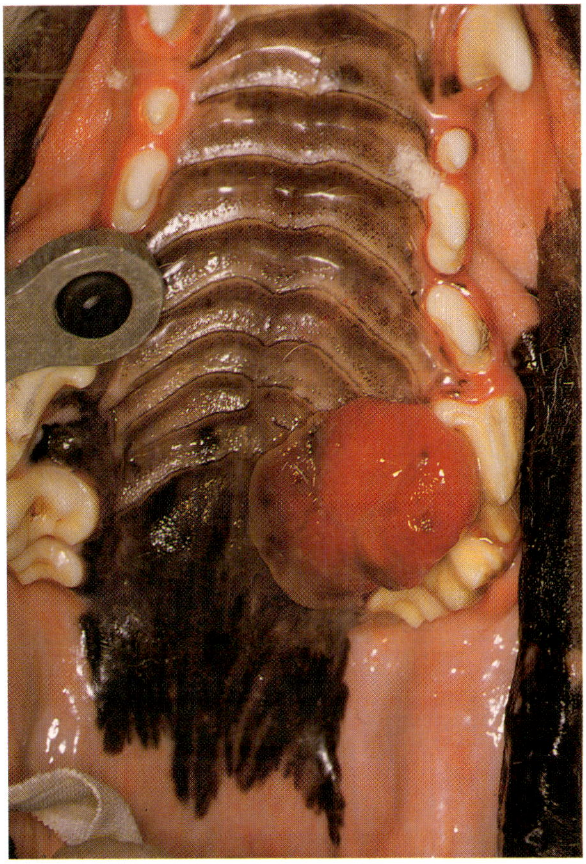

418

419 **Malignant melanoma.** These may present in the pigmented or non-pigmented form and most frequently involve the gingiva. The surface of the tumour is often ulcerated and necrotic bleeding easily if damaged. Bone involvement is found in more than half the cases. Malignant melanoma is highly metastatic and as many as 20% of cases will have evidence of secondary disease in the lungs on presentation. The remainder are likely to metastasise to regional nodes or lungs eventually.

Treatment. Surgical excision is often successful in achieving local cure but does not influence the ultimate development of regional and distant metastasis. It may have a beneficial palliative role in some cases. Radiation therapy is likewise useful for management of the primary lesion but should be delivered in large doses (5–10 Gy) to achieve a satisfactory response.

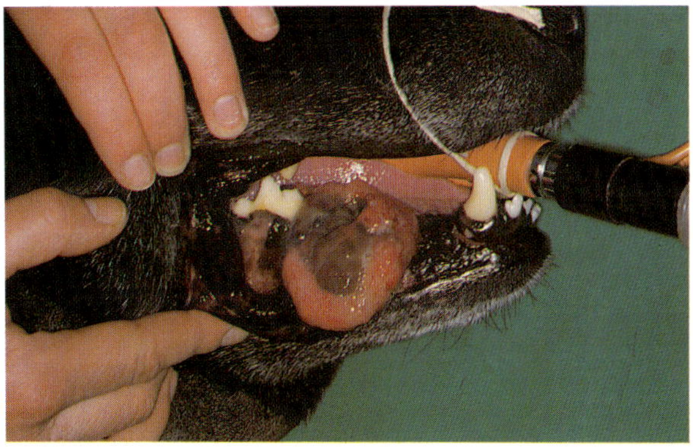

419

Treatment of oral tumours

Surgery

Surgery is indicated in the management of oral tumours:

- As the sole form of management for *benign* or *locally-invasive lesions* (e.g. peripheral odontogenic fibroma, basal cell carcinoma and ameloblastoma) and *carcinomas* in the first instance (e.g. squamous cell carcinoma).
- As part of combined modality treatment (i.e. combined with radiation and/or chemotherapy) for *sarcomas*.
- As a means of *palliating* discomfort or dysphagia and improving the patient's quality of life where outright cure is not attainable.

The selection of the *surgical margin* should be based in each case on the individual requirements of the tumour type:

- Benign or locally invasive tumours normally dictate margins of up to 1 cm.
- Carcinomas dictate margins of not less than 1 cm.
- Sarcomas dictate removal of intact anatomical compartments, which is only rarely attainable in the case of oral sarcomas.

Techniques for the surgical removal of oral tumours include:

Rostral mandibulectomy
partial
unilateral
bilateral

Hemimandibulectomy
horizontal body only
vertical ramus only
total

Partial maxillectomy
rostral
oral
nasal

Patient preparation

Patients should be prepared for surgery with the head firmly positioned and the oral cavity freely accessible by means of appropriate gags. Remote anaesthetic circuits should be used to improve the surgeon's access to the patient. The pharynx should be packed off carefully with gauze tapes to prevent aspiration of blood or debris during the surgery.

There are strong arguments for using pre-operative antibacterial agents (e.g. metronidazole) to reduce the bacterial load within the oral cavity. Peri-operative antibiotics might be considered as a means of reducing the incidence of sepsis, although in practice postoperative oral infection is rare.

Rostral mandibulectomy

420

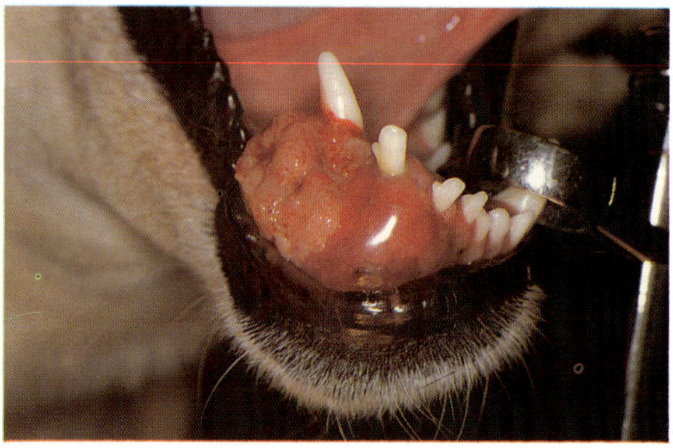

420 Rostral mandibulectomy — Case 1a. This technique may be used to deal with small tumours that involve the lower incisor teeth and associated alveolar bone (partial rostral mandibulectomy) or larger tumours that involve one hemimandible (unilateral rostral mandibulectomy) or which cross the mandibular symphysis and involve both hemimandibles (bilateral rostral mandibulectomy). In the case illustrated, a basal cell carcinoma is seen involving the rostral right hemimandible.

421

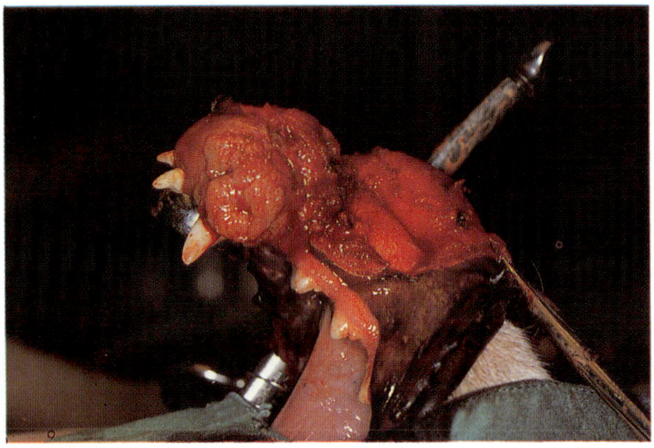

422

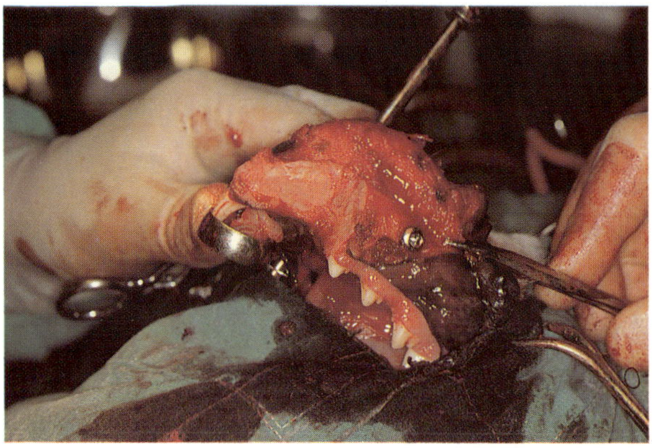

421 Exposure of symphysis — Case 1b. With the patient positioned in dorsal recumbency, the lower lip is detached from the gingival mucosa and reflected ventrally, exposing the mandibular symphysis. Stabilisation of the two hemimandibles, if required, should be performed at this stage by means of a single cortical screw or Kirschner wires.

422 Amputation of rostral segment — Case 1c. The rostral hemimandible is now amputated and the vessels within the mandibular canal carefully ligated or coagulated by diathermy. The symphysis is then split to allow removal of the tumour fragment. Where there is any possibility of the tumour extending across the symphysis, additional resection of incisor alveolar bone is performed. Where the tumour invades both sides of the symphysis, bilateral amputation is performed.

23

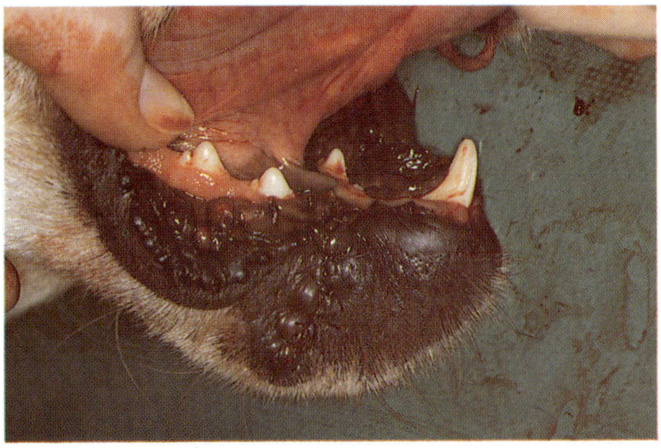

424

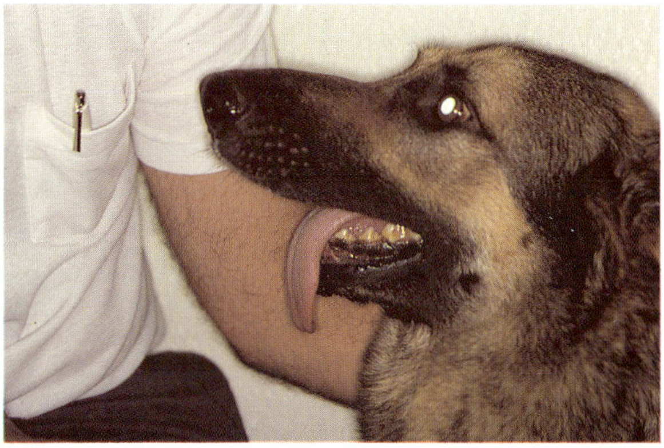

423 Immediate postoperative appearance — Case 1d. The lower lip is replaced over the amputation site and anchored directly to the gingival mucosa with simple interrupted absorbable sutures. Excess labial tissue may be excised in order to achieve a cosmetic result and avoid a drooping lip.

424 Long-term appearance. Bilateral rostral mandibulectomy performed at mid-molar level. Although the tongue may appear periodically unsupported the functional results of this and other types of rostral mandibulectomy procedures are excellent. The prehensile function between the tongue and premaxilla remains unimpaired.

425
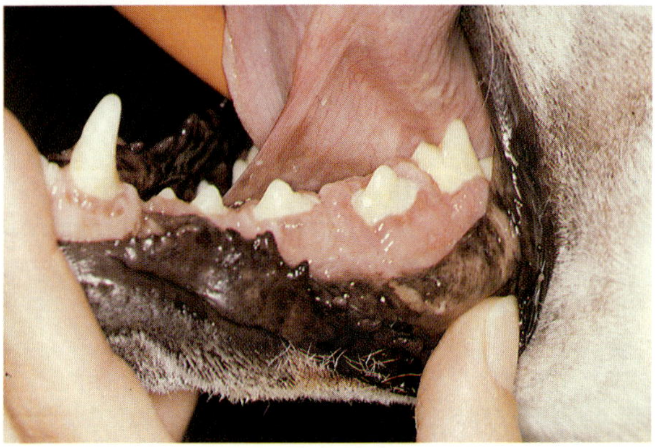

425 Hemimandibulectomy (horizontal) — Case 2a. Localised tumours involving the body of the mandible, such as this well-differentiated squamous cell carcinoma, may be amenable to management by a resection limited solely to the body of the mandible.

426
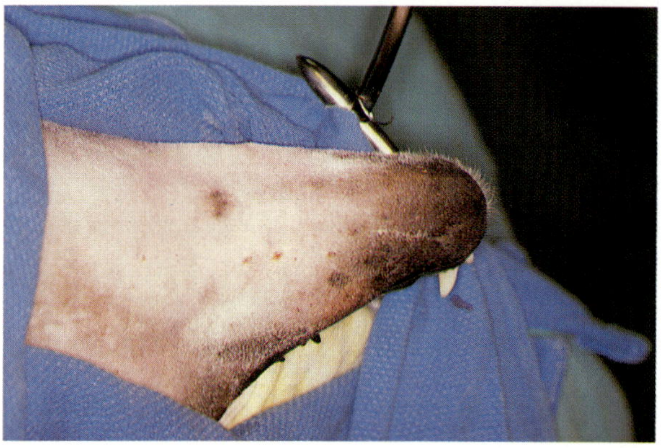

426 Extra-oral approach — Case 2b. This resection may be performed either via the oral cavity or, as in this case, via a ventral approach.

427
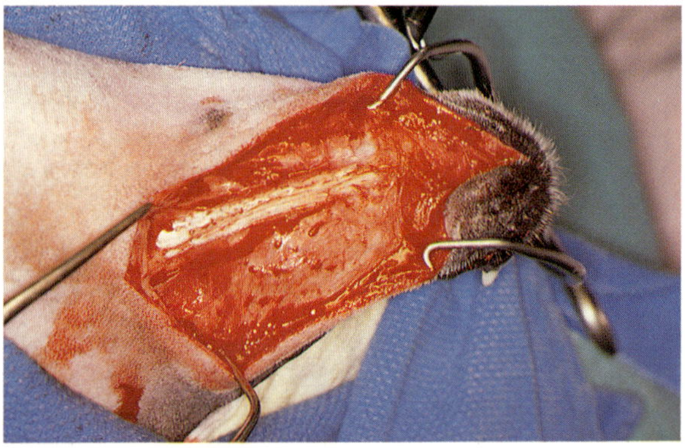

427 Exposure of the mandible — Case 2c. The body of the mandible is exposed by reflection of the lingual muscle attachments medially and the gingival mucosa laterally.

428
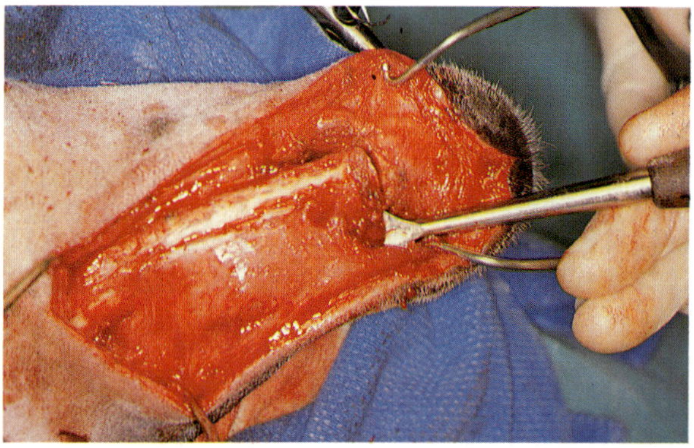

428 Rostral amputation — Case 2d. The hemimandible is freed rostrally either by splitting the mandibular symphysis or by amputation of the body distal to the canine tooth. Bleeding from the exposed mandibular vessel is controlled and the hemimandible dislocated laterally once the resection of the gingival attachments is complete. Care should be taken to salvage the sublingual salivary ducts in the base of the tongue without damage.

429

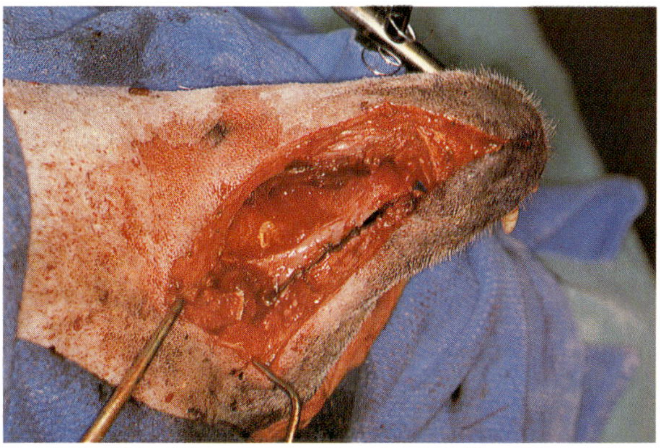

429 Caudal amputation — Case 2e. Once dislocated, the caudal aspect of the hemimandible is amputated at the level of the masseteric fossa. The mandibular artery is ligated and the tumour fragment removed.

430

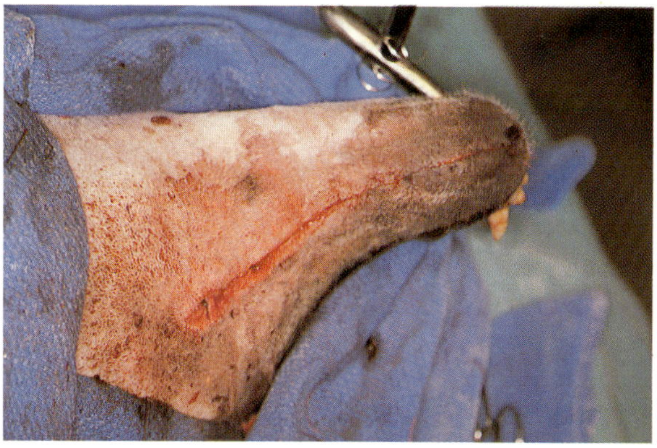

430 Primary closure — Case 2f. The oral mucosa is repaired in the ventral aspect of the wound and any minor defects can be corrected later via the oral cavity (see **426**). The remaining soft tissues (primarily lingual muscle) are then carefully closed with absorbable sutures to minimise the risk of seroma development, which may impair oral function in the postoperative period.

431

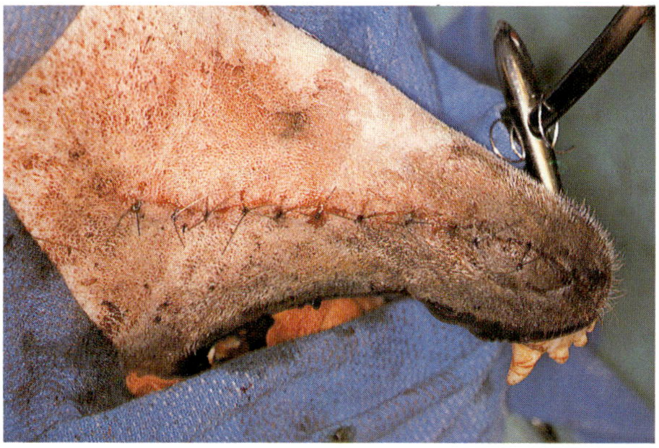

431 The skin wound is closed routinely — Case 2g.

432

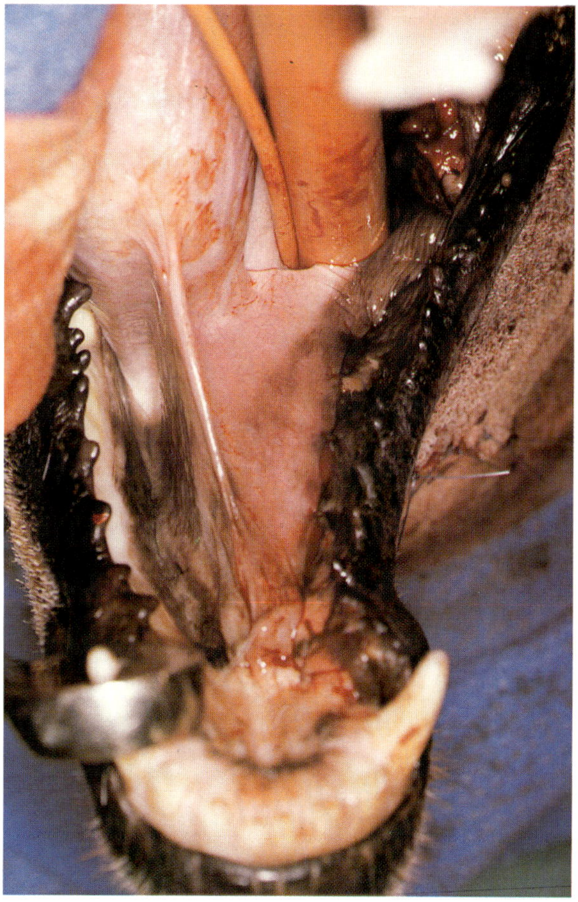

432 Intra-oral closure — Case 2h. The oral result is inspected. Any minor defects in the mucosal wound are closed and the sublingual salivary duct carefully inspected to ensure that it has not become entrapped in the mucosal repair.

433

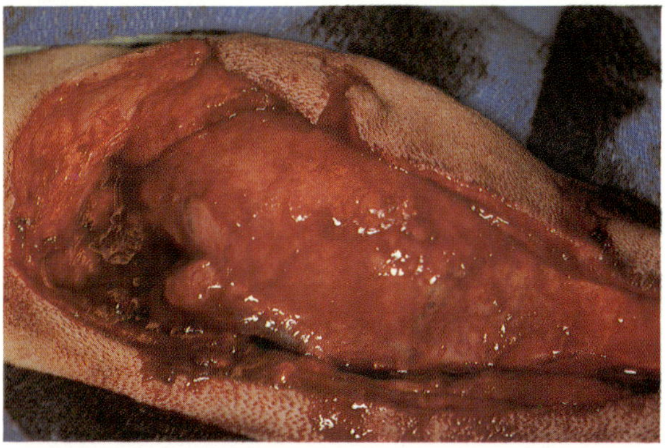

433 Ventral exposure of mandible — Case 3a. Extensive tumours involving the body of the mandible or the ramus may be managed by resection of the entire hemimandible. The hemimandible is approached ventrally, as for resection of the body, but the exposure is continued dorsally over the temporomandibular joint and zygoma as far as the temporal muscles.

434

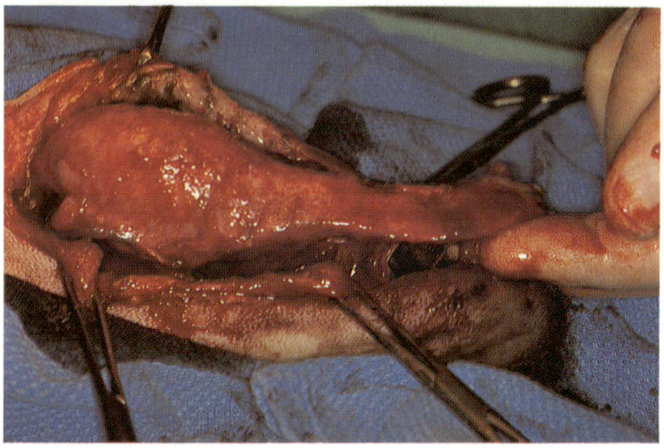

434 Symphysial split — Case 3b. The symphysis is split to allow lateral dislocation of the hemimandible once resection of the soft tissues is complete.

435

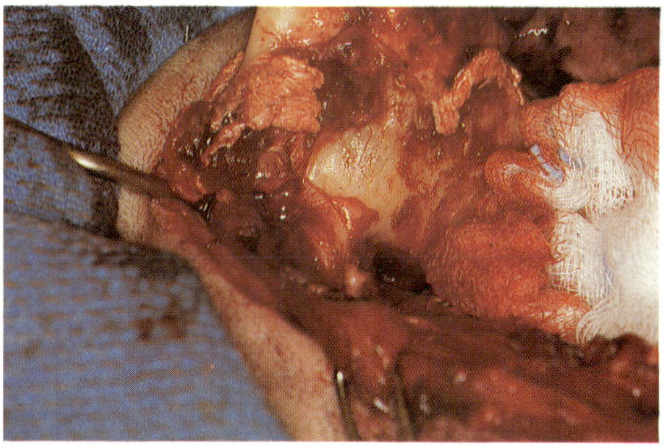

435 Freeing the ramus — Case 3c. The temporomandibular joint is disarticulated and the temporal muscle detached, freeing the ramus.

436 Excised hemimandible — Case 3d. The total hemimandible containing the tumour is removed.

436

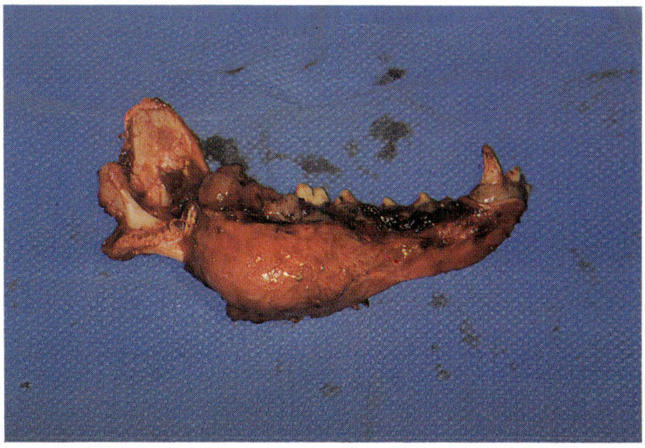

437 Skin closure — Case 3e. The oral wound is repaired before closure of the temporal dissection and the lingual muscles. The skin is closed routinely. The oral wound is inspected via the mouth and any additional repairs are completed.

437

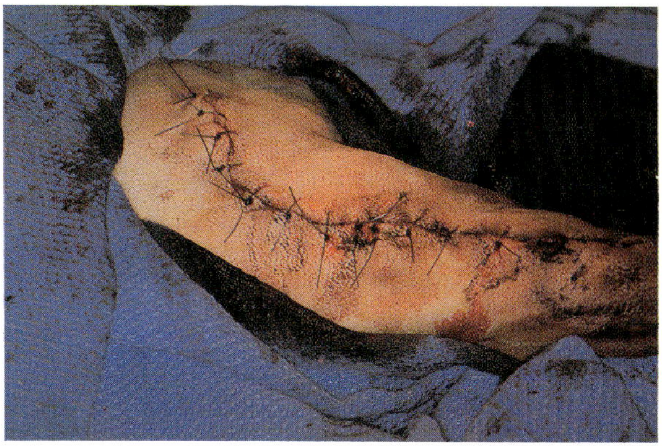

Partial maxillectomy (rostral)

438 Pre-operative appearance — Case 4a. This operation may be performed either unilaterally or bilaterally (premaxillectomy) for tumours such as this squamous cell carcinoma affecting the incisive and rostral palatine process of the maxilla.

438

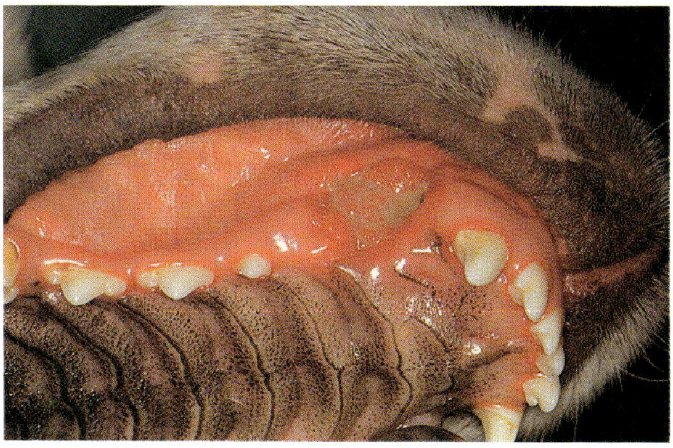

439

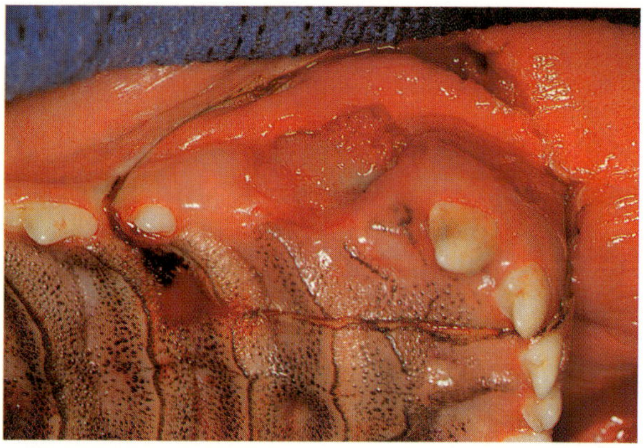

439 Extent of incision — Case 4b. The gingival mucosa and palatine mucoperiosteum are incised, allowing an appropriate margin of normal tissue surrounding the tumour.

440

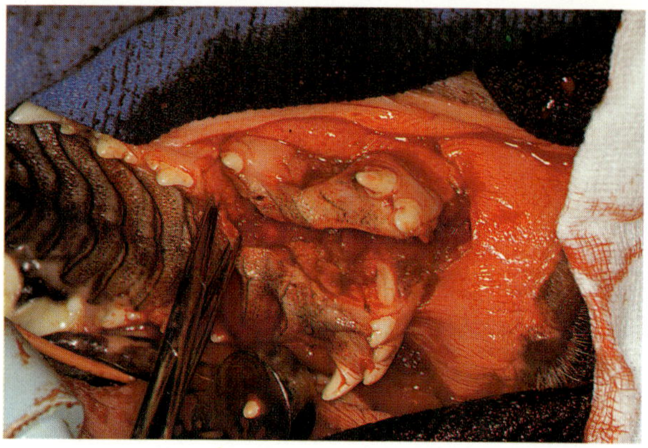

440 Dissection of amputated segment — Case 4c. The incisive bone is amputated on its oral and lateral aspect using an oscillating saw or osteotome. The rostral major palatine artery (arteries in the case of premaxillectomy) is ligated or coagulated carefully. The tumour fragment is freed from its soft-tissue attachments and removed.

441

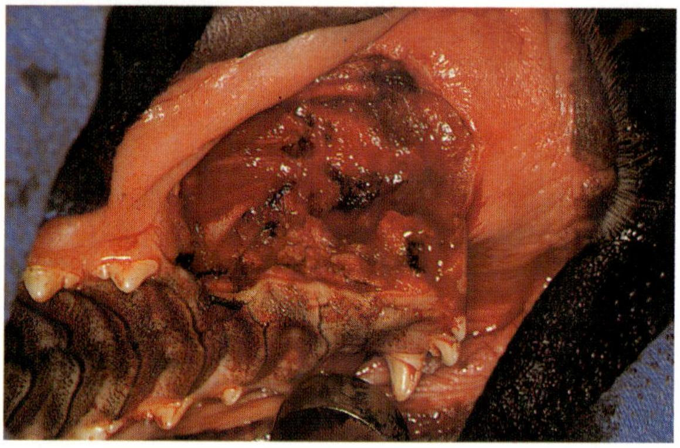

441 Appearance of defect — Case 4d.

442

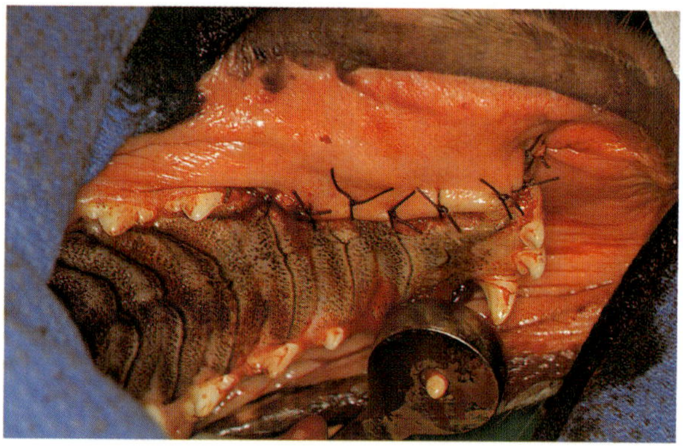

442 Closure of gingiva — Case 4e. The maxillary defect is closed by means of a pedicle flap created from the labial mucosa and underlying muscle. The flap is anchored to the palatine mucoperiosteum with simple interrupted absorbable sutures.

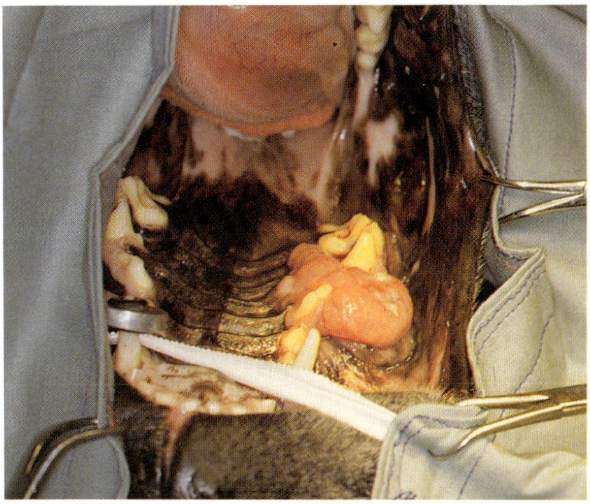

443

443 Pre-operative appearance — Case 5a. This procedure may be used to remove tumours, such as this fibrosarcoma, from the palatine process and molar region of the maxilla. Patient positioned in dorsal recumbency

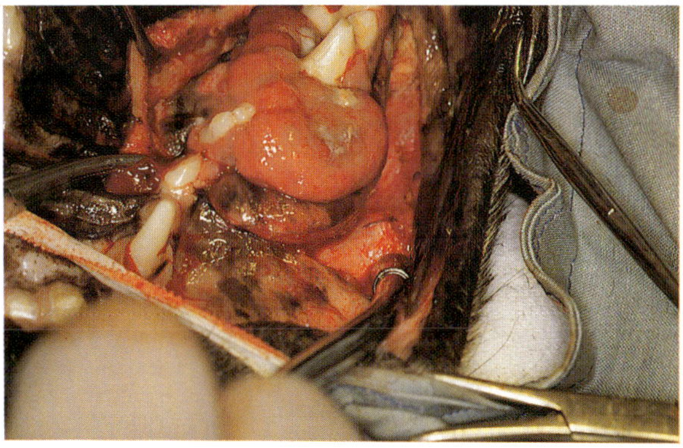

444

444 Extent of incision — Case 5b. The palatine mucoperiosteum and labial mucosa are incised with appropriate surrounding margins.

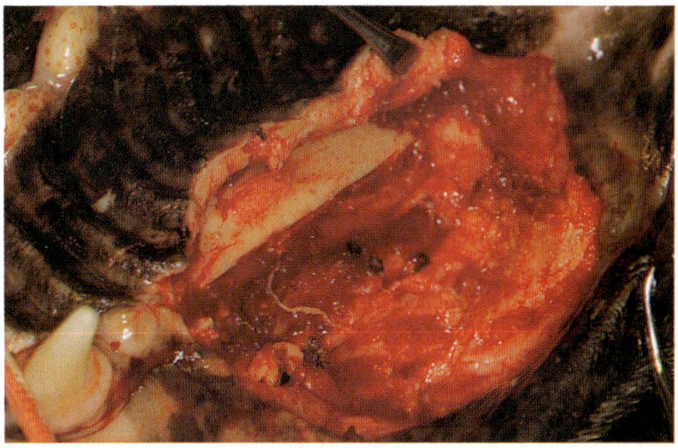

445

445 Defect before closure — Case 5c. The palatine process is resected, using an oscillating saw or osteotome following which the lateral aspect of the maxilla is resected rostrally and caudally. The tumour fragment is dislocated laterally, allowing the dorsal aspect of the maxilla to be resected and freed. The sphenopalatine artery within the nasal sinus is ligated and any additional turbinate haemorrhage controlled by temporary packing with gauze sponges. Diathermy should not be used to control turbinate bleeding since it may fragment the delicate cartilaginous structures, leading to further bleeding.

446

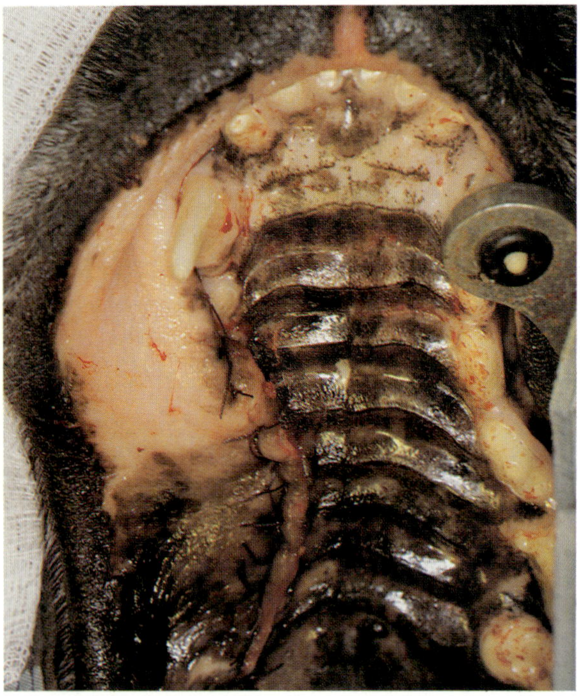

44

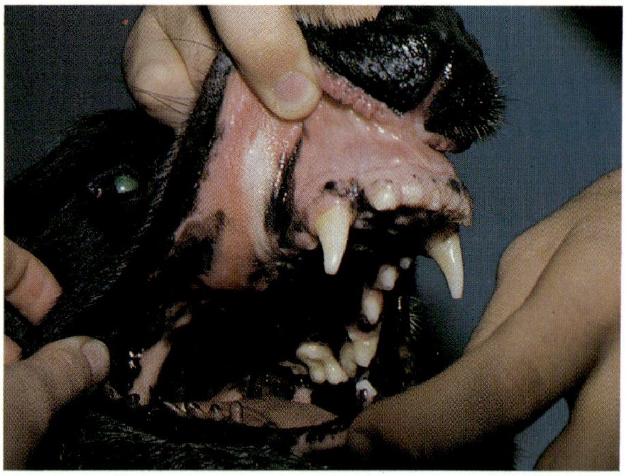

447 Postoperative appearance (one month after surgery) — Case 5e.

446 Closure of defect — Case 5d. The maxillary defect is closed by means of a labial pedicle flap, as for rostral maxillectomy. Dead space within the nasal sinus can be temporarily obliterated with absorbable gelatin sponges to allow improved anatomical restoration.

Partial maxillectomy (nasal)

448

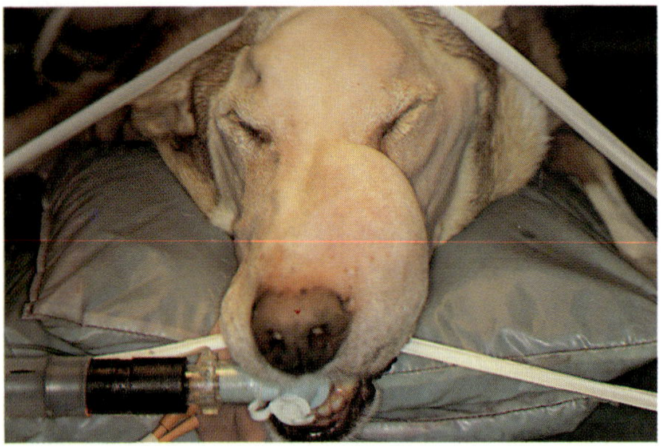

44

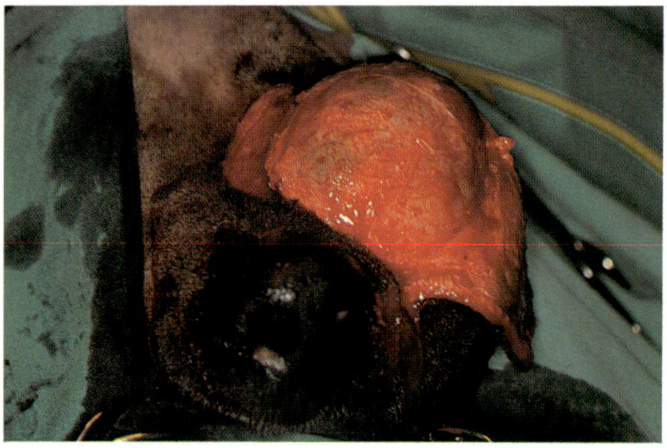

448 Pre-operative appearance — Case 6a. This approach is indicated in the removal of some nasomaxillary masses, such as this large neurofibroma that extends into the roof of the oral cavity.

449 Flap reflected — Case 6b. A dorsal approach is used, employing a facial 'fold-away' flap based on the infra-orbital artery. The tumour mass is removed by resection of the nasal bone in the dorsal midline, the maxilla laterally and the palatine process ventrally.

450 **Completed resection — Case 6c.** The palatine mucoperiosteum in the lower aspect of the wound is repaired to seal the roof of the oral cavity, gelatin sponges are used to limit the potential for haemorrhage within the nasal sinus and to allow accurate anatomical restoration of the overlying facial flap.

450

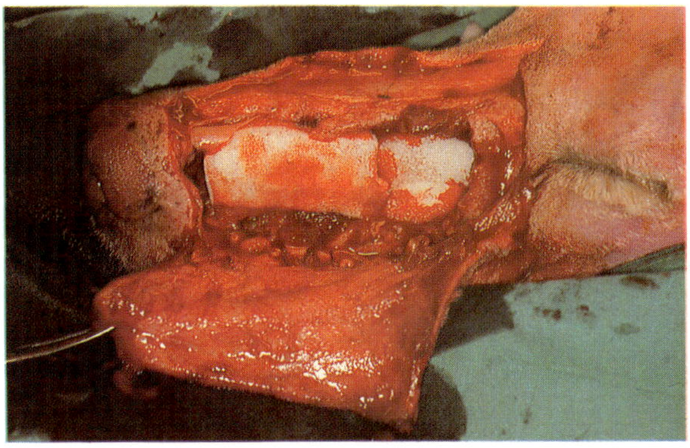

Postoperative care

Depending on the type of surgical procedure, most patients will begin to eat normally again within 24 hours of surgery. For those in which feeding is delayed, adequate provision for non-oral alimentation should be made, including, if necessary, tube gastrostomy feeding.

Seromas and, occasionally, the development of sublingual mucoceles may initially contribute to poor oral function. The latter normally resolve within 4–5 days and may require drainage although they should not warrant sialoadenectomy.

Radiation therapy

Radiotherapy is indicated in the management of oral tumours:

- As an alternative management for some *carcinomas* that are not amenable to surgical excision.
- As part of a *combined modality* approach to *sarcomas*.
- As a means of *palliating* discomfort or dysphagia and improving the patient's quality of life where outright cure is not attainable.

Teletherapy rather than brachytherapy irradiation techniques are more suited to the treatment of oral malignancy. Superficial lesions can be satisfactorily irradiated using orthovoltage X-rays although bone-involved masses are better managed by means of megavoltage sources.

Chemotherapy

Few oral tumours respond to chemotherapeutic management, although lymphomas — which are occasionally found involving the tonsils — are best treated by a medical approach.

451

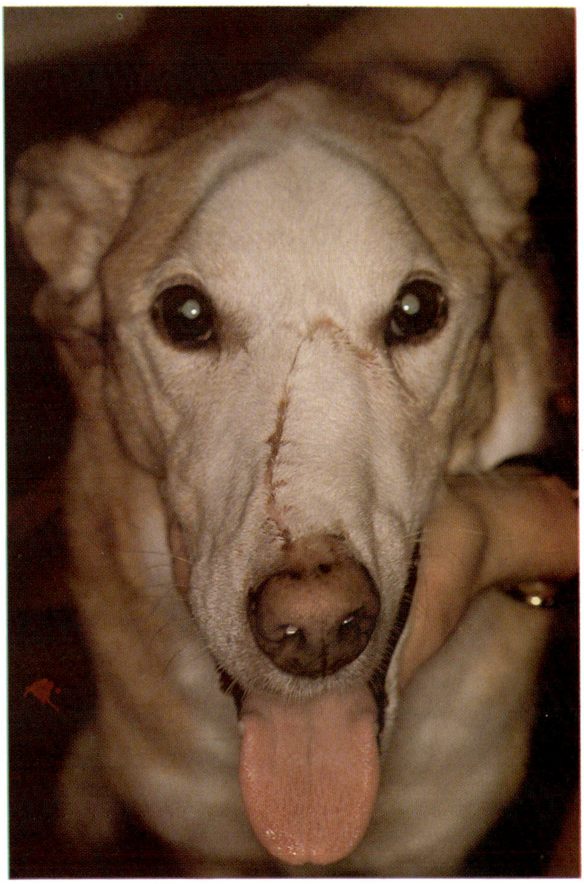

451 **Postoperative appearance — Case 6d.** The long-term (9 months) postoperative appearance of the procedure.

452 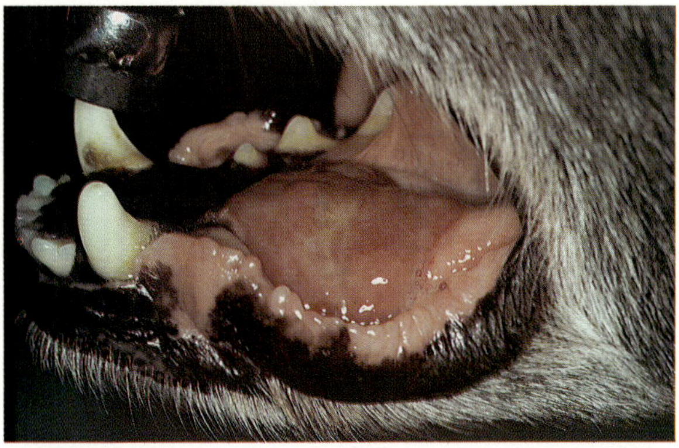

452 Pre-treatment — Case 7a. Poorly differentiated fibrosarcoma of the mandibular body.

453 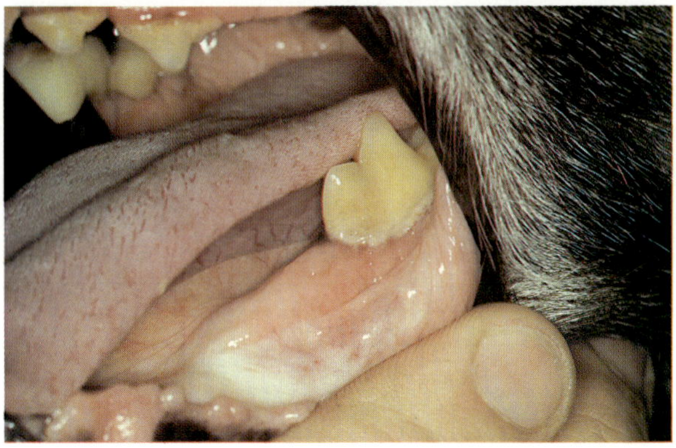

453 Post-treatment — Case 7b. Appearance of fibrosarcoma three months after irradiation with 4400 cGy (300 keV) X-rays.

13 Equine Dental Surgery

Introduction

In Western society, the role of the horse has changed over the last 100 years from being the principal mode of transport and being used in agriculture to its present day role, which is primarily for leisure. Horses are of considerable economic value as performance animals — in horseracing, eventing, show jumping, etc. — and, subsequently, for breeding.

In the wild, periodontal disease is a common cause of demise in horses, and the maintenance of dental health is a major consideration for domestic equids.

Approximately 10% of the veterinary surgeon's professional involvement in the routine care of horses is for the prevention or treatment of dental disorders. Good husbandry of horses demands that they be regularly examined for uneven occlusal tables and that preventative dentistry be instituted to control enamel pointing of the molar and premolar teeth and the correction of any malocclusions of the cheek teeth. Dental considerations also apply when the veterinary surgeon is involved in the accurate differential diagnosis and treatment of facial, antral and nasal disorders.

During pre-purchase examinations, an estimate of the animal's age and an assessment of its dental health are important.

The extraction of diseased teeth in the horse can be a traumatic procedure for the animal and can carry significant postoperative repercussions.

For the purpose of this chapter the molar and premolar teeth are grouped together as the 'cheek teeth', and numbered 1–6; in each arcade, cheek teeth (CT) numbers 1, 2 and 3 are premolars and 4, 5 and 6 are molars. The vestigial maxillary first premolar, the wolf tooth, is not included in this convention. In equine surgery *arcade* is a collective term for all the cheek teeth and their associated periodontal tissues in any one quadrant of the mouth.

Dental anatomy and the infundibulum

The dentition of the horse is classified in the *heterodont* group of animals. The teeth are *anelodont* and fall into the *hypsodont* subdivision. A detailed explanation of these terms, and their significance is presented in Chapter 4.

The infundibulum

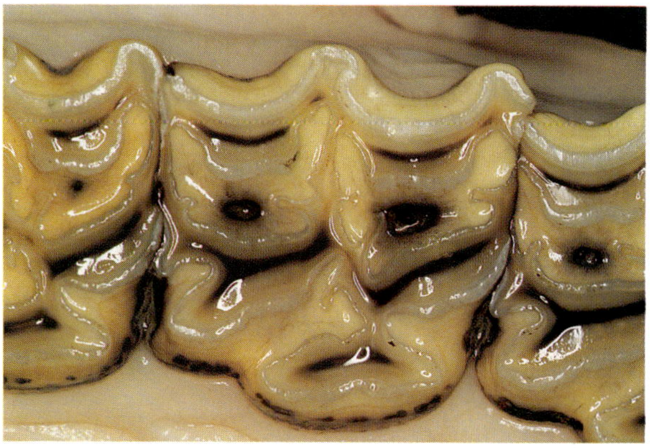

454

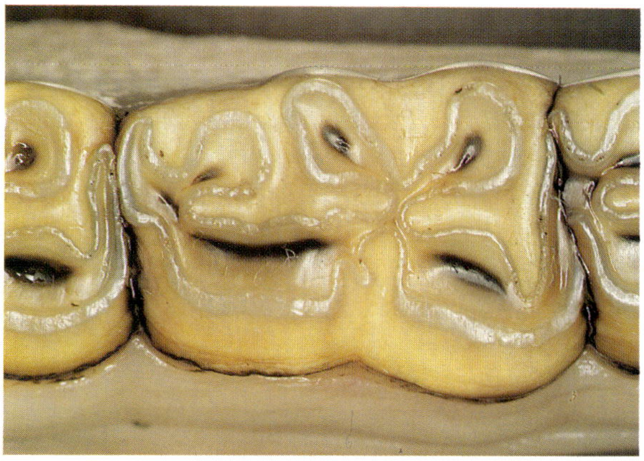

455

454, 455 Occlusal anatomy of the cheek teeth. In the horse, enamel ridging of the cheek teeth is partly achieved by longitudinal infolding of the enamel and cementum, which in the upper arcades is increased further by the formation of an infundibulum where a pocket of enamel and cement is inverted from the coronal surface (**454**). The evolutionary reasoning for infundibula in the upper cheek teeth only is not clear, but the overall effect is that the mandibular cheek teeth are smaller than their maxillary counterparts and the creation of a series of interdigitating enamel ridges in the longitudinal axis of the arcades makes for an efficient grinding mechanism. The incisor teeth of both jaws have infundibula; however, the function of the infundibulum is less obvious in these prehensile teeth. From the veterinary standpoint, the infundibula of the incisors provide a valuable aid in the ageing of horses.

Diagnostic techniques

Signs of dental disease

456 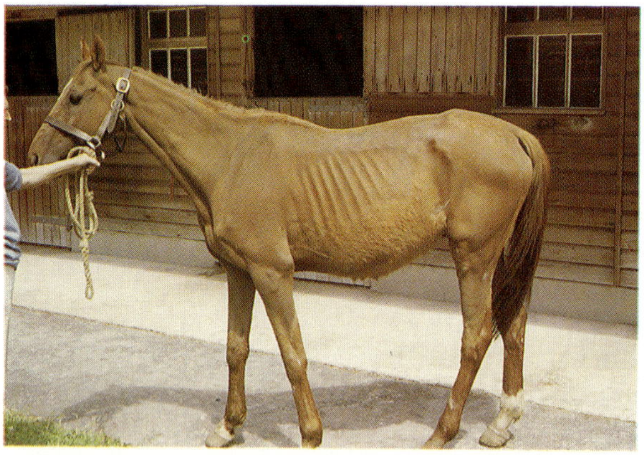

456 Poor bodily condition. Cachexia can be indicative of chronic dental disease. The products of quidding — the dropping of clumps of semimasticated food — are often seen outside the boxes of animals that are suffering with oral discomfort. The condition is frequently caused by enamel pointing of the cheek teeth provoking buccal and/or lingual ulcerations.

457 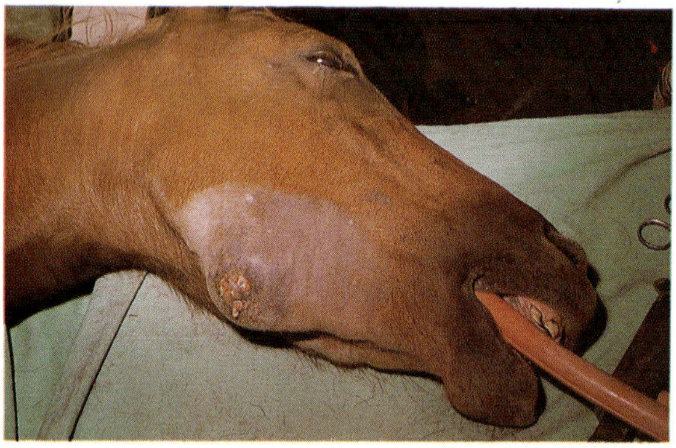

457 Mandibular abscess. Dental periapical infection must be considered in the differential diagnosis when a jaw swelling is presented with or without a discharging sinus tract. This is usually at the ventral border of the body of the mandible. Comparable abscesses of CT 1–3 in the maxilla produce swellings rostral to the facial crest.

458 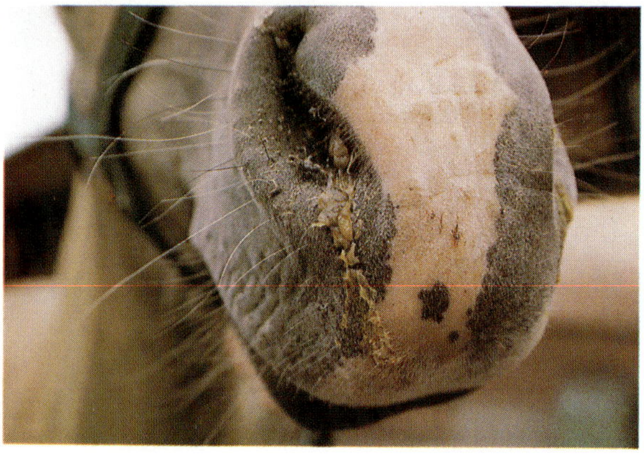

458 Fetid unilateral nasal discharge. This may be caused by a dental disease that involves any of the maxillary CT 3–6 but can equally be a sign of primary empyema of the paranasal sinuses and nasal chambers.

Clinical examination

Evaluation begins with an external examination of the face and jaws, but examination of the mouth of the conscious animal using tongue restraint or a gag has limited value. The use of Haussmann gags on conscious horses is controversial because of the potential danger to attending personnel. Detailed examination of the dental crowns, gingivae and interproximal areas can only be performed under general anaesthesia and is greatly enhanced by endoscopy. An endoscopic examination of the nasal meati can also be helpful in the differential diagnosis of nasal discharge.

Other signs of oral discomfort include:

- Dorsal displacement of the soft palate. A tendency to breathe through the mouth at exercise may result from dental discomfort, which in turn can cause 'choking up' during exertion.
- Abnormal bit behaviour.
- Shaking of the head.

Radiography

The excellent contrast which exists between dental tissues, the background of air, connective tissue, cartilage and cancellous bone renders radiography a highly rewarding diagnostic medium. The technique can provide useful information on erupting crowns, the spacing between teeth, alveoli, roots and associated paranasal sinuses, where applicable.

Useful projections

459

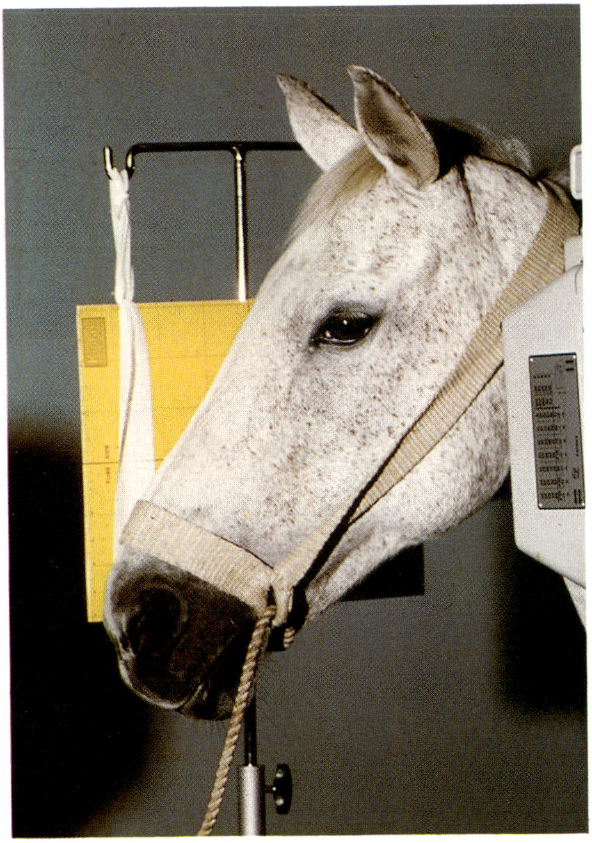

459 Erect lateral. This is the preferred means of identifying free fluid within the paranasal sinuses; radiodensities within these air spaces can also give an indication of whether periapical dental disease is involved.

460

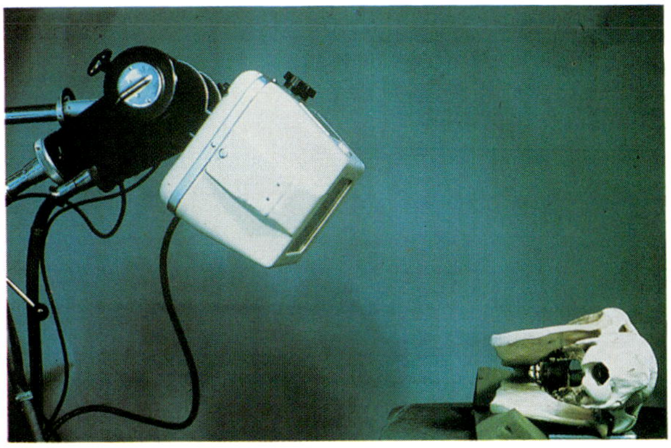

460 Lateral oblique — position of the skull in relation to the X-ray tube. With modern sedatives and due attention to radiation safety measures, this projection can be taken in the standing horse; however, it is recognised that the best results are obtained with the patient anaesthetised.

461

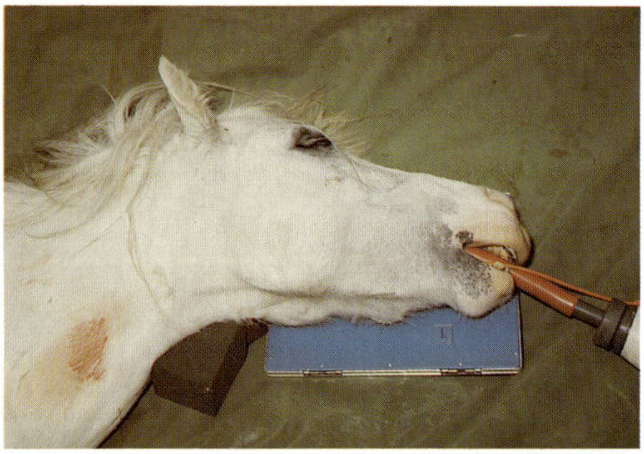

461 Lateral oblique view of a mandible. This photograph demonstrates the projection that is obtained from the X-ray tube in radiography of the mandible, so that the ventral border of the jaw and roots nearest to the tube are skylined away from the other arcade.

462

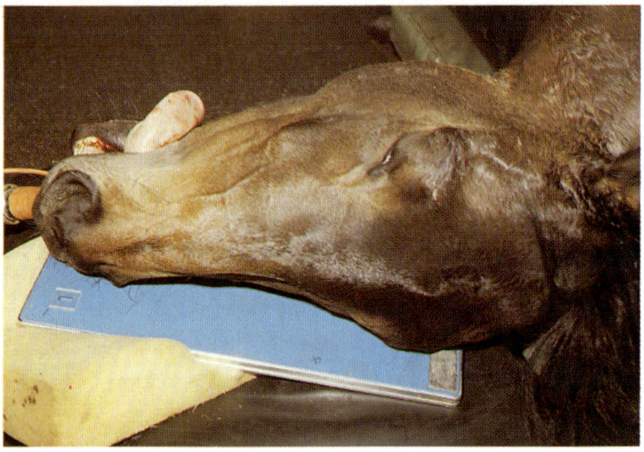

462 Lateral oblique projection of a maxilla. X-ray tube's 'eye view' of a maxilla.

463

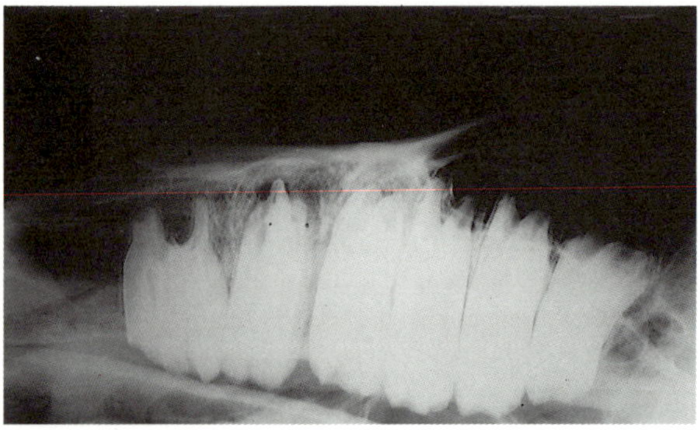

463 Lateral oblique radiograph. This radiograph of a maxilla demonstrates a periapical radiolucent area at CT 2 connected with dental disease. There is also abnormal spacing between CT 2 and 3.

464 Intra-oral occlusal — position of the patient. This view is particularly useful for incisor teeth.

465 Intra-oral occlusal radiograph. Eight permanent lower incisors are visible in the radiograph, including two supernumerary teeth.

466 Ventrodorsal position of the patient. A whole skull projection can be helpful where the X-ray beam is parallel to the periodontium and can skyline lesions arising from this structure, particularly in the maxilla. Intranasal complications may also be seen. The endotracheal tube is removed during exposure in this view.

467 Ventrodorsal radiograph. This radiograph demonstrates a periapical granuloma at CT 2 that has extended into the nasal cavity.

464

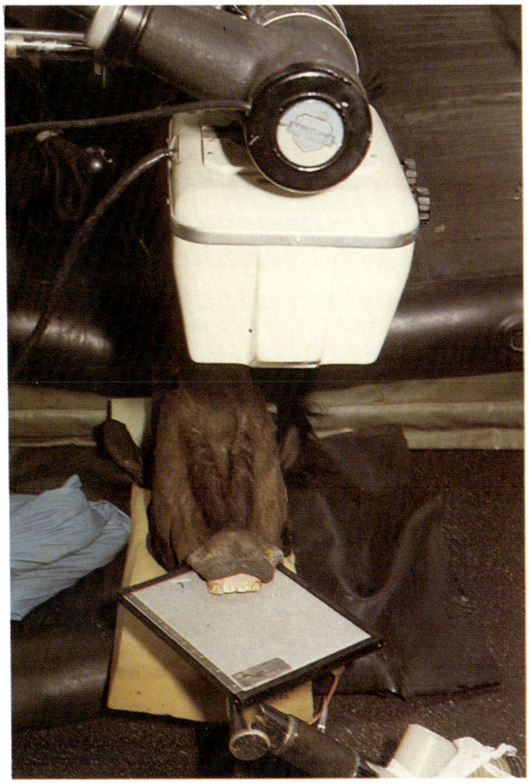

465

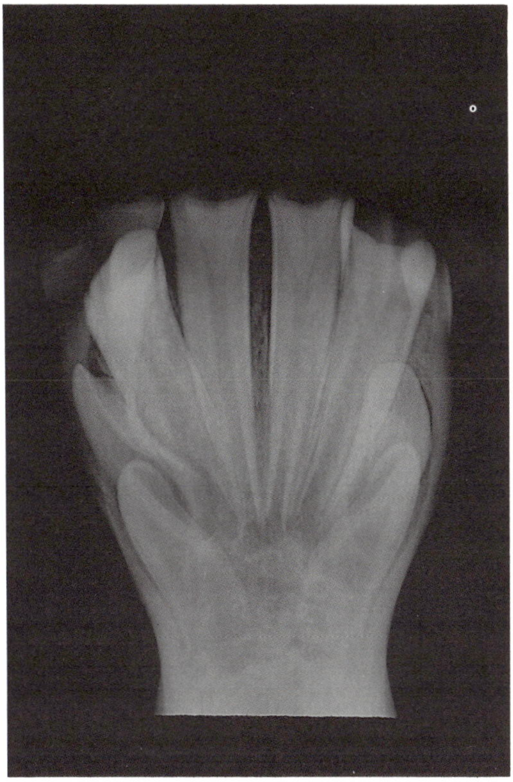

466

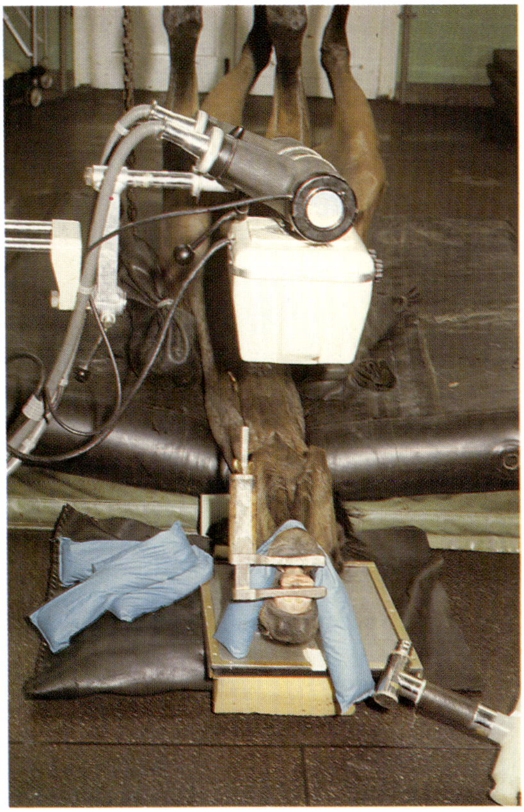

467

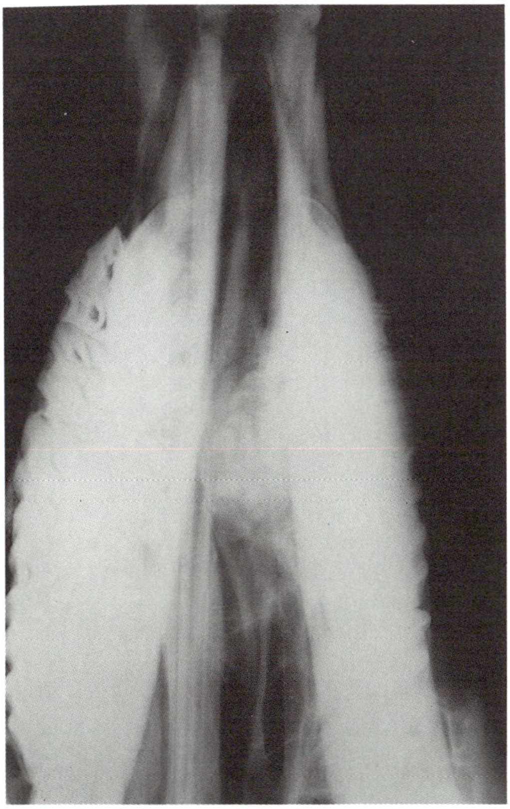

Signs of disease include sclerosis of the surrounding bone, endosteitis, divergence of the lamina dura and periapical 'halo' formation. Occasionally, dental suppuration will extend to produce metaplastic calcification of the conchal cartilages, so-called 'coral formation', as illustrated in the dorsoventral view shown in **473**. It is important to note that the dental sac of the immature tooth appears as a radiolucent area (**468, 470**) and this should not be confused with the rarefaction of periapical infection or a draining sinus tract arising at the apex of a lower cheek tooth (*see* **487**).

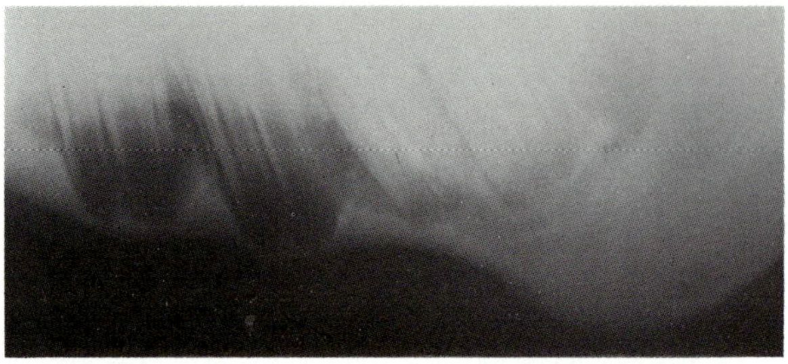

468 Radiograph of mandible. Close-up of dental sacs in the mandible.

469

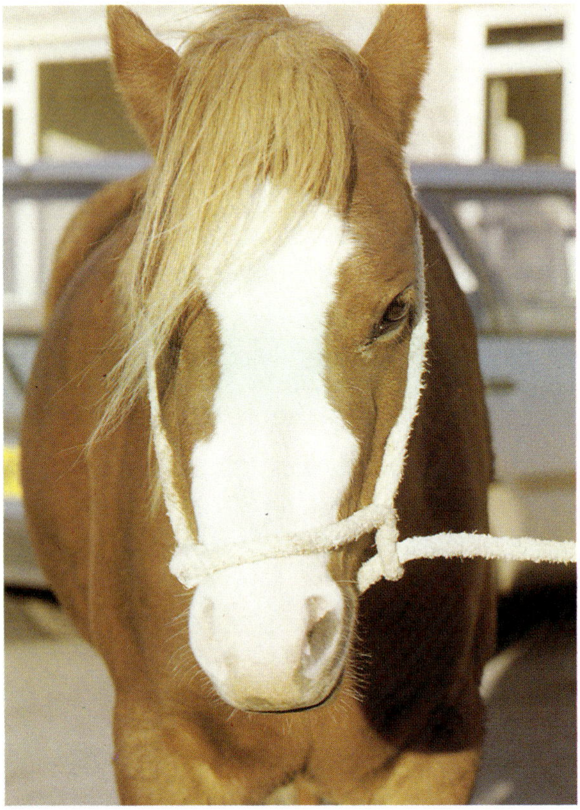

469 Frontal view of pony with swelling — Case 1a. Facial appearance associated with dental sacs in the upper jaw of a Welsh Mountain pony gives a 'boxed' facial conformation.

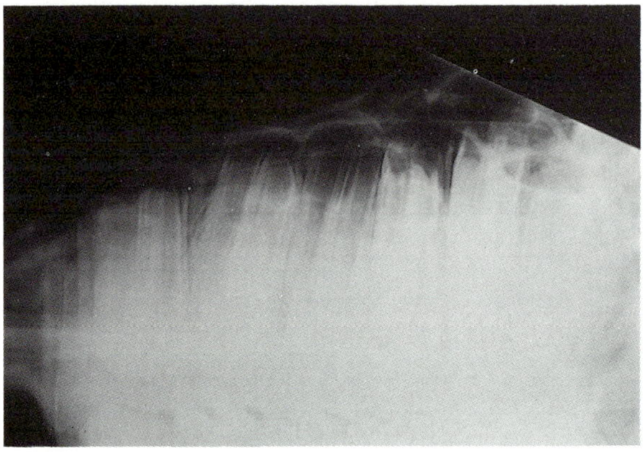

470 Radiograph of maxilla — Case 1b. Close-up of dental sacs in the maxilla associated with **469**.

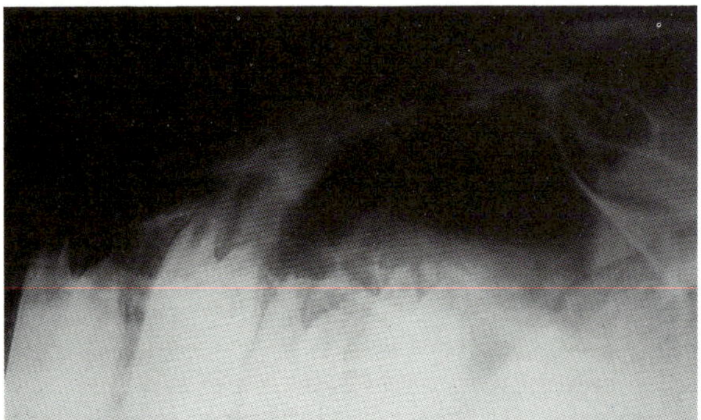

471 Radio-opacity in maxillary sinus. A radio-opaque area indicates endosteitis extending into the maxillary sinus, caused by an area of chronic periapical infection. This contrasts with the radiolucent appearance of the surrounding structures. An area of cementosis is also visible in the periapical tissues as a cement 'pearl' between the roots of CT 5.

472

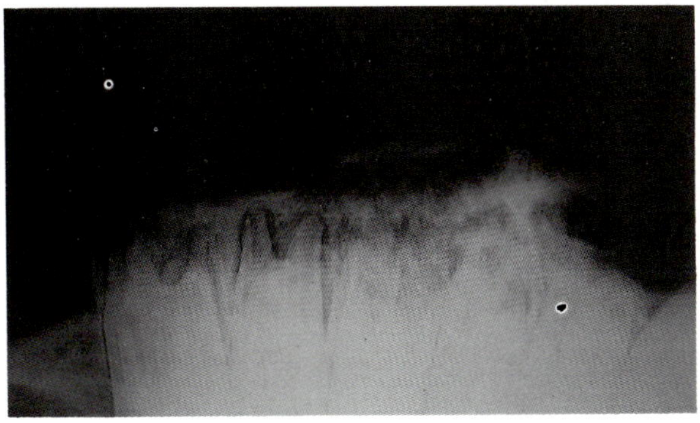

472 **'Coral formation' — Case 2a.** In this lateral oblique view, chronic periapical infection can be seen to have extended into the nasal chambers, producing metaplastic calcification of the conchal cartilages.

473

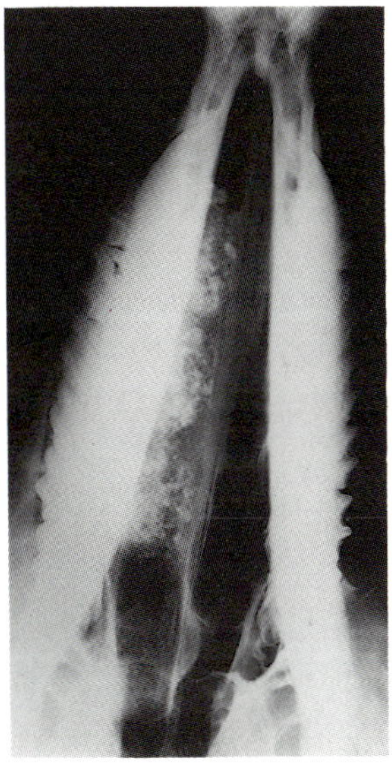

473 **Dorsoventral view of the case shown in 472 — Case 2b.** 'Coral formation' is evident in the conchi.

Dental disease

Developmental diseases

Developmental dental anomalies that occur in the horse include supernumerary teeth; odontomas, odontogenic cysts and tumours, including temporal teratomas; impactions; absent teeth; wolf tooth; retention of primary teeth; maleruption, malocclusion and malposition of teeth; and the developmental absence of infundibular cementum.

474

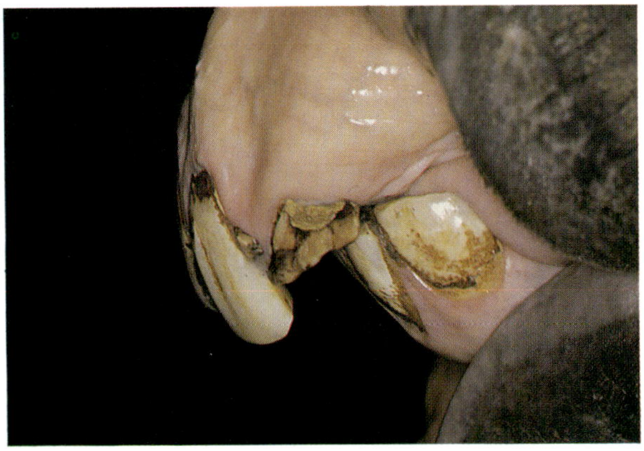

474 **Parrot mouth.** Skeletal abnormality demonstrating malocclusion of the incisor teeth. Some workers have attempted to correct these gross abnormalities. As the breeding of sound progeny is the major consideration of the bloodstock industry, serious ethical questions must be addressed as such treatments might encourage the perpetuation of the condition.

475

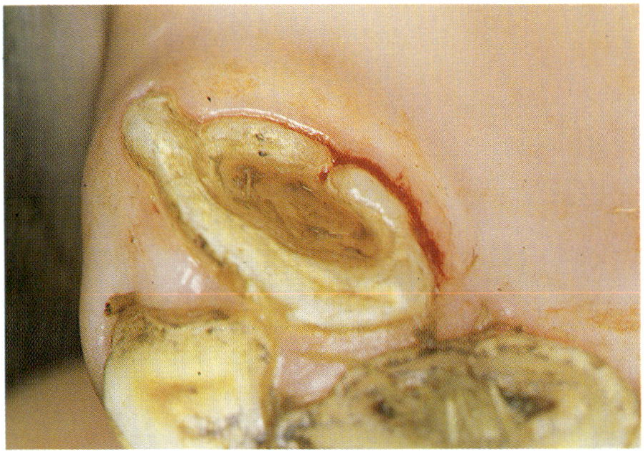

475 **Absence of infundibular cementum — lower third incisor.** Although the absence of cementum can lead to periapical lesions, especially in the cheek teeth, due to limited access these defects are not usually diagnosed before gross changes have occurred. In the incisor teeth, where the condition is more easily diagnosed and treated, prophylactic restoration of the empty infundibular space with modern dental materials can prevent caries and necrosis of the pulp tissue.

476 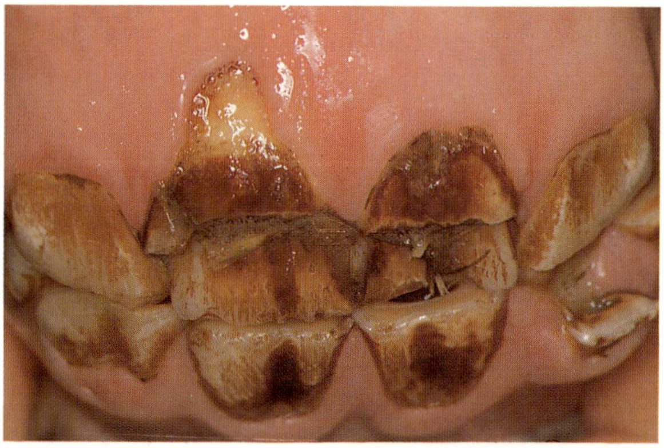

476 Fractured upper incisors. Trauma to the anterior teeth is not common in horses, but if it does occur the loose fragments should be removed and the remaining root surface carefully examined for pulpal exposure.

477 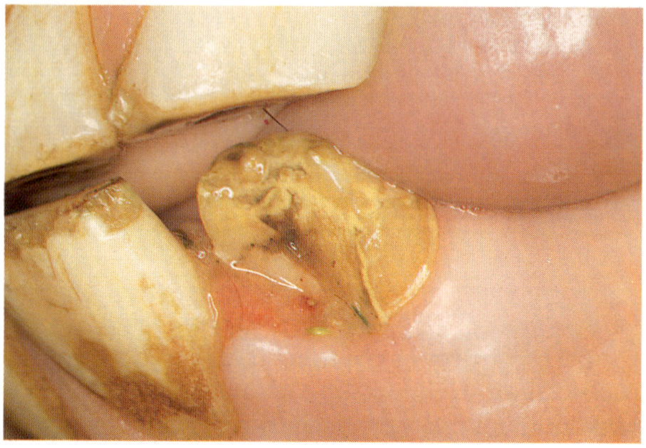

477 Pulpal exposure — lower incisor. In the event of pulp exposure endodontic treatment of the root canal, which can be 70 mm in length depending on the size and age of the animal, can provide a predictable treatment option. By maintaining periapical health, eventual tooth loss and the resultant occlusal discrepancy is prevented.

478 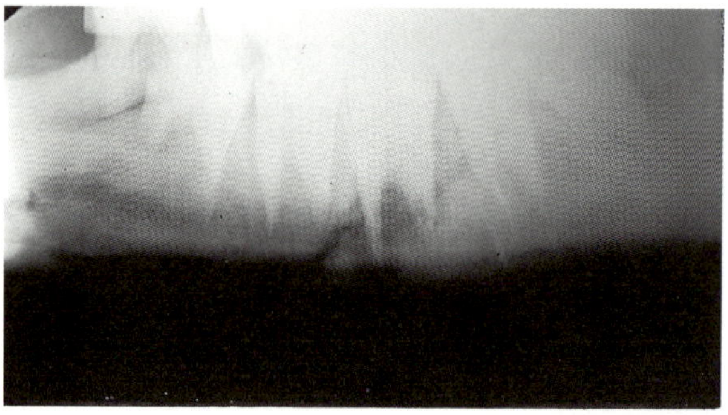

478 Fractured mandible. Fractured mandible must always be considered in the differential diagnosis of swellings associated with the lower jaw. In this case the CT 3 involved in the fracture line was extracted. This decision must be carefully assessed in the light of tooth mobility and displacement of the fragments as well as the age of the animal.

479

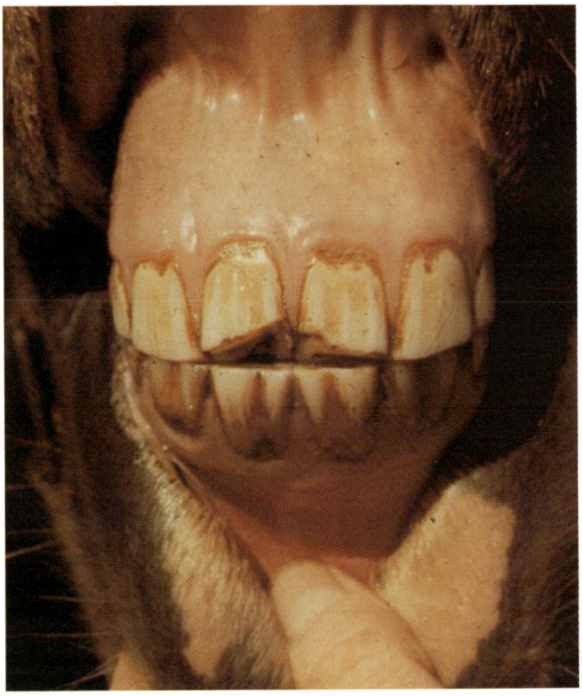

480

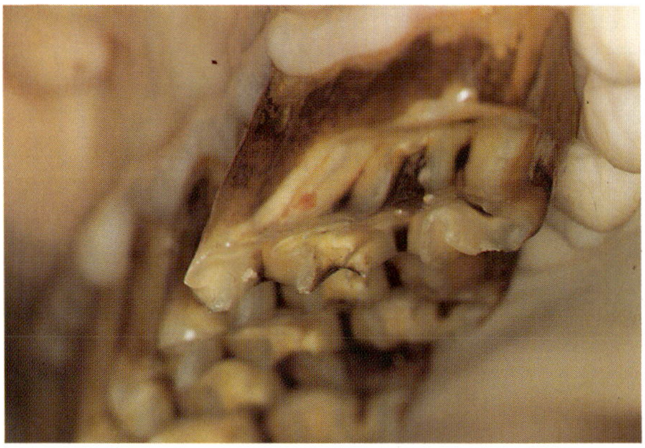

480 Enamel points on the buccal aspects of the maxillary arcade.

479 Abrasive wear — crib-biting. Abnormal tooth wear may manifest itself in attrition, enamel pointing or abrasion, as in crib-biting. Crib-biting is usually associated with aerophagia (wind-sucking), which can be detrimental to the health of a horse.

481

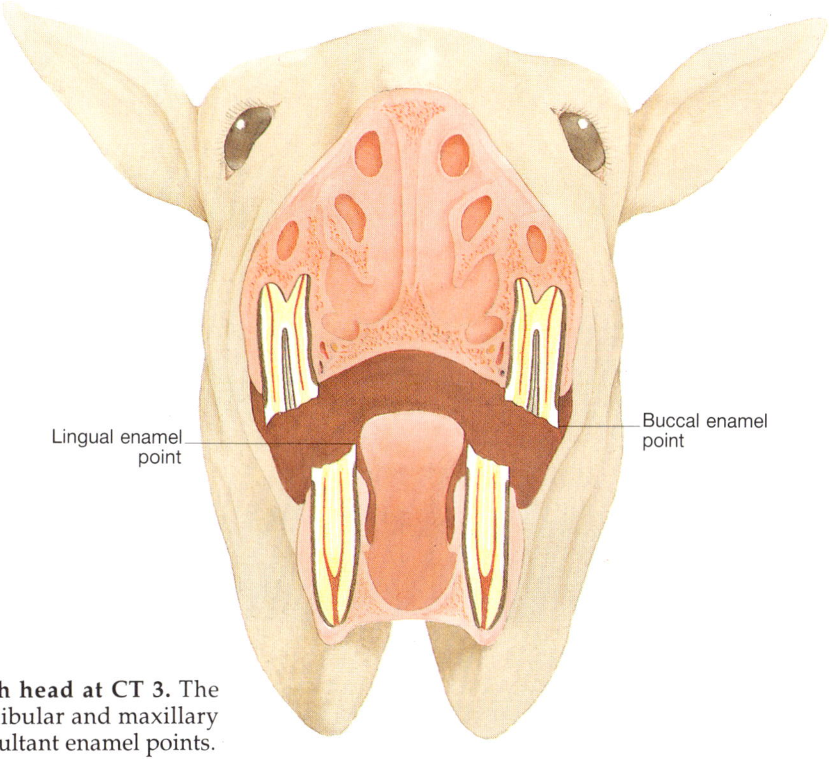

481 Transverse section through head at CT 3. The occlusal relationship of the mandibular and maxillary teeth is demonstrated with the resultant enamel points.

Periodontal disease

All horses are anisognathic. A skeletal discrepancy exists in that the width of the mandible is invariably less than that of the maxilla, at all levels of the cheek teeth. Even in 'normal' horses this amounts to 30%, but in some animals, generally described as 'shear-mouthed', the disparity is even greater. The overall effect is that natural attritional wear in horses results in the formation of sharp enamel projections on the buccal aspects of the maxillary cheek teeth and at the lingual aspect of the mandibular arcade. Normal preventive dentistry in the form of regular rasping (floating) of the cheek teeth aims to remove these sharp projections and should be performed at approximately six-monthly intervals in all horses once the full complement of permanent teeth is in wear. The role of rasping in younger horses is more questionable, but may contribute to the displacement of the primary cheek teeth, often referred to as 'dental caps', from the coronal aspect of the erupting permanent premolars, which might otherwise cause discomfort.

Neglected enamel pointing, especially in shear-mouthed animals, leads to painful ulceration of the buccal and lingual mucosae. Oral pain inhibits thorough mastication, leading to quidding and unthriftiness. The normal movement of ingesta in the mouth is inhibited and stale half-chewed food material tends to become impacted at the gum margins of the teeth. This pattern of events typifies the aetiopathogenesis of periodontitis in the horse.

482

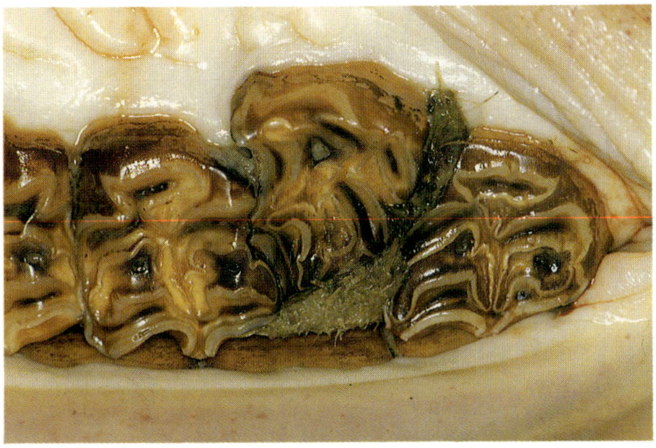

482 Occlusal view of a horse with periodontitis. Intra-oral picture demonstrates food packing between rotated molars that was responsible for periodontal disease and gross secondary sinus contamination.

Maleruptions and malalignment of the wearing surfaces can have similar consequences (see **482**). Periodontitis is a painful condition and is the most frequent cause of dysphagia involving the oral phase of deglutition in the horse. The condition is to some extent preventable by regular rasping, but once established can only be treated by extraction of the offending teeth. This solution is not often a practicable remedy.

Battery operated, mechanical equine floats are becoming commercially available and should ease the physical tedium of the rasping procedure and enhance the efficiency of this important preventative technique.

Degenerative dental diseases

48

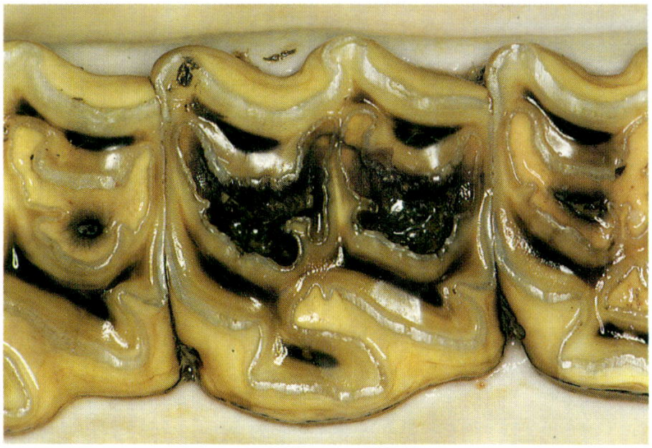

483 Infundibular necrosis. The cement in the infundibula has been lost and 'decay' of the cement lakes has taken place to the extent whereby these structures are almost joining up as a single lesion in the mesiodistal direction. Once such defects have been formed, they create a weakness through which longitudinal fractures of the teeth can easily occur.

Dental extractions

The most common teeth extracted are the vestigial first premolars — the wolf teeth. It is believed by many owners that they cause abnormal bitting behaviour. Although elevators are a great help in their removal, extreme care is required to prevent inadvertent damage to the palatal artery should the instrument slip and traumatise the soft tissues palatal to the dental arcade. This extraction is performed with the horse standing and possibly sedated. Infiltration of local anaesthetic can also be used if necessary.

The second most common teeth where extraction may be needed are the upper canines, which can cause bit resentment, especially when unerupted, partially erupted or positioned caudally in the interdental space. The canine is a significant tooth with a long root, and a general anaesthetic is required for its removal. Direct access is possible through a labial approach. With a planned procedure utilising a mucoperiosteal flap and buccal bone removal according to the basic principles of oral surgery (see Chapter 9), the extraction can be rendered a reliable technique.

Extraction techniques

484

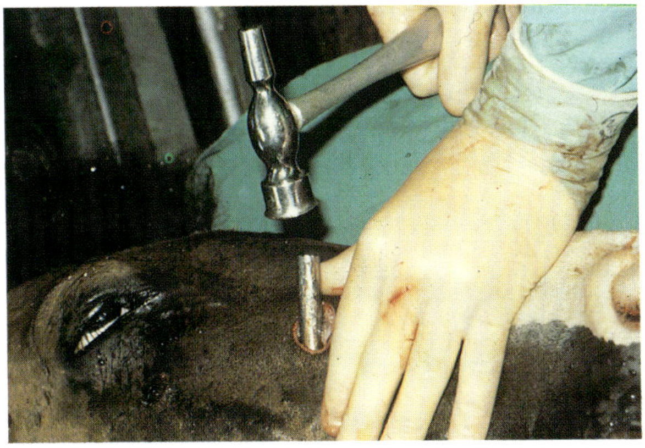

484 Repulsion of upper cheek tooth. The risks associated with extracting teeth through the trephine and repulsion technique are numerous. The procedure is most traumatic in the maxilla where it often involves penetration of the paranasal sinuses and prolonged and unpredictable aftercare of the resultant oro-antral fistula. Iatrogenic damage may be created to adjacent structures especially neighbouring teeth, the parotid duct, the palatine artery, the nasolacrimal duct, the infra-orbital nerve, the facial nerve and the linguofacial artery and vein. Other complications that may occur are:

- Incomplete removal of teeth.
- Retained roots.
- Alveolar infection/sequestration.
- In the lower jaw, fracture of the mandible.

485

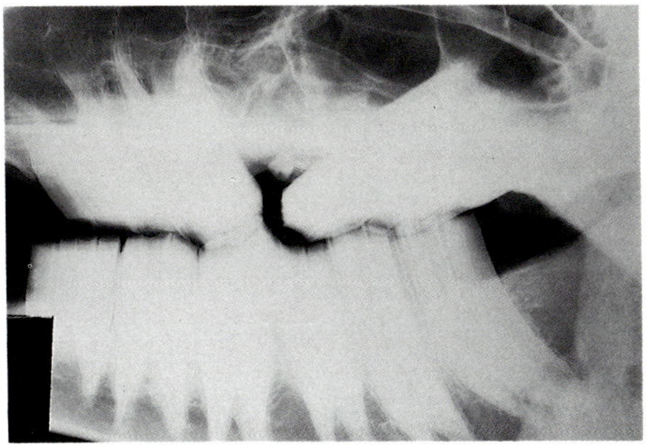

485 Collapsed dental arch. A significant disadvantage of the removal of a cheek tooth of a horse is that the tooth in the opposite jaw will continue to erupt into the space left by the extracted tooth, contributing to gross unevenness of the arcade and the wearing surfaces. At best this will require regular attention with rasping. Inevitably there will also be drifting of teeth in the arcade to close the gap left after extraction; this opens the interproximal spaces, leaving them vulnerable to food impaction and periodontitis. Thus, treating the involved teeth in situ to maintain the integrity of the dental arcade is worth considering. Active conservative treatment has proved effective in certain mandibular teeth. The authors are convinced that future trends in equine dental surgery will strive towards conservation of teeth in situ.

486

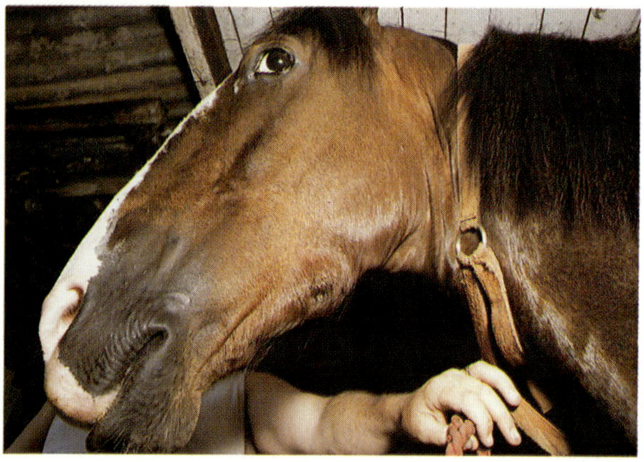

486 Mandibular sinus tract — Case 3a. In the differential diagnosis of a discharging mandibular sinus tract, pulpal necrosis, periodontal disease, fractured mandible or a fractured tooth must be taken into consideration. In this case the condition was through a periapical infection of CT 3, which is not uncommon in the permanent mandibular CT 1–3 of animals aged between two and five. The aetiology of the condition is still unclear. It is interesting to note that on examination of the affected teeth, necrosis of the pulp is not always seen. Simple curettage of the periapical space is contrary to the basic principles of dental surgery. Such an approach will devitalise any remaining pulp, and necrosis of that tissue will take place. Devitalised pulp tissue or a root canal containing necrotic material will inevitably perpetuate the suppuration (see Chapter 8, endodontic treatment section).

487

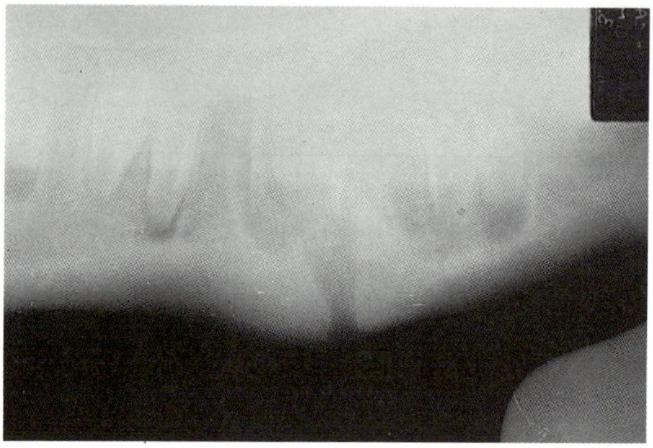

487 Radiograph of draining periapical suppuration — Case 3b. The radiograph of the lesion demonstrates destruction of the lamina dura and of the cortical bone apical to the tooth in question. Endodontic treatment of the affected tooth through a retrograde approach has in some cases proved successful in eliminating chronic infection and promoting resolution of the sinus tract. An orthograde oral approach is impossible as well as unnecessary as there is usually no direct oral communication into the pulp chamber. Treatment is achieved through the ventral border of the mandible. The structures to be avoided are the external maxillary vein/artery and the parotid duct, which cross the ventral border of the mandible at the rostral margin of the masseter.

488

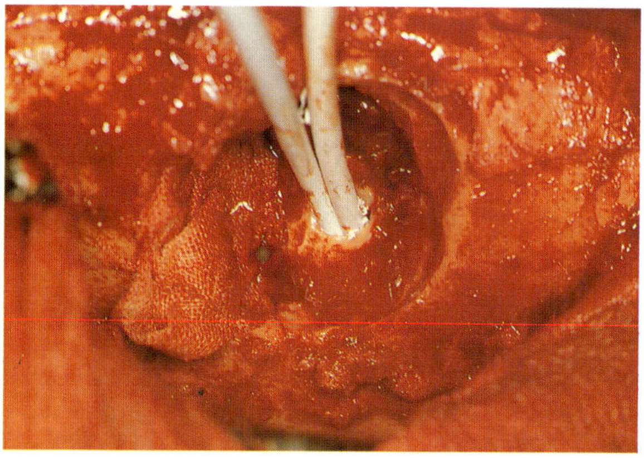

488 Exposure of apex — Case 3c. Skin and periosteum are reflected to expose the osseous defect. By following the sinus tract the apex of the correct tooth is relatively easy to find, but must be confirmed. Periapical granulation tissue needs to be curetted and the apices resected to the extent where the root canals and relatively thick canal walls are visible. Any vital or necrotic pulp must be removed, the canals debrided with sufficiently long endodontic instruments, then irrigated and dried. The canals are filled with a sealer and custom-rolled gutta percha points. The photograph illustrates the gutta percha points extruding from the resected distal root.

489 Retrograde amalgam — Case 3d. If condensation of the gutta percha is difficult because of the size of the root canals, retrograde amalgam fillings are also placed to assure an adequate seal. A completed distal canal and a still untreated mesial canal are shown.

489

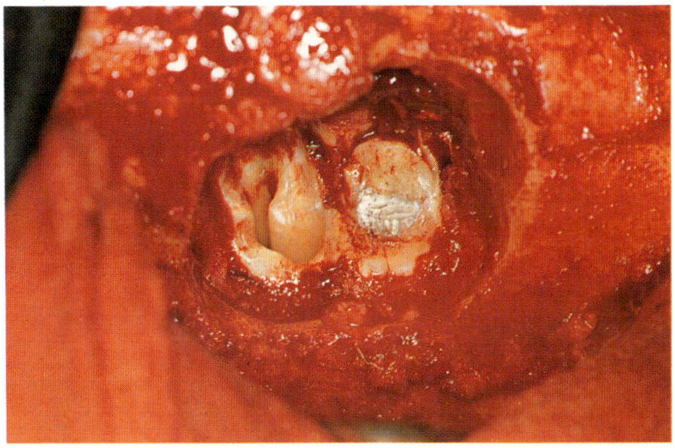

490 Retrograde amalgams — Case 3e. Two completed canals with retrograde amalgam fillings.

490

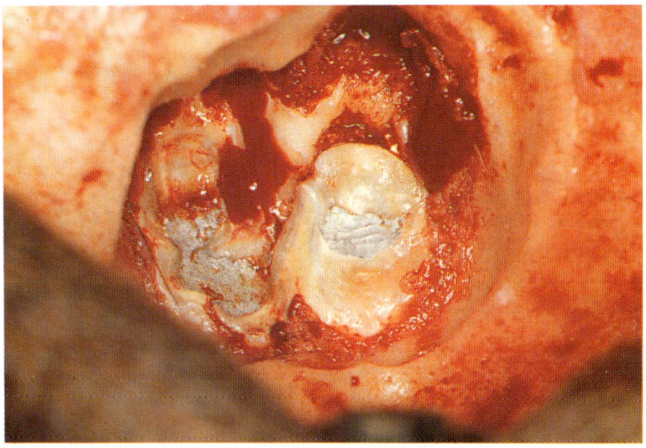

491 Postoperative radiograph — Case 3f. This radiograph taken four months after surgery demonstrates the retrograde amalgams, apical healing and resolution of the sinus tract.

491

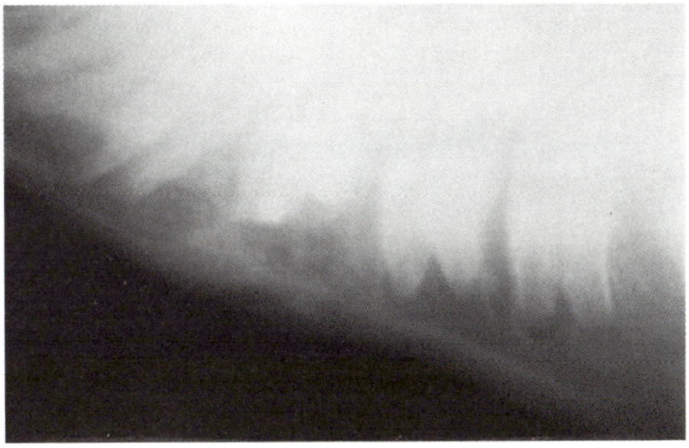

492

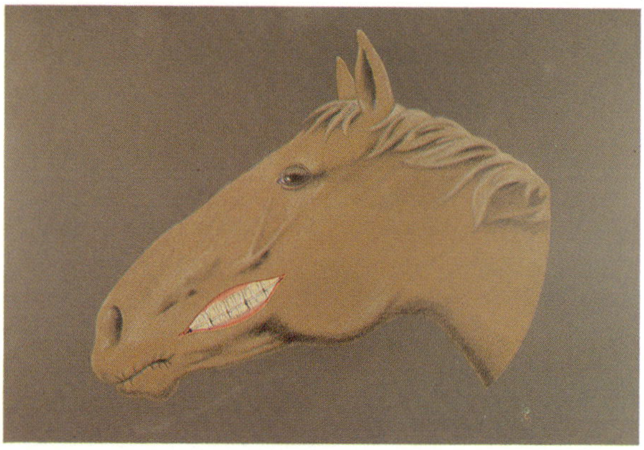

493

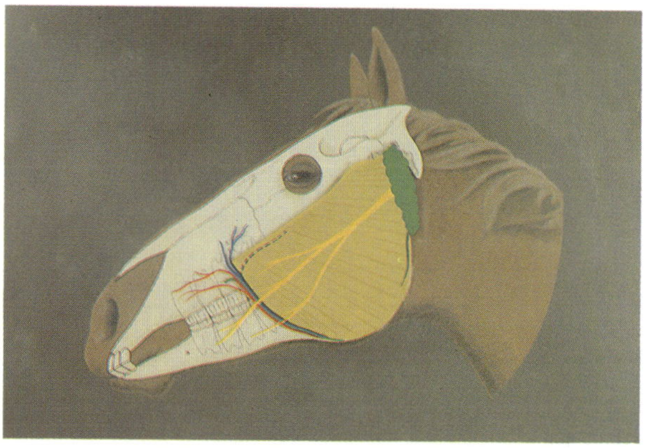

492 Diagrammatic illustration of a buccotomy. The lateral buccotomy approach to dental extractions is based on techniques used on other types of animals. It affords direct vision to remove the buccal alveolar bone before sectioning the tooth and delivery of the segments. The advantages of this approach are the safety of adjacent teeth and the simplicity of aftercare.

493 Regional anatomy. It is important that operators have an intimate knowledge of the surgical anatomy of the area as vital structures often obstruct a direct approach to the tooth that requires extraction. The technique becomes progressively more difficult the more caudal the tooth to be extracted and thorough familiarisation with the anatomical relationships and instrumentation is required before it is attempted. Structures to note include the branches of the facial nerve, the parotid duct, especially in the region of CT 2–4, the facial branches of the external maxillary artery and vein and the buccal venous plexus.

494

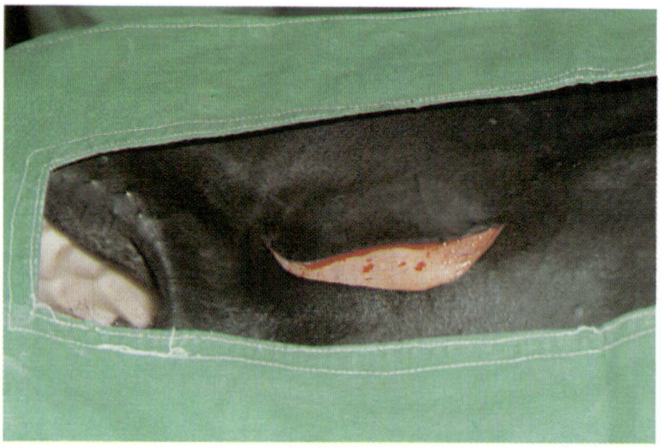

49

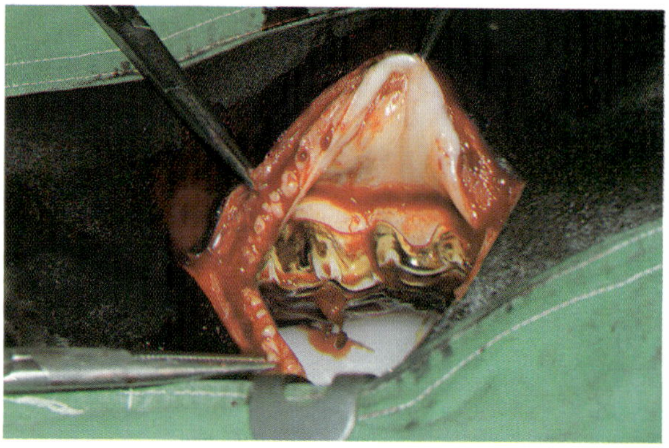

494 View of buccotomy skin incision — Case 4a. Note that **467** applies to this case.

495 Buccinator muscle incised, teeth exposed — Case 4b.

496 Mucoperiosteal flap — Case 4c. The vertical relieving incisions of the flap could have been made more remote to the borders of the socket in this case (for design of flaps see Chapter 10).

496

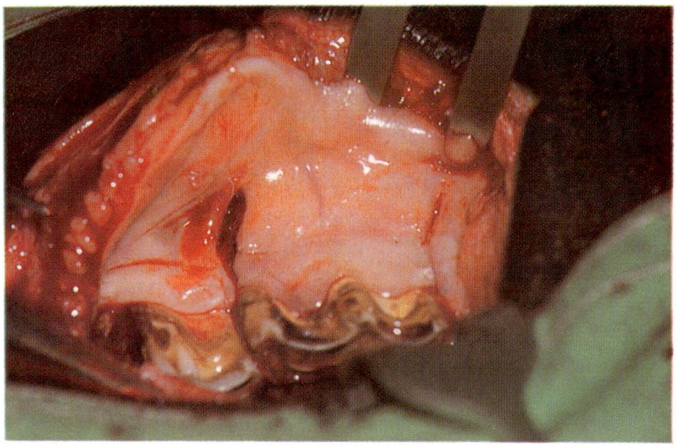

497 Buccal bone removed — Case 4d. Buccal bone is removed either with a drill or an osteotome. Depending on the age of the animal and the stage of development of the tooth, it often needs to be sectioned longitudinally to eliminate the retention of the divergent roots. Rotary instruments combined with osteotomes can be used to create an intersegmental space. Large dental elevators can separate the segments and aid in the extraction.

497

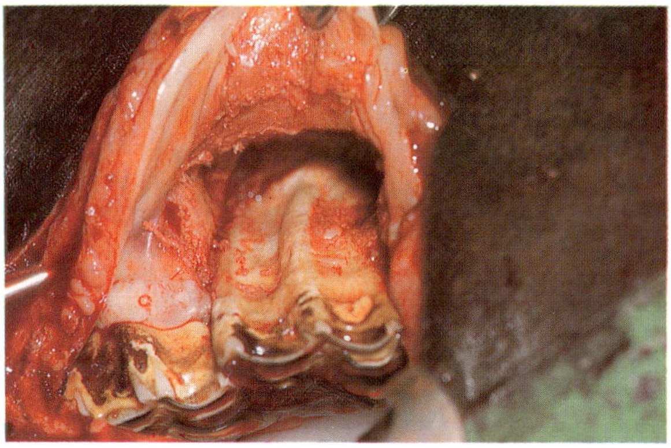

498 Post-extraction socket — Case 4e. The extracted tooth needs to be closely inspected for retained root apices. The socket should be carefully investigated, if necessary, for apices and loose pieces of alveolar bone as these are often in close proximity with the floor of the maxillary sinus and a fistula can easily be created through careless instrumentation. Intra-operative radiographs are invaluable for identifying fragments of dental tissue.

498

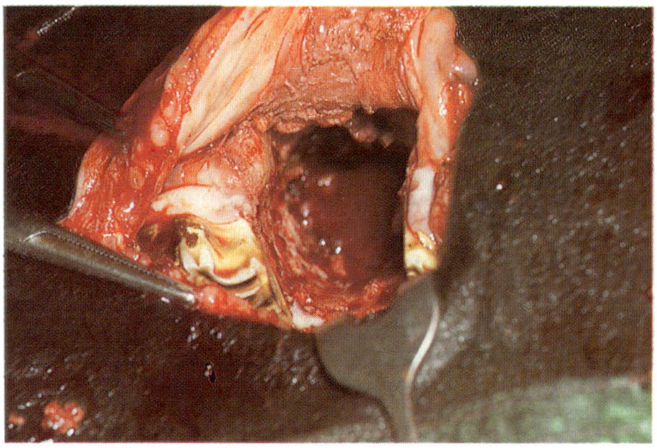

499

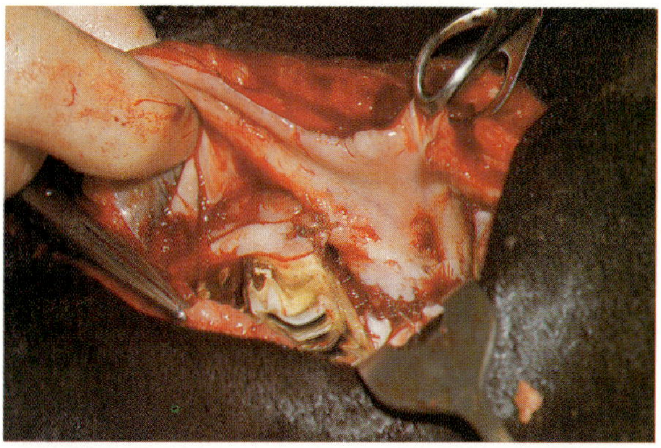

499 Flap sutured — Case 4f. The mucoperiosteal flap can be sutured to encourage primary healing and minimise food packing. The socket in this case was packed with ribbon gauze impregnated with bismuth iodoform paste. This was removed piecemeal through a stab incision on the face in the first 10 days after surgery.

500

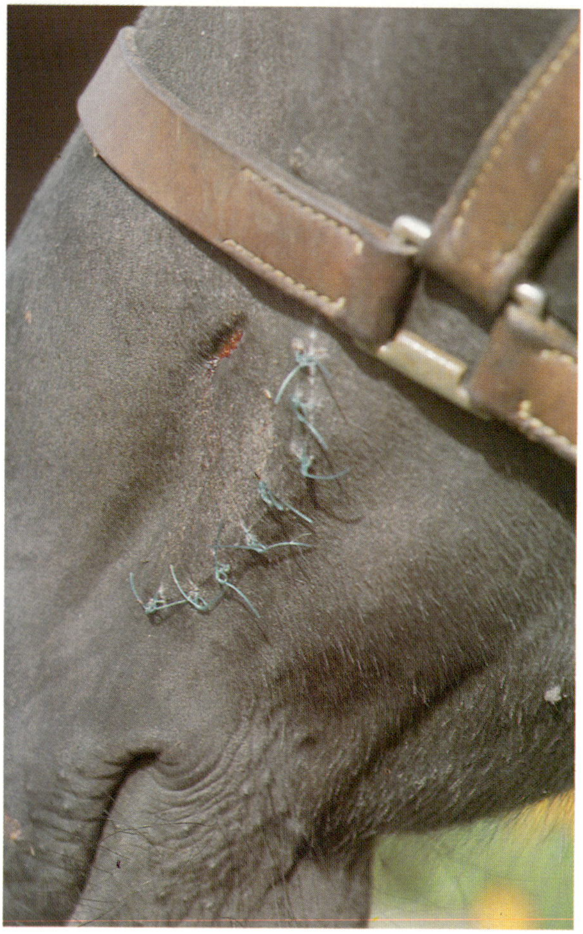

500 Two-weeks postoperative view — Case 4g. The ribbon gauze pack has been removed through the stab incision. Healing was uneventful, without the need for further general anaesthetic to attend to alveolar osteitis, dental sequestration, etc. The horse was shown successfully within six weeks of surgery.

14 Dental Diseases and their Treatment in Captive Wild Animals

As discussed in Chapter 1, the awareness and treatment of dental disease in captive wild animals, as well as its repercussion on their general health, is not a recent phenomenon. Most of the animals cannot be handled regularly and many lesions often do not become apparent until they are advanced. A preventative approach and an early assessment of dental diseases must be encouraged in order that conditions are treated before resultant general debility increases the anaesthetic risks.

Veterinary surgeons involved in the treatment of these animals are increasingly becoming experts in immobilisation and advanced anaesthetic techniques; hence, treatment often involves a joint effort between various professionals. The specialist dental team plays a vital role in this area of zoo animal medicine.

The dental treatment of wild animals is a demanding discipline for many reasons:

- It involves treating animals of different sizes, anatomy and physiology.
- Treatment is often performed in a less than ideal environment, but one must still be equipped and prepared for all eventualities.
- With the varying sizes of animals encountered it is often necessary to modify existing instrumentation, devise and manufacture special ones or utilise industrial tools.
- Treatment must be performed to the highest standard in the minimum of time.
- The dentist involved in such work must be aware of the priorities and needs of the veterinary surgeons and animal keepers and vice versa.
- On many occasions examination, diagnosis, treatment planning and treatment must be completed at the same time.
- Many of the animals are already stressed, which adds to the anaesthetic risks.
- To minimise the anaesthetic period the operator should have the help of dental assistants who are experienced in the subject and who have a thorough understanding of the needs of the operator.
- Postoperative care usually cannot be monitored as with domestic animals due to the lack of regular handling opportunities.

It is important that any operator in this field should have wide experience, knowledge and skills in all aspects of human and small animal dentistry. This branch of veterinary dentistry demands absolute dedication, especially in the investment of time in the study of regional anatomy and the design and funding of instruments and equipment, and is not to be embarked upon by professionals who are looking for a 'fun' day of their working week. Operators should also be able to interpret fundamental dental principles, according to the anatomy and physiology that one meets in the different types of animals, and must be able to diagnose and treat successfully the unexpected and unusual conditions that regularly arise. At the same time it is vital to appreciate the animal's true dental needs and that performing the highest quality of work on animals does not mean trying to mimic human dentistry. To ensure long-term success any treatment must be the most predictable and at the same time the least-invasive, creating the minimum of stress. The primary objective must be to assure that the animal's life is free of dental pain and infection.

The dental treatment of wild animals in this chapter has been arranged according to the classification of the dentitions shown in Scheme 1 of Chapter 4. In cases where different types of teeth exist in one species, the teeth are discussed separately in the appropriate section. In the relevant sections for each of the animal families illustrated, a representative dental formula is given.

Homodonts

Pathology and treatment of homodont dentitions is relatively unusual when compared with the diverse range of dental problems encountered among the heterodonts.

Monophyodonts

Order Cetacea

Delphinidae — Dolphin family

Toothed cetaceans have been reported to have suffered from periodontal disease and alveolar bone loss. The aetiology is unclear, but vitamin deficiency or advanced nephritis has been suspected in some cases.

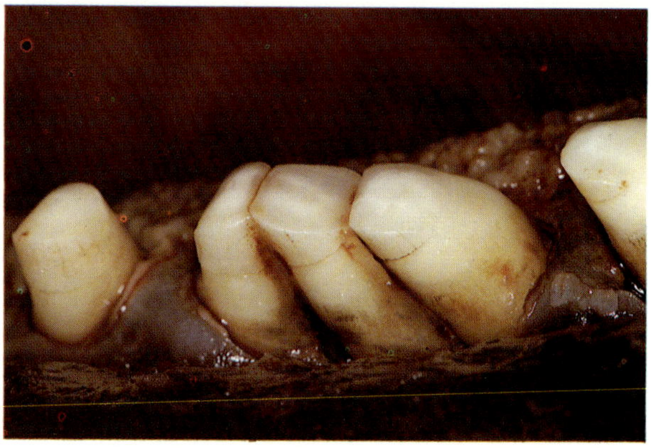

501 Supernumerary teeth — bottlenosed dolphin — wild. Normally 20–23 teeth per quadrant are present. The regular diastemas of the monophyodont dentition were disrupted in this specimen by supernumerary teeth in the mandible.

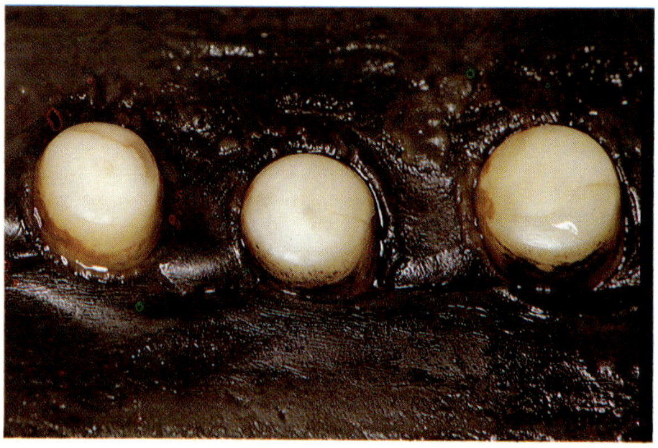

502 Attrition — bottlenosed dolphin — wild. Attrition of the dentition of odontocetes takes place in the wild and in captivity.

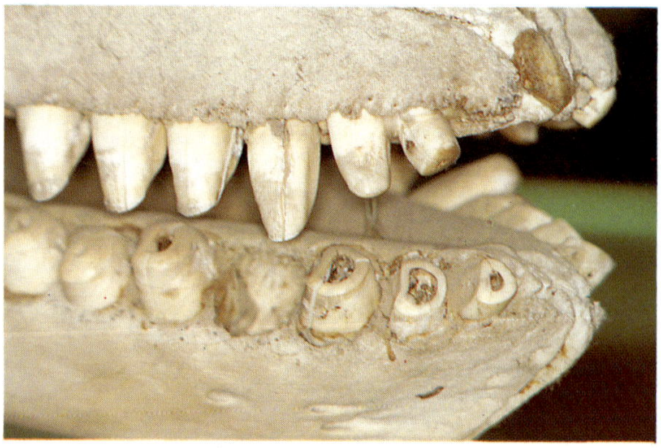

503 Pulp exposures — killer whale — wild. Normally up to 15 teeth per quadrant are present. Pulp polyps, pulp necrosis, mandibular abscesses and raised white cell counts have been reported in captive odontocetes suffering pulp exposures. This skull illustrates how a tip-to-tip malocclusion, instead of the normal interdigitation, has resulted in attrition and exposure of the pulp chambers in this relatively young animal. (Captured by fishermen 1872 — Bristol Channel, UK; Oxford University Museum No.14465.)

504 Porpoise — tooth cross-section for ageing. Secondary dentine, which is deposited throughout the life of toothed cetaceans, can be a guide to the life history of an individual. The dentine is deposited in growth layer groups (GLGs), which occur at a rate of one per year in several species examined, and can be used directly in age determination of the individual. The cementum also has GLGs, and has been widely used in the age determination of terrestrial mammals as well as cetaceans. The GLGs are best seen in longitudinal, decalcified and stained sections of only 25–30 µ thickness. This slide illustrates a 30 µ decalcified section stained with haematoxylin. The GLGs and associated accessory laminae are believed to be associated with intra-seasonal growth rhythms of the individual, fluctuations in food availability, breeding and other stressors. Mineralisation anomalies can be recognised in cetacean teeth, apparently related to species, age, geographical origin, sex, maturity, health and environmental factors. Age determination using GLGs is a highly specialised procedure and worldwide only a few individuals with relevant experience are able to interpret them accurately.

504

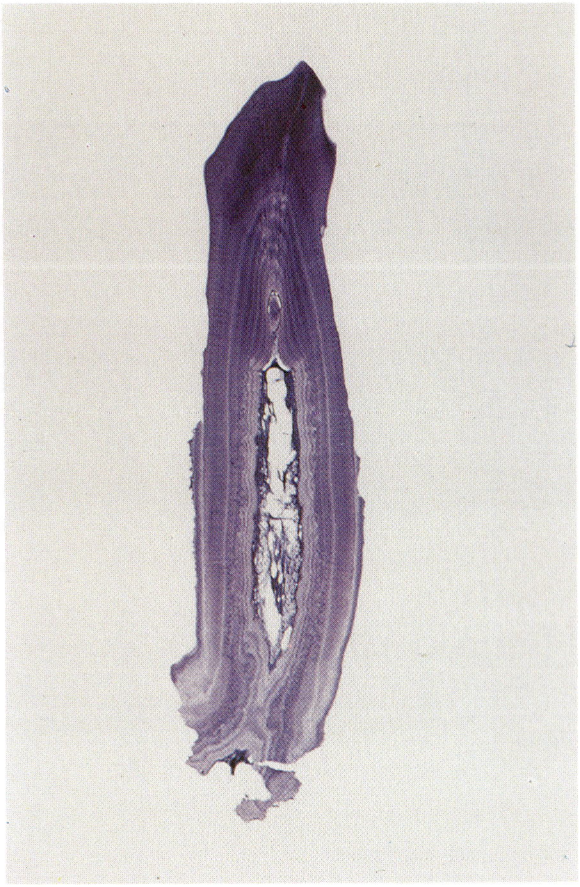

Polyphyodonts

Order Crocodilia

Alligatorinae — Alligator and Caiman subfamily

505 Discoloured dentition of a Caiman. Six-year-old animal was found to have a uniform intrinsic discolouration of its dentition. On closer examination it was noticed that the next set of teeth were erupting a normal colour. X-ray micro-analysis of an exfoliated tooth detected the consistent presence of calcium, phosphorous, copper and zinc, and a variable presence of aluminium, iron and chlorine. It indicated that the disclouration was due to salts of metals, especially copper, and it is most likely that the animal ingested a piece of copper, possibly in the form of coins, at the period when the discoloured dentition was being formed.

505

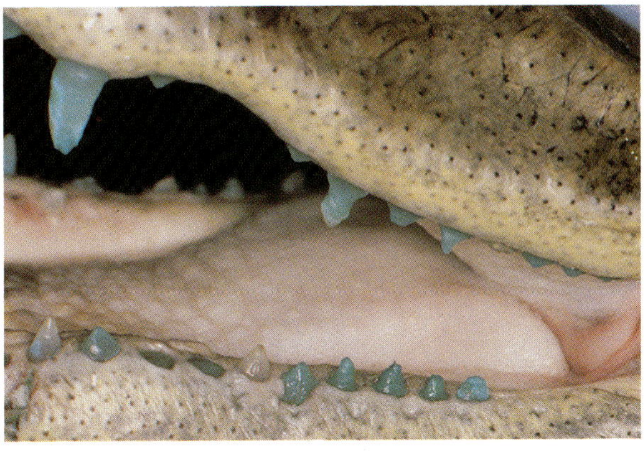

Order Carcharhiniformes

Carcharhindae — Requiem shark family

506 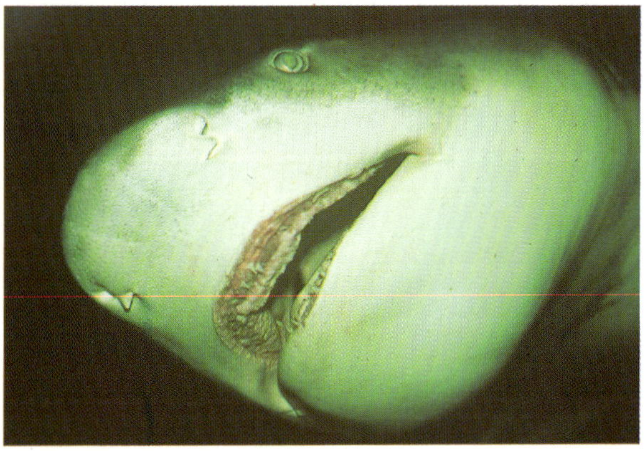

506 Necrotising gingivitis — lemon shark — captive. Sharks in captivity can suffer from hypothyroidism. It is believed that high nitrate levels in the water can block the 'thyroid trap'. This condition manifests itself in a much reduced tooth production and may lead to necrotising gingivitis. Appropriate modification to the water chemistry and/or supplements of the hormone can reverse the condition.

Heterodonts

Elodonts

Order Lagomorpha

Leporidae — rabbits and hares $\frac{2}{1}:\frac{0}{0}:\frac{3}{2}:\frac{3}{3} = 28$

507 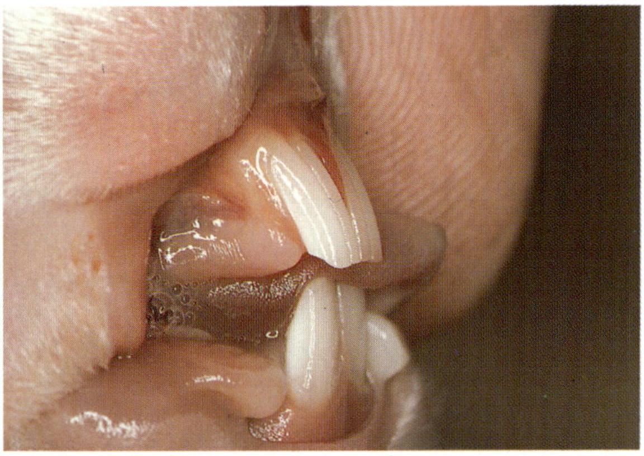

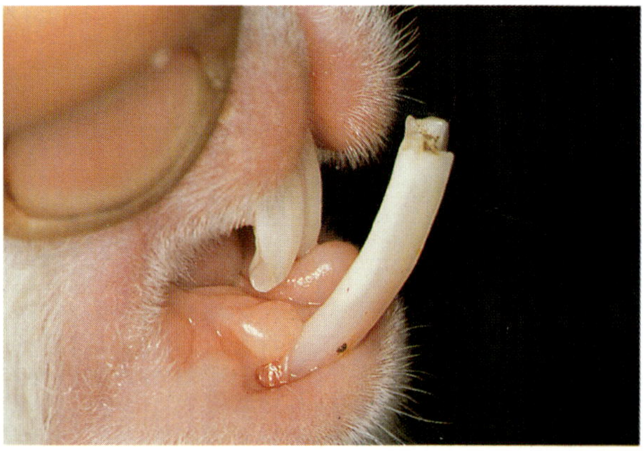 508

507 Normal occlusion. The normal edge-to-edge incisor relationship is responsible for the constant attrition that controls the length of these continuously growing teeth.

508 Abnormal occlusion. If no occlusion exists, usually as a result of a skeletal discrepancy, the incisors will become overgrown.

509 Abnormal occlusion with soft-tissue trauma. Eventually, the overgrown incisors create soft-tissue damage to the tongue, gingivae or the cheeks; the animal is unable to eat and starves to death. Tooth length reduction temporarily improves the condition, but the pulp chambers of the lower incisors are exposed by such action. As these teeth have dilated apices, they are often able to repair such exposures with secondary dentine. If that does occur, tooth overgrowth continues, often with increased abnormality in the angulation of the amputated teeth. Further treatment is necessary within a few weeks. Sometimes, secondary dentine fails to develop and pulpal necrosis occurs. Pus may discharge at the ventral surface of the mandible or through the gingival sulcus. Because of the curvature of the upper incisors, pulp exposure does not occur on amputation of the teeth to the level of the gingival margin. The speed of growth of the upper incisors also seems to be slower than that of the lowers. As a result of the regenerative power of the elodont pulp, root canal treatment on orthodox endodontic lines is not possible in the treatment of overgrown incisors. Regeneration of the pulp will take place. Extraction of the lower incisors, which can be a difficult procedure, and periodic trimming of the uppers is one option. The extraction of the upper incisors is not possible because of their curvature, and the extensive surgical trauma that would be created to the maxillae.

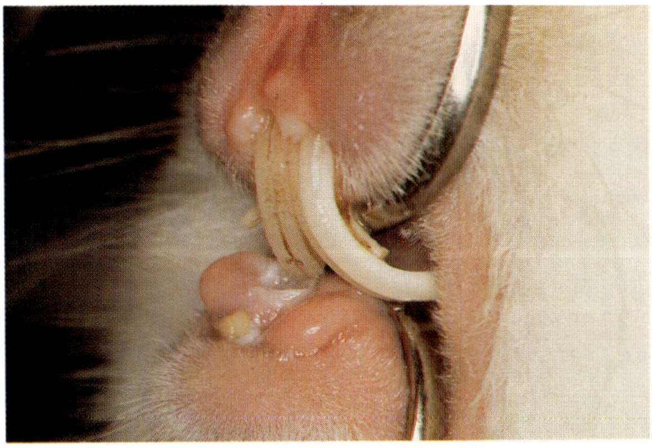
509

510 Pulp exposure — Case 1a — rabbit. Another option is to attempt to stop the growth of the lower incisors after tooth-length reduction has taken place. Although no histopathology is available to demonstrate how this occurs, partial pulpectomy and pulp mummification have been successful in controlling the growth of the lower incisors without any apparent clinical evidence of periapical infection.

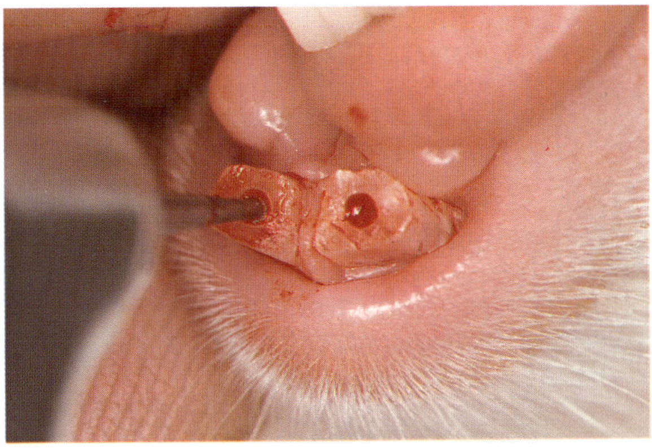
510

511 Haemostasis — Case 1b. Pulpal haemorrhage must be controlled, this may be achieved by applying very gentle pressure with the wider end of a paper point to the amputated pulp tissue in the cavity. Only rarely does a haemostatic agent need to be employed.

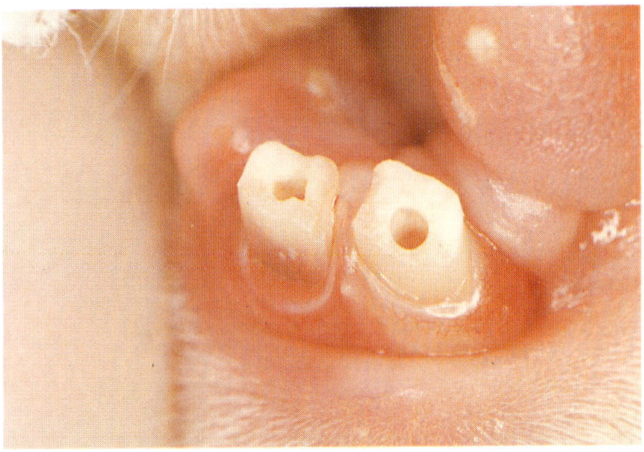
511

512

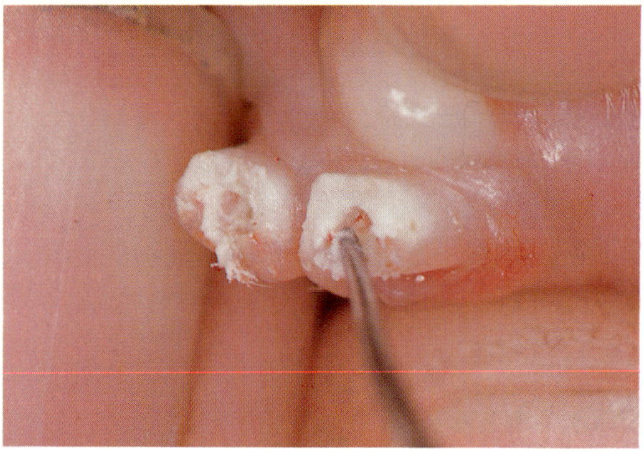

512 Mummifying material being applied to vital pulp — Case 1c. A paraformaldahyde-based product marketed for the mummification of primary human pulp tissue has proved to be successful.

513

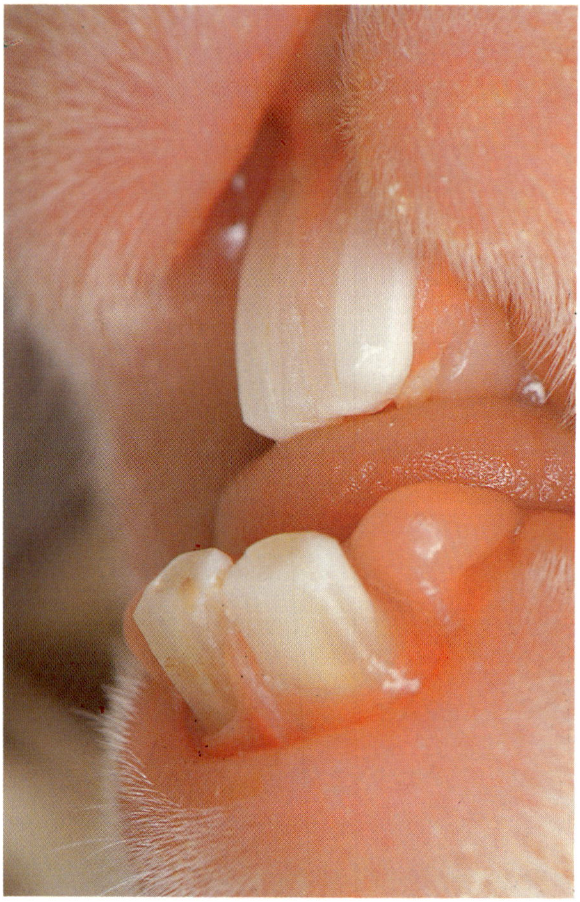

513 Final restoration and occlusion — Case 1d. After a sublining a composite filling material was placed as the permanent filling.

514 Buccal ulceration — rabbit. Rabbits often suffer from either anorexia, quidding or hypersalivation. A thorough examination of the mouth under a general anaesthetic or deep sedation is necessary to evaluate the buccal and lingual edges of the cheek teeth. The sharp enamel points on the occlusal tables of these abnormally worn teeth is usually responsible for buccal and lingual ulcerations. The aetiology may be partly dietary, but often an anisognathic malocclusion is responsible for the uneven wear. The removal of the enamel points will immediately alleviate the discomfort on a temporary basis, but they will usually reform within 12–16 weeks. Extended rotary instruments are infinitely more efficient and rapid in the trimming procedure than hand files. It must be stressed that careful retraction and protection of the soft tissues is mandatory when rotary instruments are used for adjustment, or lacerations can result.

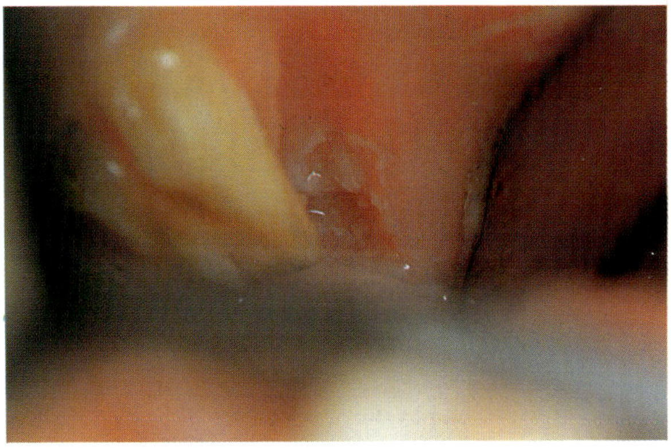
514

515 Mandibular abscess — rabbit. Rabbits also suffer from acute facial abscesses arising at the angle of the mandible. The aetiology is unclear, but there is strong indication that food packing between the teeth and, occasionally, impacted molars are responsible for the infection. Antibiotic therapy and curettage offers only short-term resolution, as the primary cause of the condition must be eliminated. Any long-term therapy must include the extraction of the teeth involved and elimination of the fibrous capsule. Even with the most careful surgical technique, postoperative losses are high among rabbits. Many respond poorly to antibiotics and postoperative stress. Intra-oral extractions of the long molars are difficult and unpredictable. On the other hand, the rabbit's mouth does not lend itself to a buccotomy approach, because it leads to contamination, necrosis, wound dehiscence and postoperative food packing between the muscle layers. The most favourable surgical approach is through the ventral aspect of the extra-oral abscess. Extractions can be made through direct vision, without invading the oral cavity. Buccal bone removal, tooth sectioning, when necessary, and gentle elevation can be easily accomplished through this route. The defect in the mandible is gently packed with ribbon gauze saturated with Whitehead's Varnish to eliminate food packing through the sockets. Replacement under sedation at two-week intervals allows granulation and healing through secondary intention.

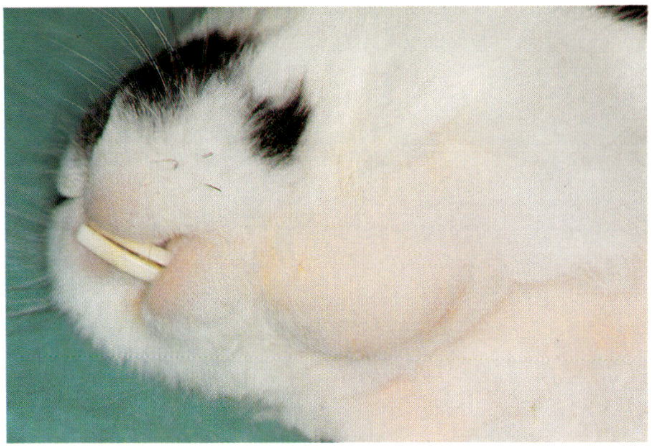
515

516 Radiograph of mandibular abscess — rabbit. Reparative bone spicules growing into the osseous defect associated with osteomyelitis are visible.

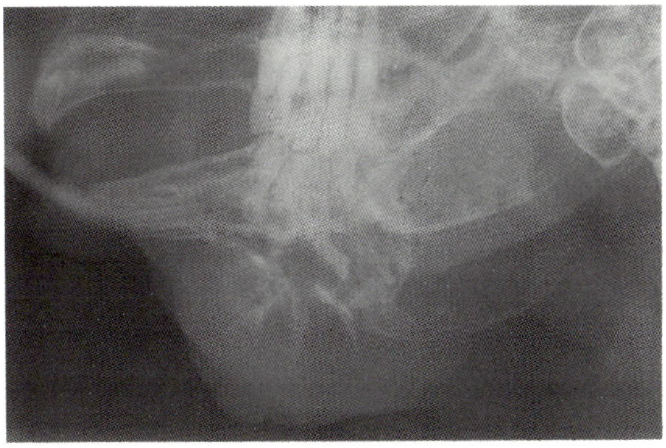
516

Order Rodentia

Chinchillidae — chinchilla family $\frac{1}{1}:\frac{0}{0}:\frac{1}{1}:\frac{3}{3} = 20$

517

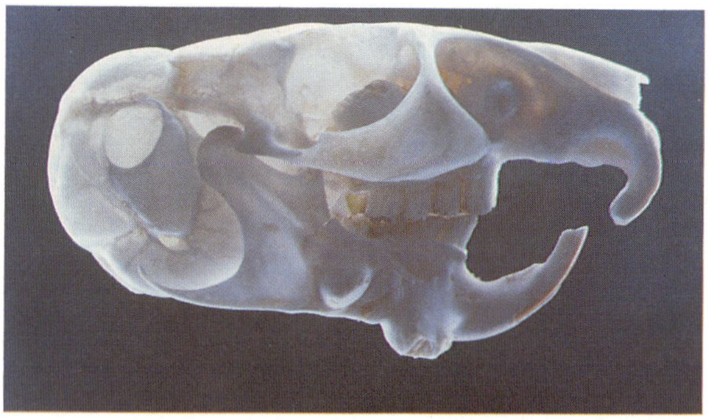

517 Chinchilla skull. Chinchillas often exhibit anorexia and ocular discharge; dental disease and malocclusion are thought to be contributing factors. Intra-oral examination often reveals no abnormalities, but the radiographic appearance can show the roots of the posterior teeth to be overgrown apically. This picture illustrates the root apices perforating into the orbit and through the cortical plate of the ventral border of the mandible. The aetiology of the condition is unclear: genetic as well as dietary factors have been implicated. It is possible that a diet lacking the necessary fibrous elements gives rise to less than normal occlusal attrition, leading to overgrowth, but in the chinchilla this may take place in an apical direction rather than the crowns extruding intra-orally.

Caviidae — guinea-pig family $\frac{1}{1}:\frac{0}{0}:\frac{1}{1}:\frac{3}{3} = 20$

518

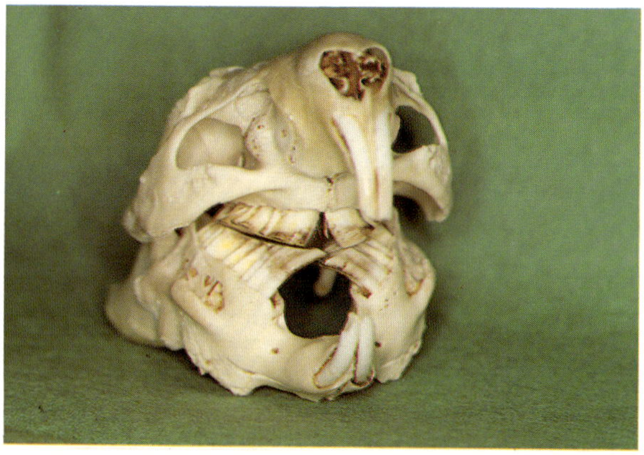

518 Malocclusion — guinea-pig. In contrast to **517**, this animal had overgrown cheek teeth to such an extent that his tongue was trapped under the lingually over-extended occlusal tables. He was also unable to shut his mouth and died of starvation.

519 Extra-oral sinus tract — Case 1a — paca. Abscess healing at the angle of the mandible.

520 Interdental food packing — Case 1b. Intra-oral view illustrating severe pocketing and food packing between the cheek teeth. Extraction of the teeth involved resolved the condition.

519

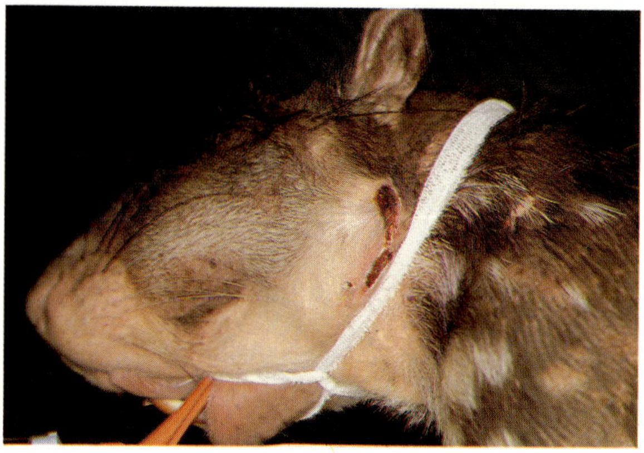

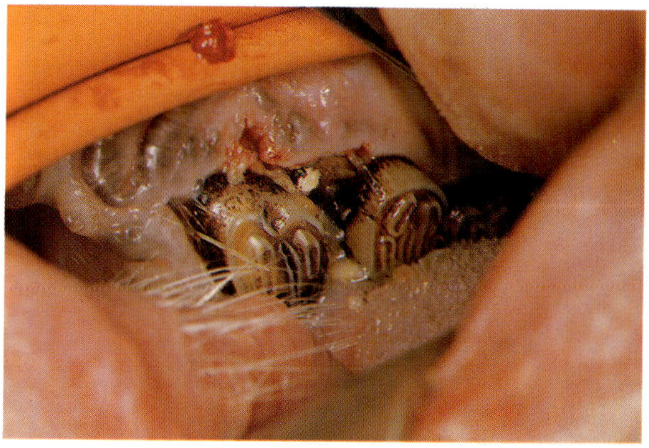

52

Muridae — rat family $\frac{1}{1}:\frac{1}{0}:\frac{1-2}{1}:\frac{3}{3} = 20-22$

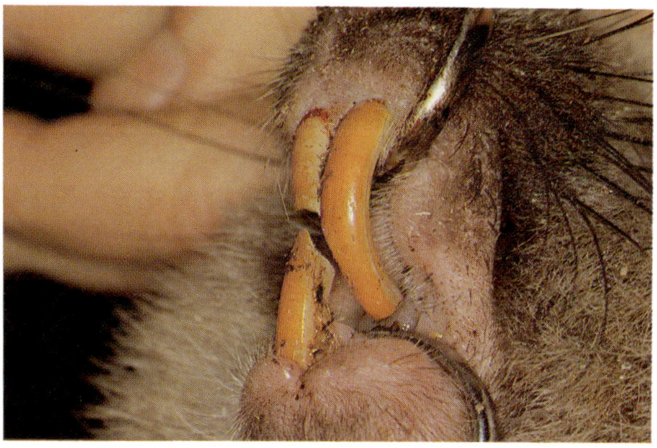

521

521 Overgrown upper incisor — Case 1a — Philippine cloud rat. This animal had to have the lower left incisor extracted because of a longitudinal fracture and resultant osteomyelitis.

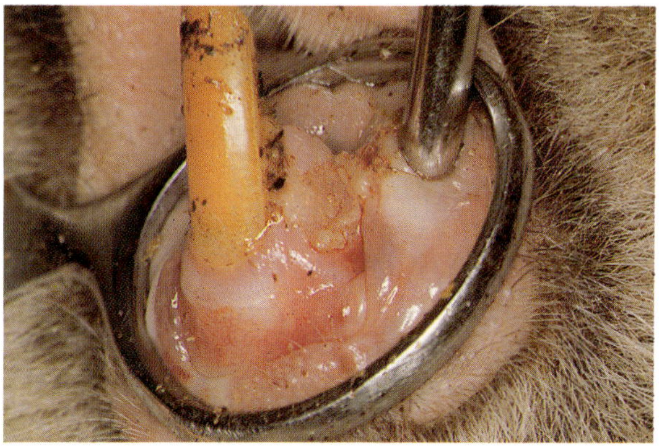

522

522 Traumatic occlusion — Case 1b. The opposing upper incisor overgrew and caused severe trauma to the gingiva overlying the socket of the extracted tooth.

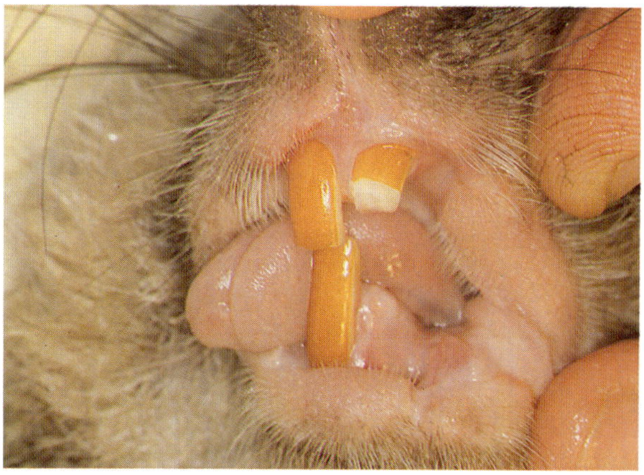

523

523 Incisor trimmed — Case 1c. Trimming the overgrowing tooth at intervals of 8 weeks maintained a non-traumatic occlusion. The operations were performed without sedation on the restrained animal using an air-rotor. The tooth was trimmed very close to the gingiva: note that no exposure of the upper incisor pulp occurred through such trimming. It was also interesting to note that the animal managed to masticate with only one posterior tooth remaining, the others having been exfoliated through ageing.

Order Marsupialia

Vombatidae — wombat family $\frac{1}{1}:\frac{0}{0}:\frac{1}{1}:\frac{4}{4} = 24$

524

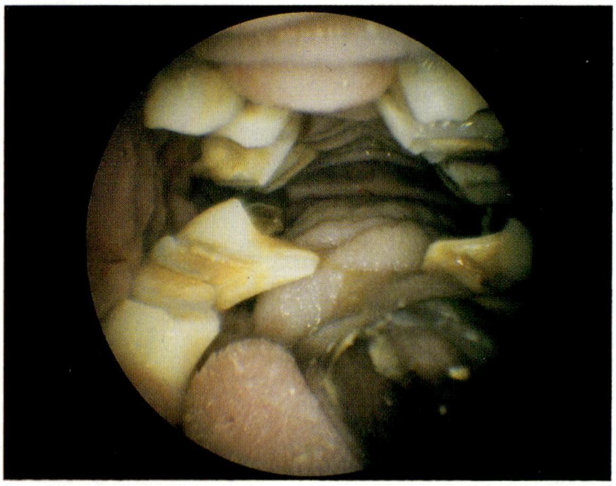

524 Molar overgrowth — wombat. Endoscopic view of protruding lingual edges of the cheek teeth. The overextended sharp buccal edges of the upper molars were ulcerating the buccal mucosa. The lingual edges of the lower molars impeded the tongue. The teeth were trimmed with the aid of extra-long tungsten and diamond drills.

Order Proboscidea

Elephantidae — elephants $\frac{1}{0}:\frac{0}{0}:\frac{0}{0}:\frac{6}{6} = 26$

Tusks — upper incisors

The treatment of elephant tusks and molars is probably the most challenging area of veterinary dentistry. The primary reason is that the dental apparatus of the elephant is quite different from that encountered in other animals. Secondly, the sheer size of an elephant requires an approach alien to orthodox dentistry; although some of the basic principles still hold true, they need to be interpreted into industrial sizes and instrumentation. Thirdly, access to the structures may be limited, which considerably hinders the visibility and instrumentation of the tusks and molars. Success in elephant dentistry requires much preparation and team effort to ensure a predictable outcome.

It is inevitable, because of their environment, that some captive elephants will suffer damage to their tusks. Some observers have also reported that as many as 5% of wild African elephants also sustain fractures to their tusks. These wild animals have been seen to be more aggressive and irritable, and parasites have been found to harbour in the pulp chambers of the injured structures. In a captive situation, pulp exposures of tusks have often lead to obvious signs of pain, aggressive behaviour, chronic and acute infections, necessity for euthanasia, or sudden death associated with septicaemia arising from the purulent tusk infection.

525

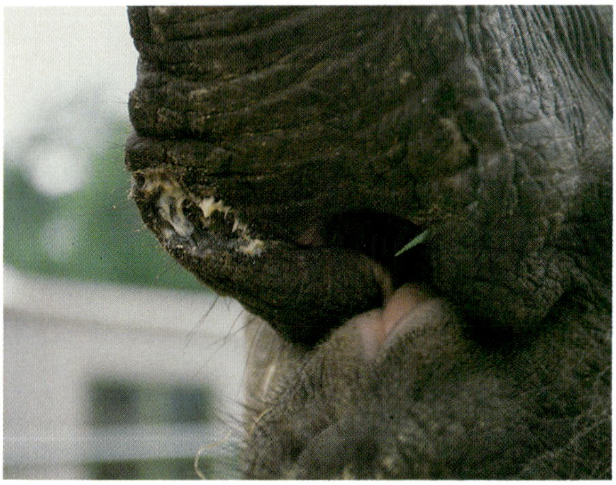

525 Pericoronitis of an erupting tusk — African elephant. Infection of the tusk sheath is common in young elephants at the time of tusk eruption. A relieving incision sometimes needs to be made to aid eruption.

526

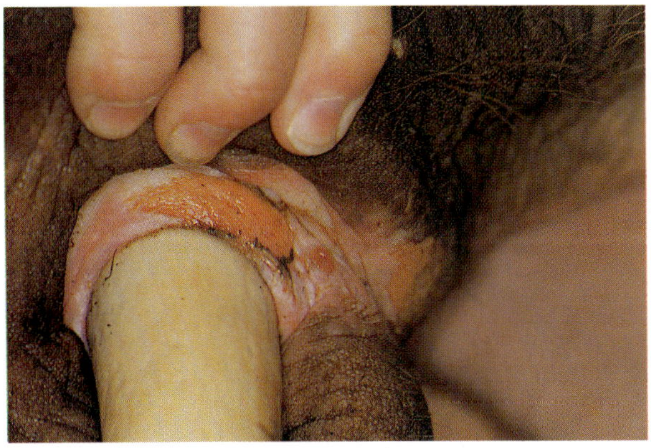

527

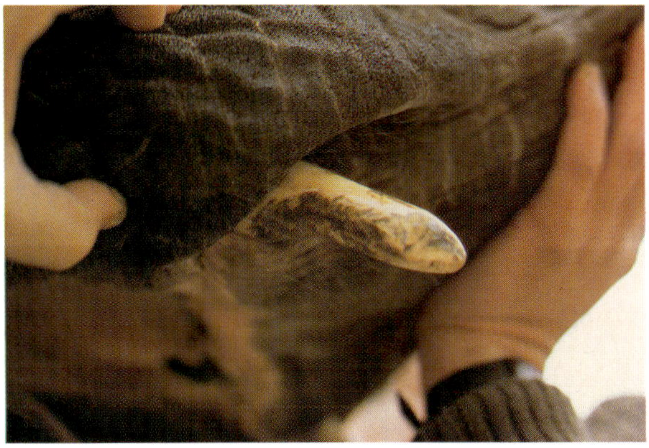

526 Pericoronitis of an erupted tusk — Asian elephant. The inflammation of the tusk's gingival margin occurs occasionally. It is usually associated with the blowing of sand and urine into the area. A thorough investigation can reveal the impaction of a foreign body in the gingival sulcus.

527 Abrasion of a tusk — Asian elephant. Because of the nature of the captive animal's environment, the natural abrasion of the tusks through rubbing is accelerated and often takes place in areas other than the coronal tip. This tusk eventually fractured without exposing the pulp. The fitting of protective rings to minimise the damage may be considered, but many animals give the foreign structure increased attention and a high failure rate can be expected.

528

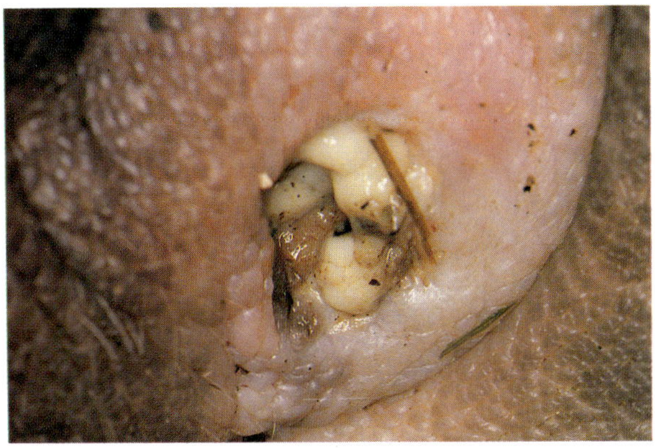

529

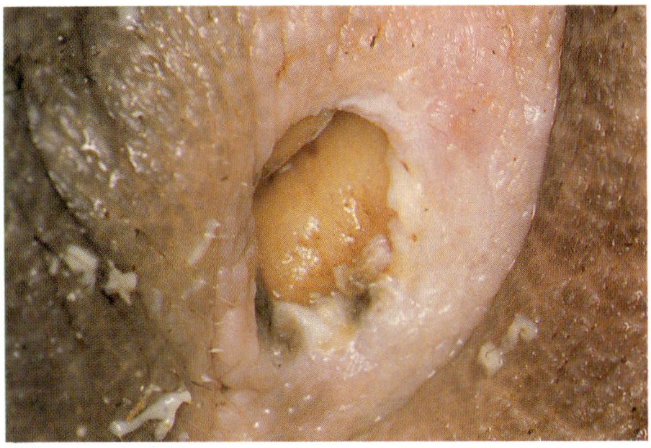

528 Subgingival fracture — Case 1a — Asian elephant. A fresh subgingival fracture in a six-year-old female is shown. Purulent discharge from the gingival sulcus is visible. Pulp chamber lengths vary between the African and Asian species. African males and females both possess canals that are close to the coronal tips of the tusks, and pulp exposures are common in cases of tusk injuries as they are among Asian bulls. In the author's experience, Asian females, even at an early age, have pulp chambers that are significantly apical to the coronal tips and do not become exposed through fractures, even if they occur at a subgingival level.

529 Pulp chamber almost exposed — Case 1b. Once the exudate had been removed, although no pulpal exposure could be elicited with a probe, the pulp was showing through the thin ivory wall as a small pink spot at the floor of the wedge-shaped defect.

530
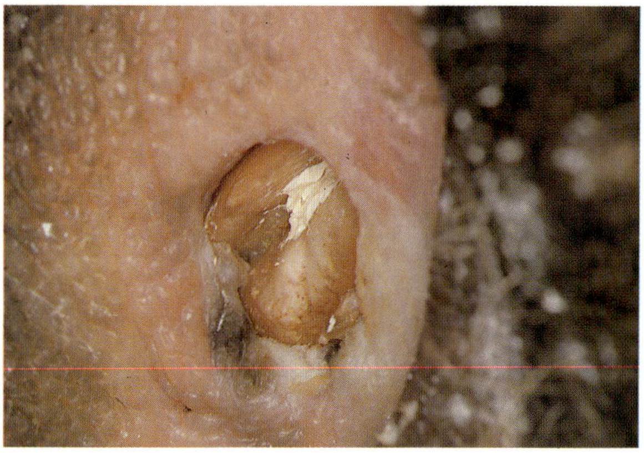

53
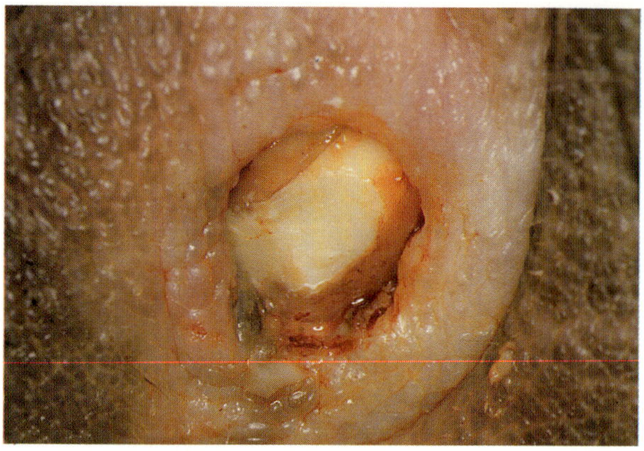

530 Lining — Case 1c. To protect the pulp before restoration, a layer of calcium hydroxide lining was placed at the base of the cavity.

531 Glass ionomer restoration — Case 1d. Glass ionomer cement was placed in the wedge-shaped cavity to prevent the animal from levering on the edges of the defect and fracturing it even further. Once the material had set, it was smoothed and the sharp subgingival margins of the tusk were rounded off with a high-speed drill.

532
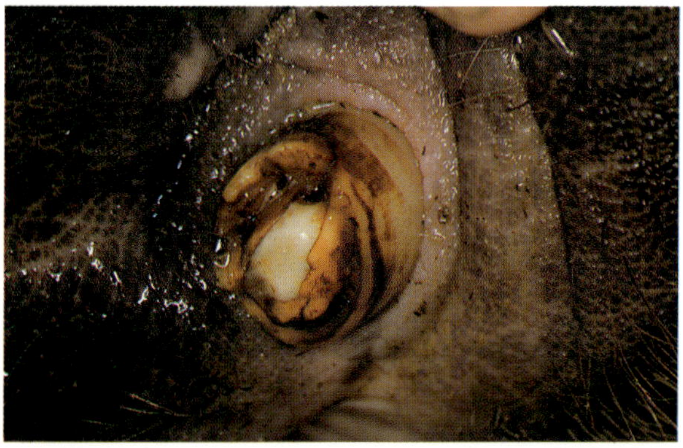

53
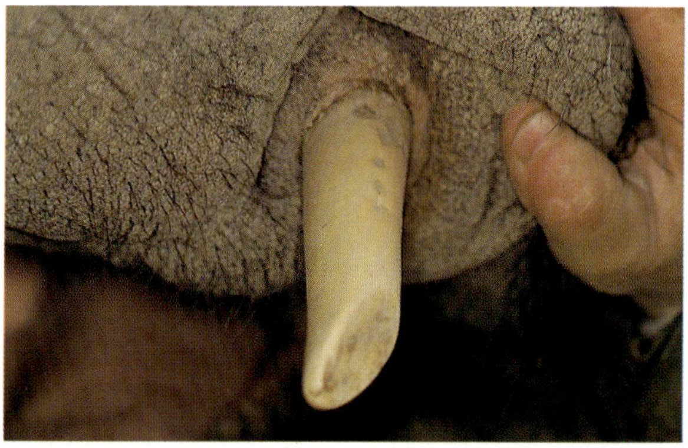

532 Six months postoperative — Case 1e. The tusk erupted at a rate of 40 mm in six months. It was subjected to abrasion immediately on eruption, but some cement remained on the tusk tip. The material possesses adhesive properties to ivory, but the importance of this feature must not be exaggerated, especially in such a testing environment. The prolonged success of the restoration was primarily due to the defect having a favourable, retentive shape.

533 Two years postoperative — Case 1f. Tusk tip attrition has been regular, with no pulpal exposure.

534

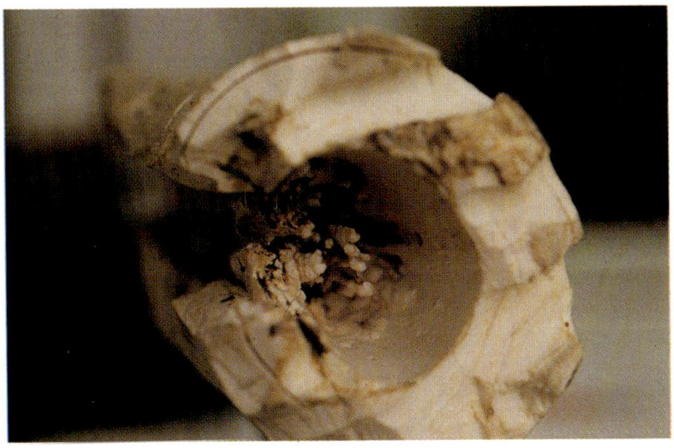

535

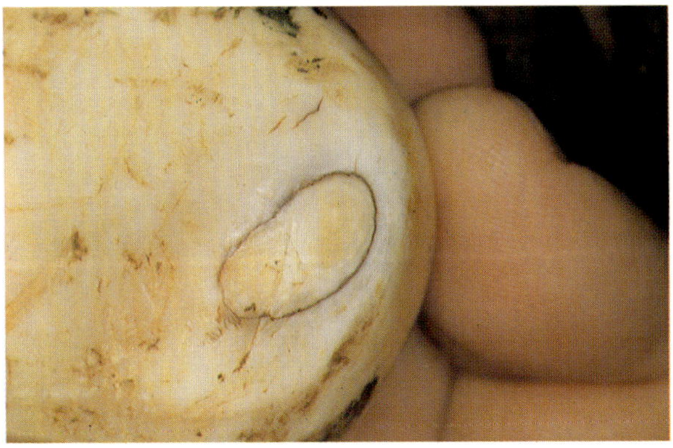

534 Secondary ivory — Asian elephant. Extracted section of a tusk demonstrates the way secondary ivory attempted to wall off an exposure to the pulp chamber in a 16-year-old bull. The irregular ivory is often termed 'ivory pearls'. In captivity a satisfactory seal to the pulp chamber often fails to form naturally in cases of exposure.

535 Secondary dentine — Case 2a — African elephant. Constant abrasion of the right tusk tip caused rapid wear in this seven-year-old bull. Secondary ivory was laid down and prevented pulpal exposure.

536

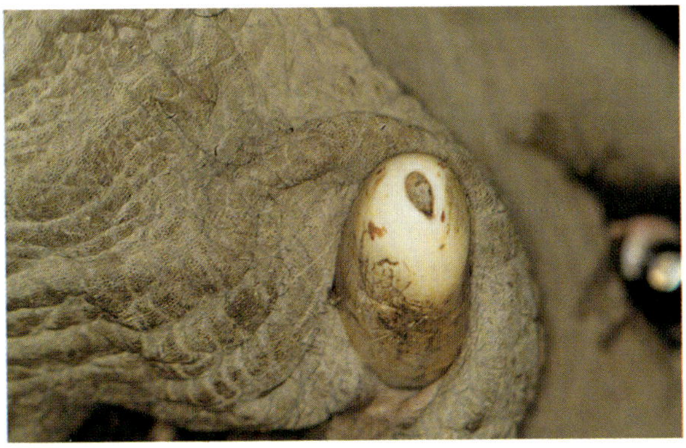

537

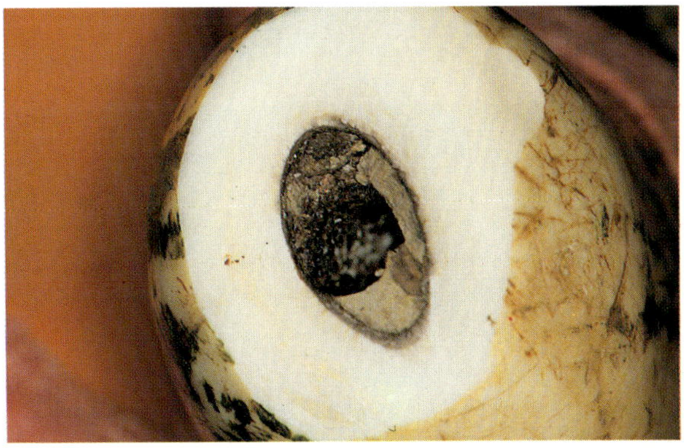

536 Pulp exposure — Case 2b. In the animal's left tusk the abrasion resulted in pulp exposure and purulent pulpitis.

537 Close-up of tusk tip — Case 2c. The tusk tip has been resected to gain better access to the pulp chamber. The animal had packed the defect with debris.

538

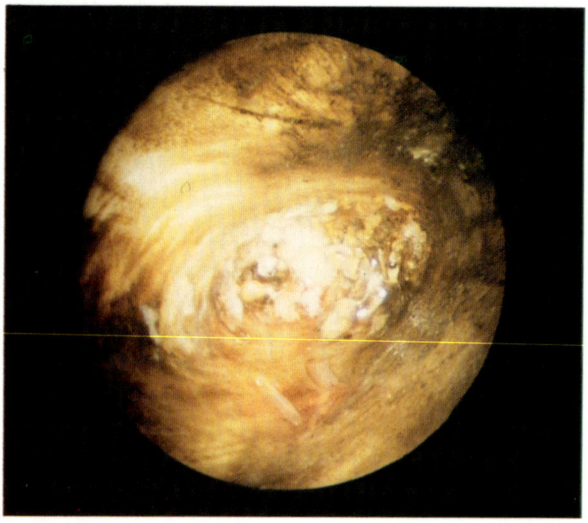

539

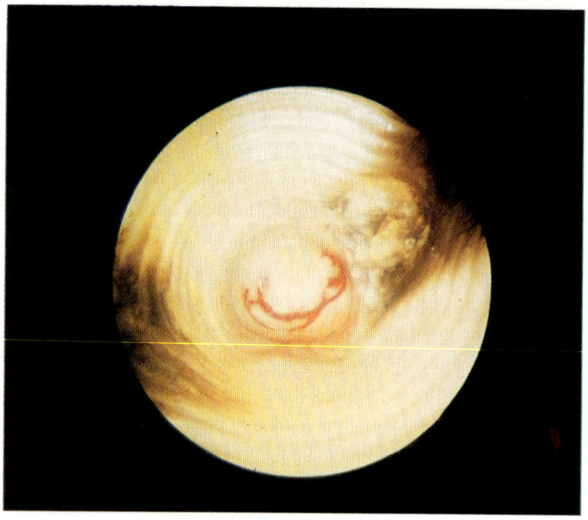

538 Endoscopic view inside a tusk — Case 2d. On debridement, necrotic material and the evidence of some secondary dentine, which attempted to wall off the exposure, was seen.

539 Endoscopic view of pulp — Case 2e. Further debridement revealed a ring of healthy bleeding pulp at the periphery of the apical extremity of the infected canal. This was interpreted as a ball of secondary ivory attempting to block off the exposure.

540

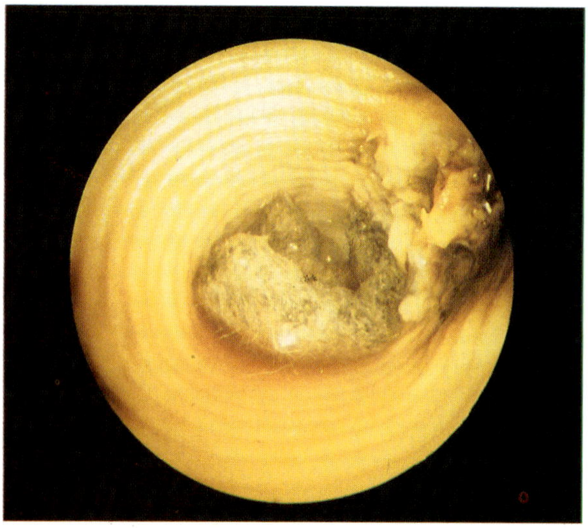

54

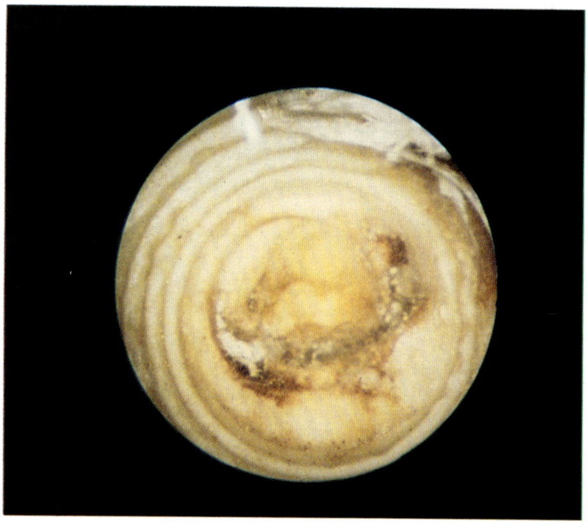

540 Dacron in place — Case 2f. The coronal 60 mm of the tusk was thoroughly debrided and irrigated. The wall of the canal was tapped to the appropriately sized thread so that it could be obturated temporarily with a threaded nylon rod while antibiotics and antiseptic dressings were placed. Surgical Dacron felt, soaked in Whitehead's Varnish and soluble penicillin, was placed at the apical end of the prepared space to eliminate the infection and encourage secondary dentine formation. Irregular secondary ivory is visible on the wall of the canal.

541 Two months postoperative — Case 2g. On re-entry, the endoscopic view indicated complete healing and secondary ivory formation. There was no sign of pulp or purulent discharge. Bacteriological culture indicated a great reduction of organisms. The coronal defect was obturated by bonding a nylon rod in the canal.

542 Seven months after sealing the canal — Case 2h. Abrasion of the tusk tip had taken place to the extent of 35 mm in seven months. The full length of the nylon screw and its threaded canal had been abraded and a healthy wall of secondary ivory wall is visible. In the same period of time, 40 mm of growth had taken place in the length of the tusk. This was ascertained by marking the position of the gingival margin on the tusk by scoring its surface and measuring the growth from that point.

Discussion: Abrasion of the tusk tip cannot be eliminated in the captive environment. Placing a cast prosthesis to protect the tip has been considered as a possible long-term measure but may prove to act as a dangerous weapon, especially if a sharp edge is created through abrasion. The case will be reviewed at regular intervals to record if tusk growth and secondary ivory deposition can keep ahead of ivory loss and pulp exposure through wear.

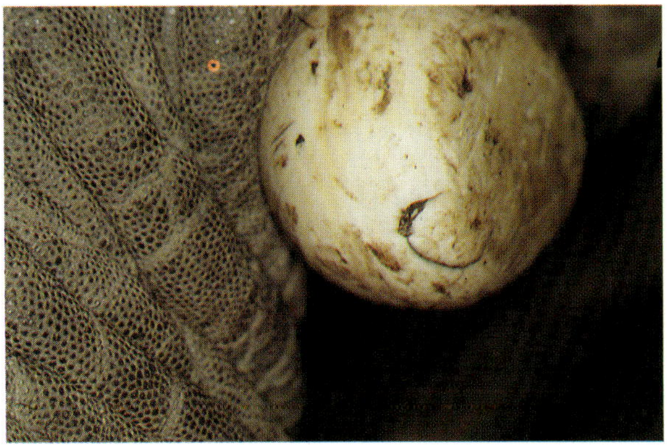

542

543 Pulp polyp — Case 3a — African elephant. 22-year-old female with a history of tusk fractures from the age of 5 years. Because of her psychotic behaviour, euthanasia was considered. Although the pulp was still alive and granulating out of the canal, there was purulent material internally and a large lateral abscess present. Tusk was extracted through the longitudinal split technique.

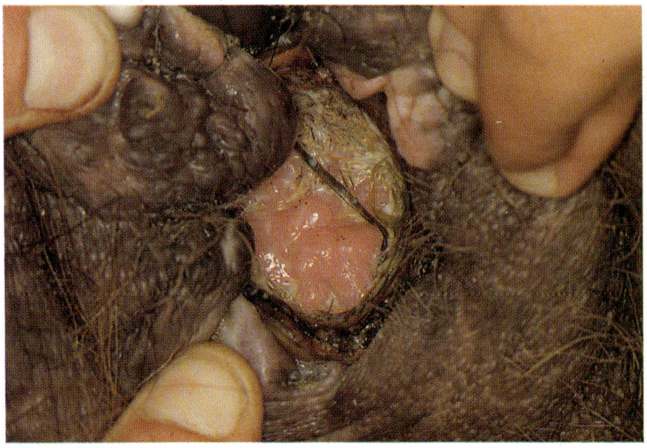

543

544 Impacted tusk — Case 3b. The left tusk of the same animal. No pulpal exposure was present but the animal was packing mud and faeces into the tusk sheath, indicating pain. The tusk tip was impacting into the soft tissues, causing a hyperplastic reaction. Wedge resection from the tusk sheath allowed immediate relief of pain and eliminated the packing behaviour. The animal's aggression and 'head banging' against the walls of her compound ceased immediately on recovery from the anaesthetic after the tusk extraction and wedge resection. She now exhibits a normal behaviour.

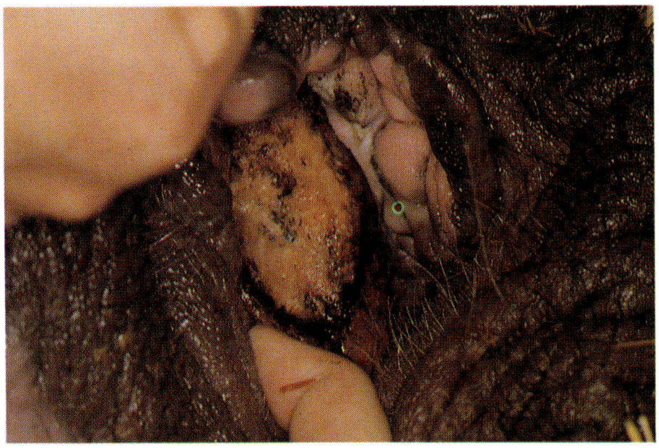

544

545

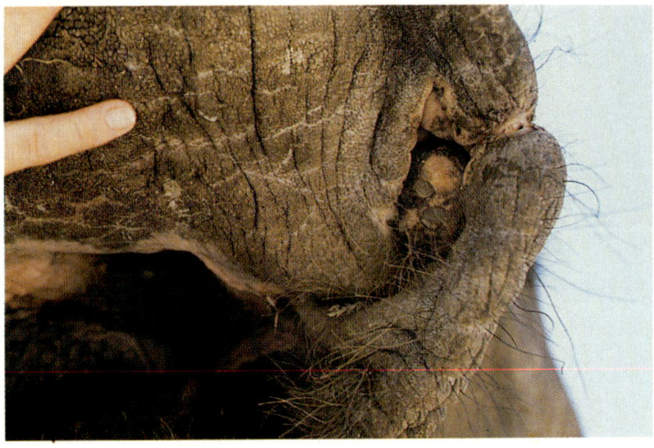

546

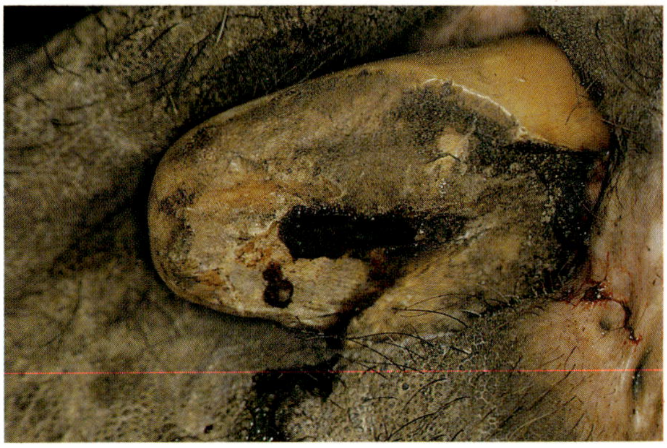

545 Six months postoperative — Case 3c. Although worn down through abrasion, the tusk has erupted past the critical stage of impaction. Nylon screws visible at the centre of the tusk were placed to fill pilot holes, which were used to investigate the condition of the tusk.

546 Fractured tusk — Case 4a — Asian elephant. 13-year-old male with a fractured tusk. Purulent material is visible discharging from the exposed pulp chamber.

547

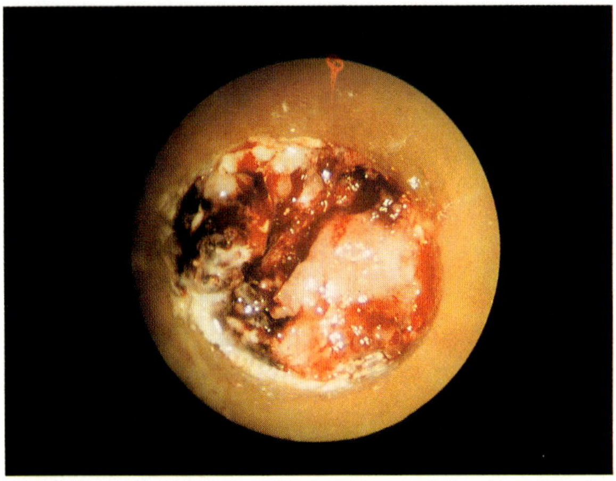

548

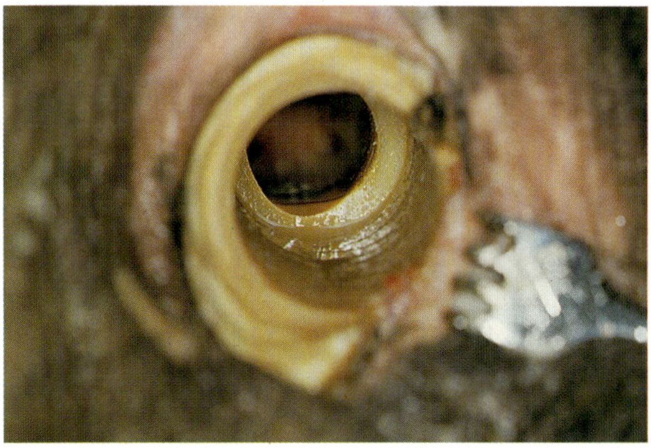

547 Endoscopic view inside a tusk — Case 4b. Granulation tissue and purulent material is visible at the apical end of the root canal. As no healthy pulp tissue remained in the tusk, extraction was the treatment of choice. The 'Welch internally collapsing' extraction technique offers the least traumatic way of extracting exposed and infected tusks. Before the technique was introduced, tusk extractions required excessive rotational forces, which often damaged the maxilla, or a highly invasive approach, where the removal of maxillary bone was necessary.

548 Thinning the tusk wall — Case 4c. Modified engineering counterbores were used to gradually increase the size of the canal, thereby thinning out the wall of the tusk for longitudinal sectioning. This early stage of the wall-thinning procedure demonstrates the smooth and regular cut that was obtained.

549 Longitudinal cuts — Case 4d. Longitudinal cuts were made to the full length of the tusk with mechanical and modified hand saws. A custom-designed tusk splitter was used to complete the longitudinal cuts to the apex of the tusk.

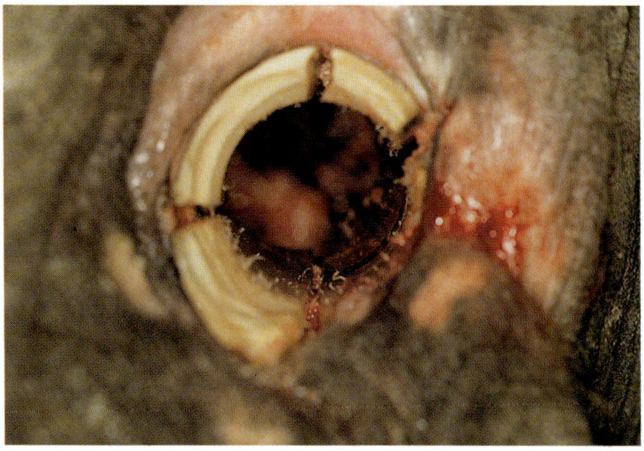

549

550 Chisels. Specially made long stainless steel chisels and elevators are used to separate segments from the alveolar bone.

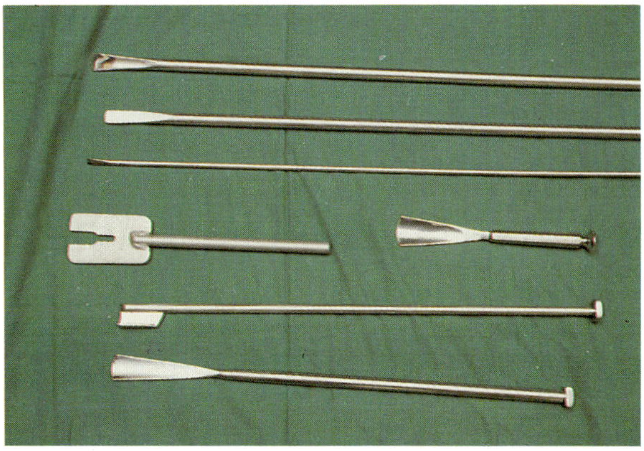

550

551 Extracted tusk segments.

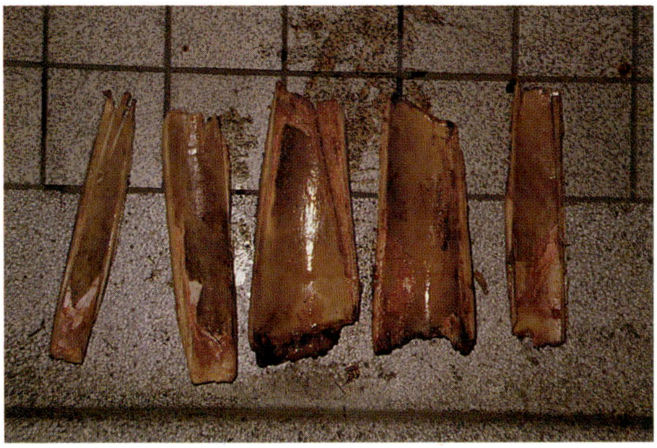

551

Order Tubulidentata

Orycteropodidae — aardvark $\frac{0}{0}:\frac{0}{0}:\frac{2-4}{2-4}:\frac{3}{3} = 20-28$

552

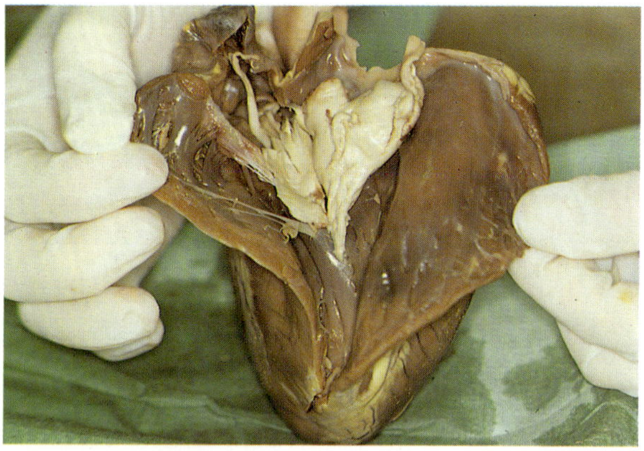

553

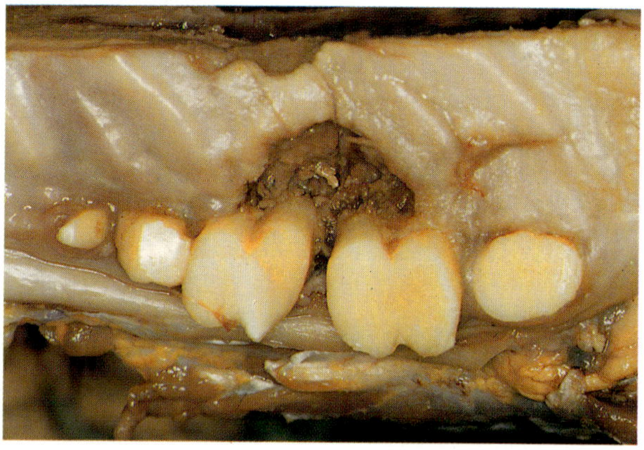

552 Cardiac thrombosis — Case 1a — aardvark. This animal was suffering from chronic dyspnoea of unknown origin. He developed epistaxis and heart failure. Postmortem examination revealed a hydrothorax and a large thrombus attached to the right atrioventricular valve which extended into the right ventricle and atrium.

553 Palatal food packing — Case 1b. On postmortem examination, food packing between the upper molars, with the presence of a deep periodontal defect, was found.

554

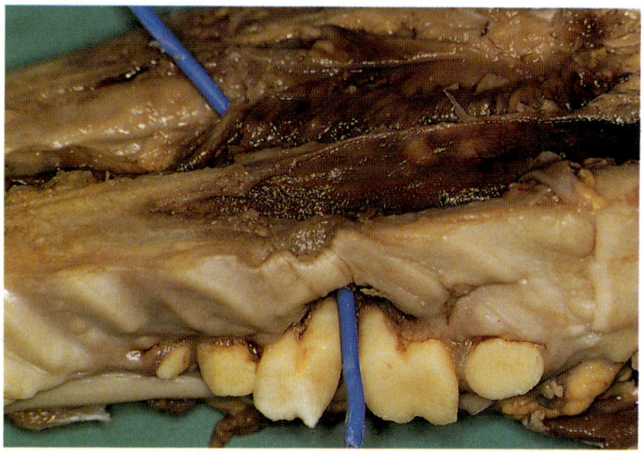

555

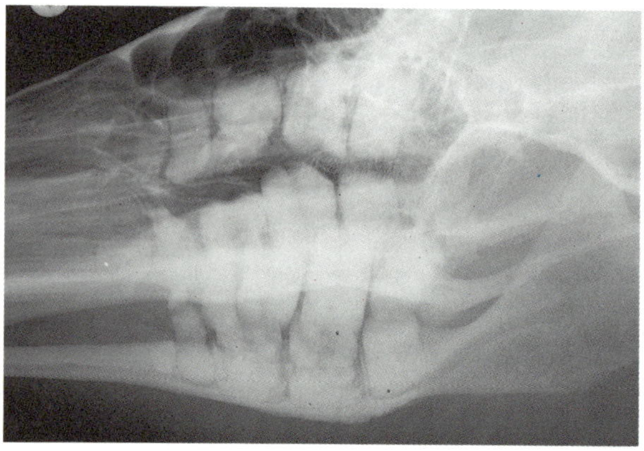

554 Probe in oronasal fistula — Case 1c. The periodontal defect penetrated into the nasal cavity and was associated with a purulent unilateral rhinitis. The pathologist indicated that the oronasal fistula and the subsequent rhinitis were most likely to have been the consequence of periodontal disease. It was also felt that the resultant bacteraemia contributed to cardiac changes that gave rise to the thrombus which in turn precipitated the heart failure.

555 Preoperative radiograph — Case 2a — aardvark. The animal developed a hard mandibular swelling with no discharge or sinus tract. Extensive remodelling at the ventral border of the mandible body was visible on the radiograph. Some of the mandibular and maxillary teeth showed irregular radiolucency, indicating resorptive lesions. Extractions of the affected teeth was the only treatment possible. Due to the highly limited access to the oral cavity, the surgery was performed through a buccotomy approach.

556

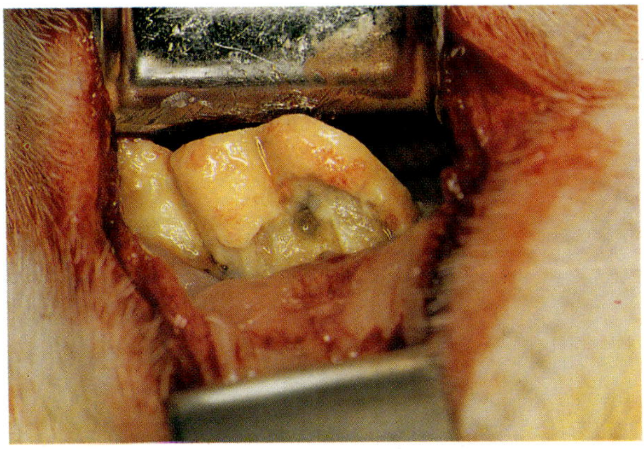

557

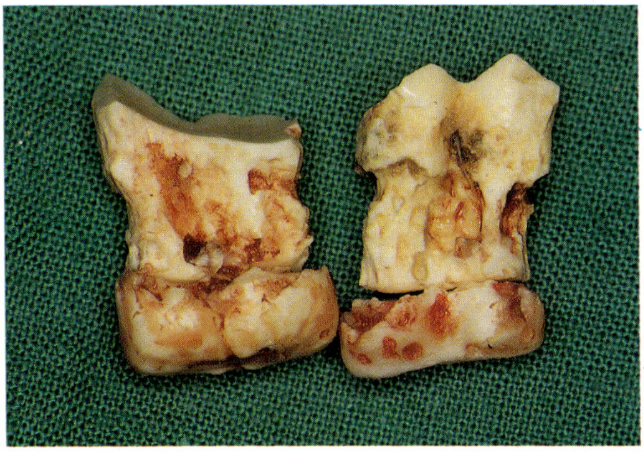

556 Molar cavity visible through buccotomy — Case 2b. This cervical cavity resembles resorptive lesions often seen in domestic cats. Due to the mesiodistal morphology of the teeth, forceps extractions were strongly contraindicated and would have resulted in mandibular fracture. A buccal mucoperiosteal flap was reflected and the buccal bone removed with great care, mainly in a guttering fashion, so as not to weaken the fragile mandible. The extracted teeth had a fetid odour.

557 Extracted teeth with resorptive lesions — Case 2c. Irregular cavities extend subgingivally, close to the apices.

558 Longitudinal section of the tooth — Case 2d (×*12*). Histological examination of the extracted teeth identified lesions close to the apical growth regions. There is strong suggestion that the cervical cavities at the gingival margin migrated from the apical area in these elodont teeth. The diagnosis was external resorption caused by odontoclastic activity associated with chronic periodontal disease. Inflammation was thought to have been produced by accumulated debris on the surface of the teeth, which may have been caused by the unnatural soft diet of the animal. No evidence of caries was found.

558

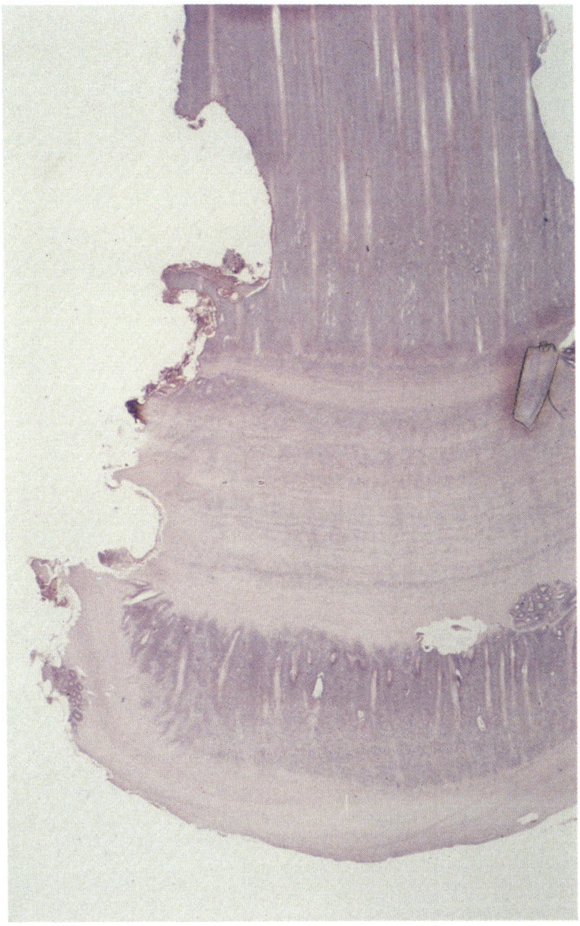

559 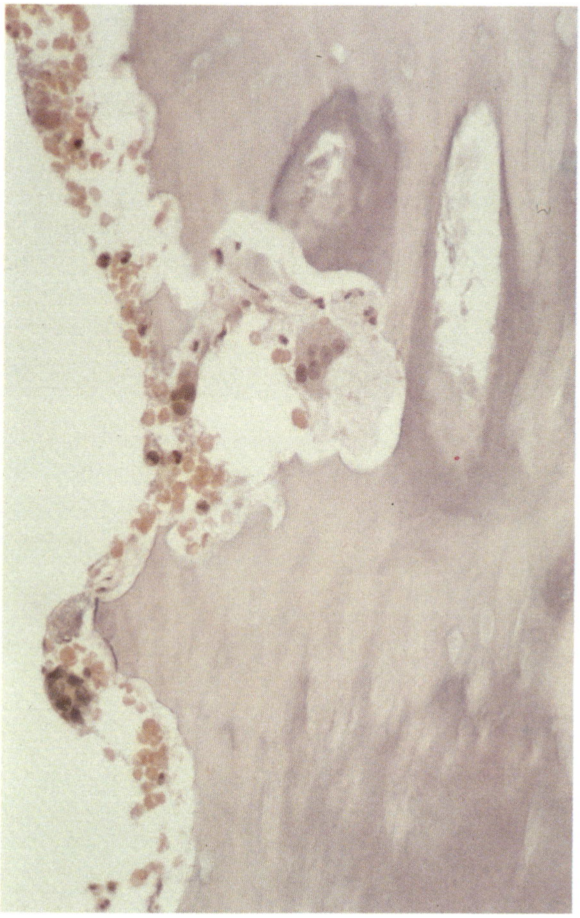

559 Close-up of section — Case 2e (*×290*). Two odontoclasts, a few mononuclear inflammatory cells and debris are seen in the resorption cavity.

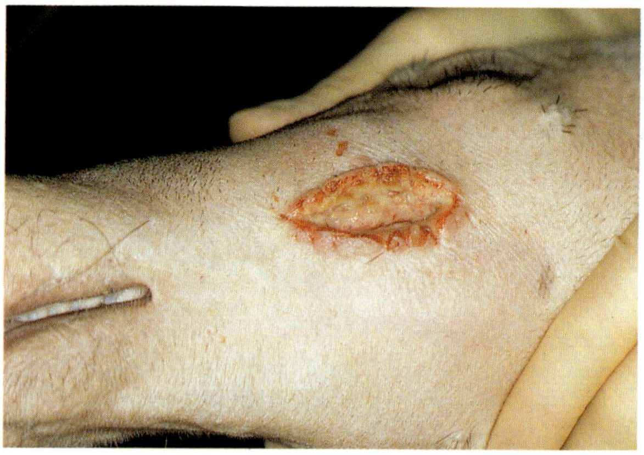 560

560 Infected incision one week postoperative — Case 2f. Due to contamination by the paste-like diet the closure of the buccotomy broke down resulting in a fistula. The extraction sockets also became infected. The sockets were irrigated and dressed with ribbon gauze soaked in Whitehead's Varnish and changed at two weekly intervals under sedation. The animal was treated with systemic antibiotics for a period of four weeks.

561 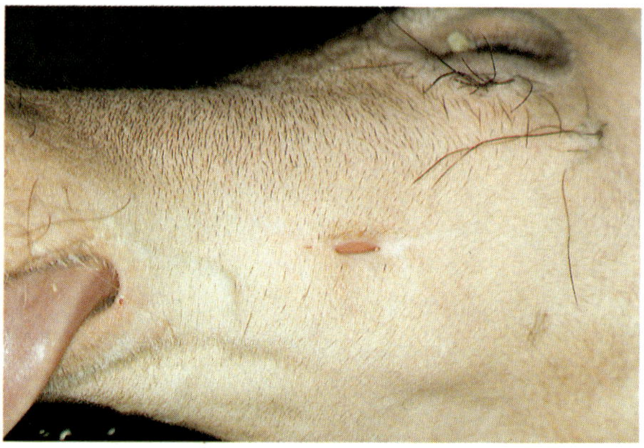

561 Six months postoperative — Case 2g. Healing of the sockets was complete in four weeks. The fistula healed through secondary intention, but a 10 mm long defect remained which was closed surgically. Teeth on the opposite side also had to be extracted and a buccostomy was prepared during surgery to facilitate aftercare. The extraction sites were gently packed with ribbon gauze soaked in Whitehead's Varnish for a period of two weeks and systemic antibiotics were given. Food was withheld for two days postoperatively and the animal was maintained on water only to minimise the possibility of alveolar contamination. Healing of the sockets was uneventful and the buccostomy was surgically closed four weeks after the extractions.

Anelodonts: hypsodonts

Order Artiodactyla

Camelidae — camels and llamas $\frac{1}{3}:\frac{0-1}{0-1}:\frac{2-3}{2}:\frac{3}{3} = 28 - 34$

562

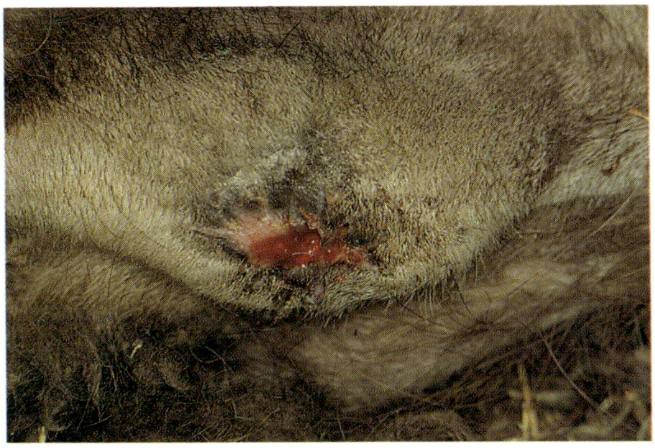

563

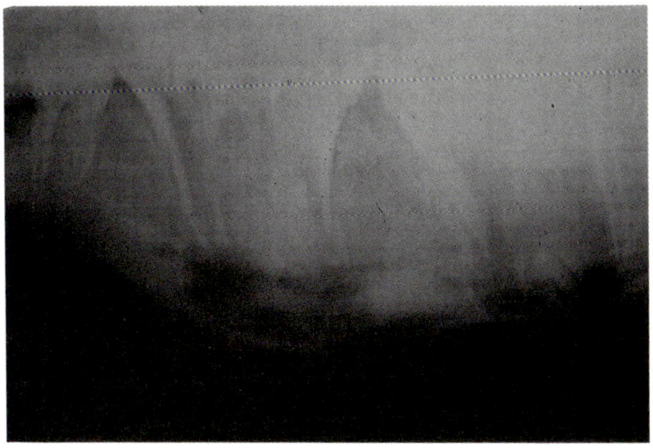

562 Submandibular swelling — Case 1a — Bactrian camel. A hard swelling at the ventral border of the mandible of an 18-month-old camel is shown. Although some osseous remodelling had taken place, the spongy consistency of the superficial tissues indicated a considerable soft-tissue oedema. A relatively small amount of discharge, in relation to the size of the lesion, was present.

563 Radiograph of mandible — Case 1b. Radiography revealed a radiolucent periapical area involving the second lower primary molar.

564

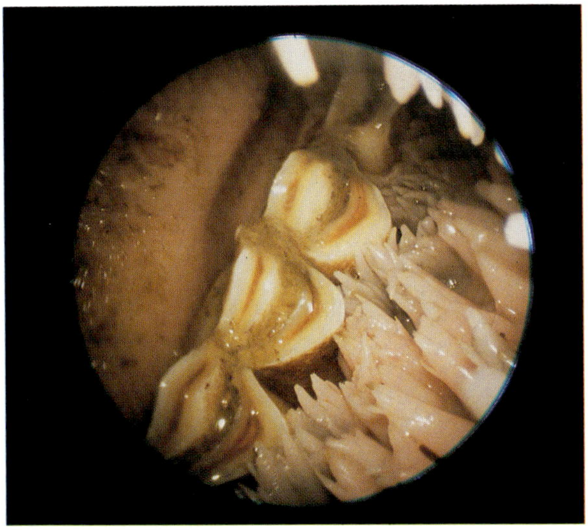

564 Endoscopic view — Case 1c. Intra-oral examination with a rigid 50° angled laparoscope demonstrated that the tricuspid primary molar lacked infundibular cementum and there was a direct communication into the pulp chambers, which were packed with food debris. This contributed to pulp necrosis and periapical abscess formation. The absence of infundibular cementum and perforations in the molars of camelids is not uncommon. In young animals the aetiology is developmental, while in old animals it may be degenerative. In the author's experience, primary molars with this defect are more likely to give rise to clinical symptoms.

565

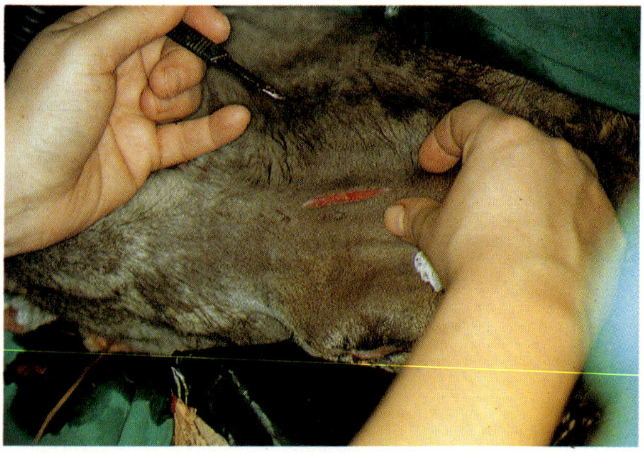

565 Incision line — Case 1d. Because of the relatively long, fine, divergent root formation, the extended mesiodistal dimensions of the crown and the brittle consistency of the teeth, forceps extraction is not possible on these teeth. The root morphology is quite different from that of the horse, and the teeth are not suitable for repulsion from an apical direction. A buccotomy approach is the treatment of choice. It is important to note the position of the rostral border of the masseter lies more caudal in the camelids and bovids than in the equids. This allows for easier access to the first permanent molars through the buccotomy approach before encountering the external maxillary vessels and parotid duct.

566

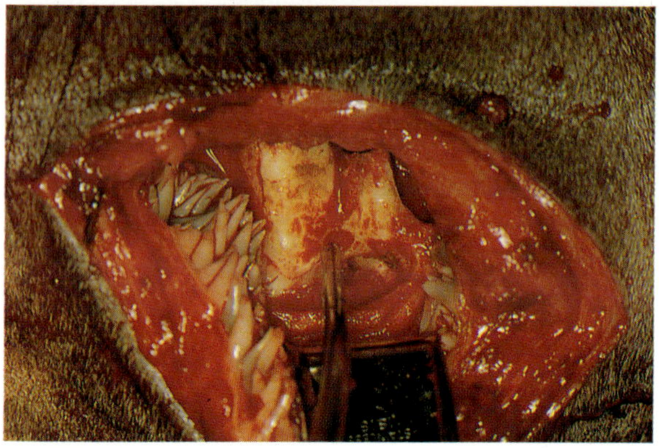

566 Mucoperiosteal flap reflected — Case 1e. Once inside the oral cavity, normal oral surgical principles are followed. In young animals, mandibular sockets heal without packing although some food will collect postoperatively. Packing of the sockets in older animals and large maxillary defects is recommended for a period of two weeks because of the risk of antral/nasal involvement.

567

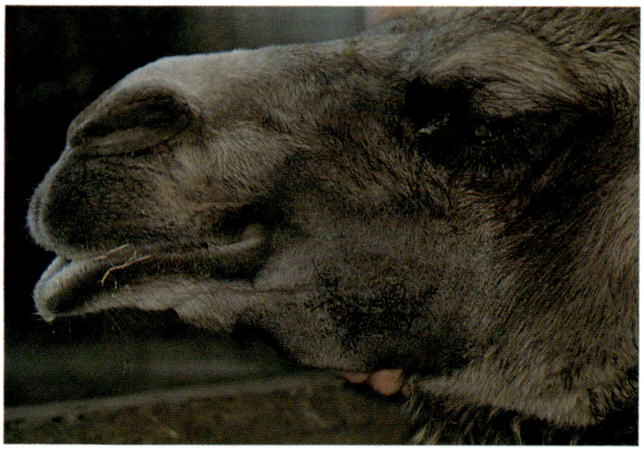

567 Postoperative healing. Typical healing pattern of a different animal one week postoperatively. Skin healing was complete.

568

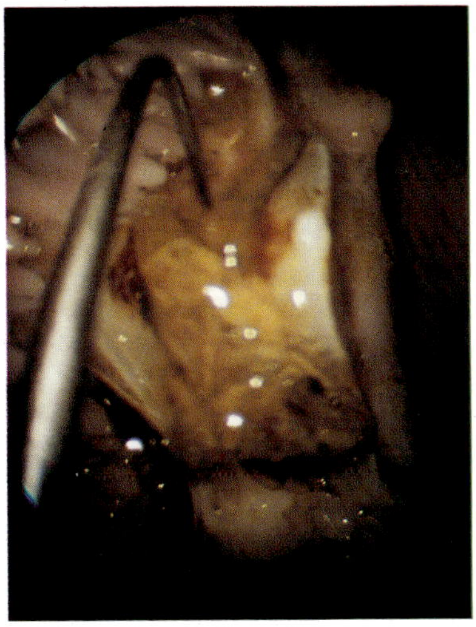

568 Endoscopic view of a permanent molar — Case 1f. Food debris being probed away from the infundibulum of the first lower permanent molar.

569

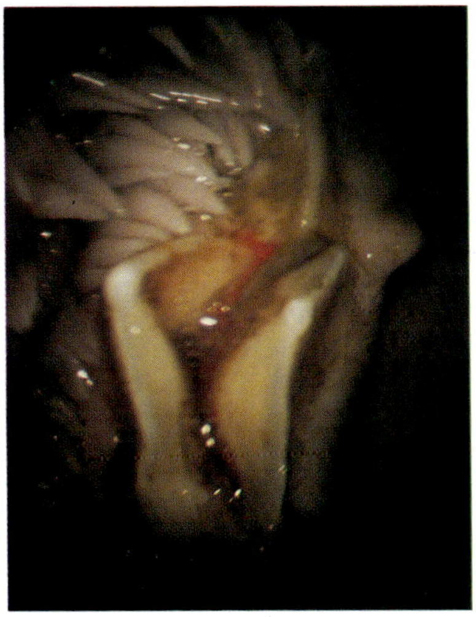

569 Endoscopic view of a pulp exposure — Case 1g. The tooth was at the eruption stage. No infundibular cementum was present and there was a direct communication into the pulp chambers. Pulp was still vital and bleeding.

570

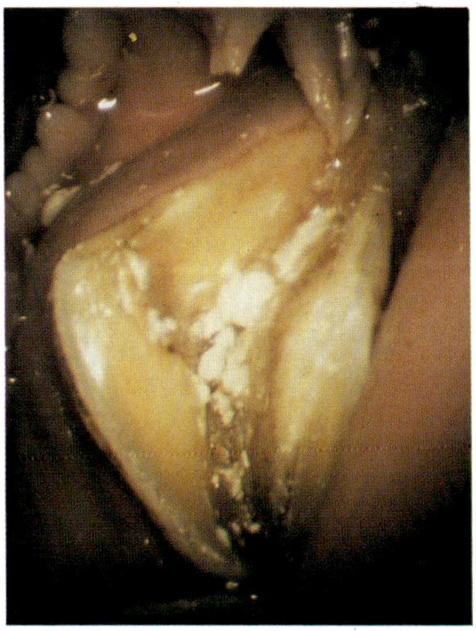

570 Partial coronal pulpectomy — Case 1h. Access to the posterior teeth of herbivores is highly limited and a buccotomy cannot be justified for restorative treatment. To prevent pulp necrosis and periapical infection, partial coronal pulpectomy was performed and a calcium hydroxide dressing was placed via a labial approach.

71

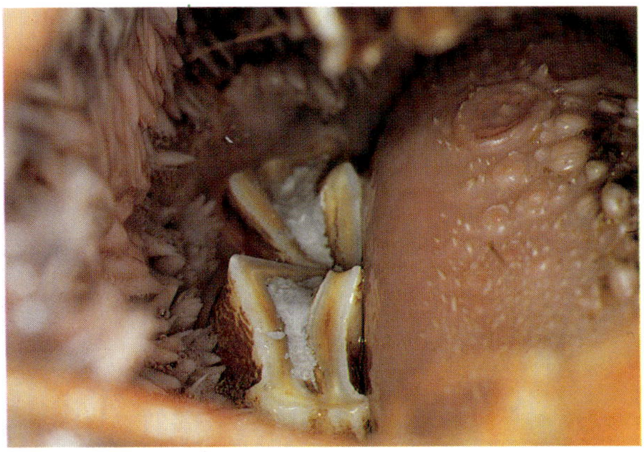

571 Final restorations — Case 1j. Occlusal amalgam restorations in place.

572

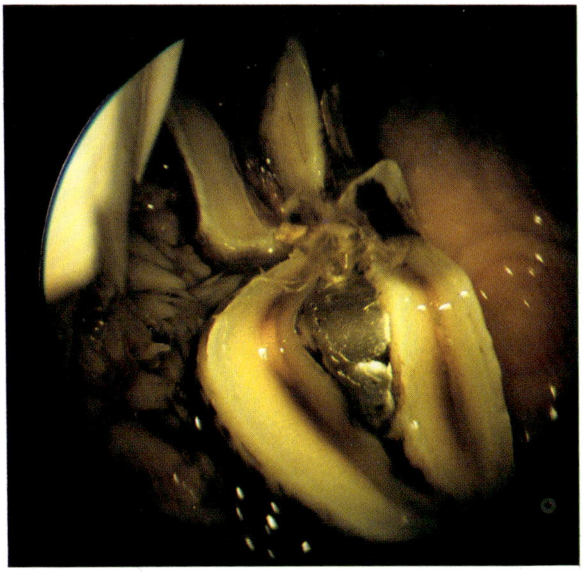

572 Postoperative view at two years — Case 1k. Even though the amalgam restorations survived well in this destructive environment, the long-term prognosis of such a procedure must be guarded. A more radical pulp resection may have been helpful in allowing the placement of a deeper occlusal restoration.

573

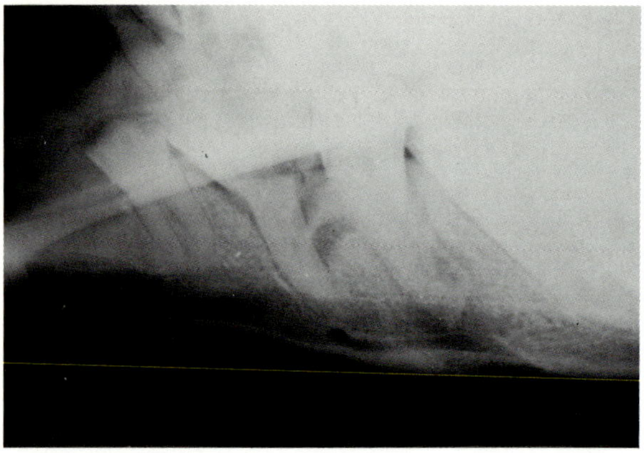

573 Radiograph of a lower primary molar — Case 2a — Bactrian camel. Mandibular swelling with a discharge can also be caused by dental trauma. In this case the second lower primary molar was fractured through the bifurcation in a one-year-old animal. The food packing in the fracture line and the resultant chronic infection caused osteolysis. The increased mobility this created and the midline fracture allowed the roots to be rotated separately and extraction through a labial approach with equine forceps was possible.

574

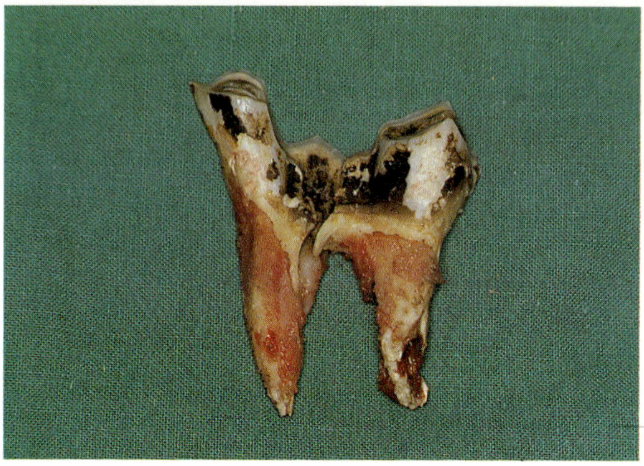

574 Extracted tooth — Case 2b. The relocation of the extracted segments demonstrates the fracture through the furcation.

575

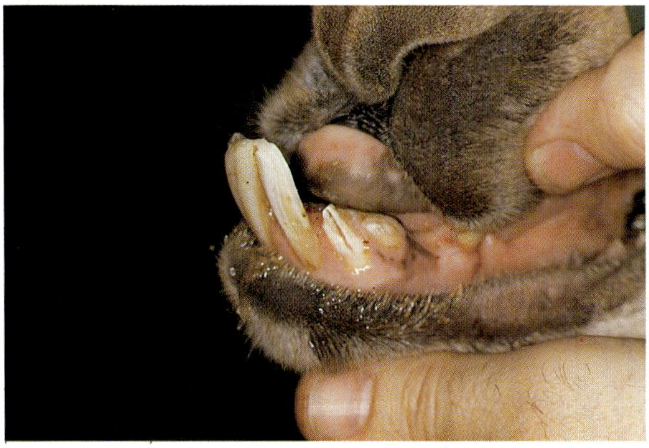

576

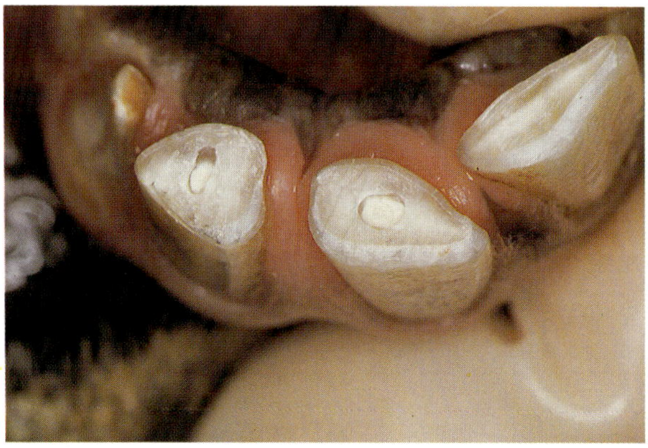

575 Overerupted lower incisors — Case 3a — llama. The incisors of the camelid family are anelodont teeth, although different species appear to have a different age at which apical maturity occurs and amelo- and dentinogenesis ceases. These overerupted incisors, caused by a skeletal discrepancy, hindered prehension of food and placed abnormally large forces of leverage on the roots and the periodontal tissues. This leverage can contribute to excessive mobility and early tooth loss.

576 Incisors reduced with air rotor, pulp exposed — Case 3b. Reduction of the length of the incisors is acceptable as long as basic dental principles are followed. If any appreciable length of crown height is removed the pulp is usually exposed. These teeth do not possess the healing potential of elodont teeth, and pulp necrosis and its sequel follow root canal exposures.

577

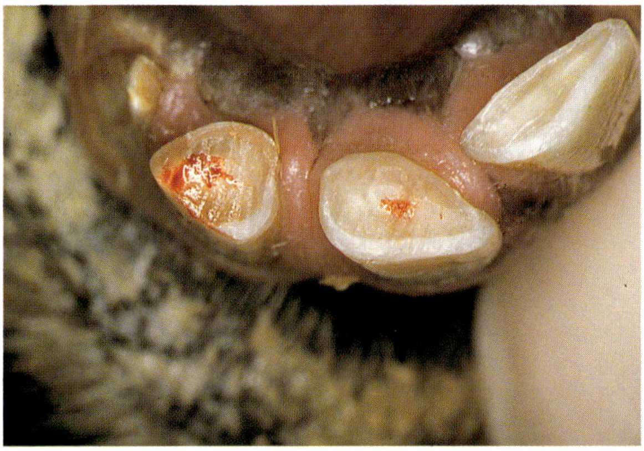

578

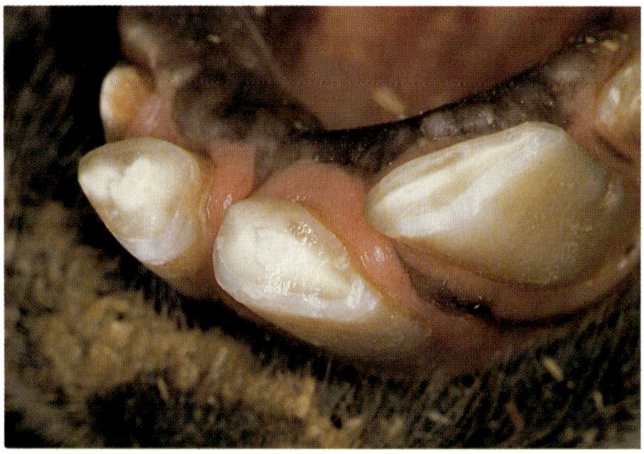

577 Partial coronal pulpectomy — Case 3c. Partial coronal pulpectomy is performed on the same lines as with other animals. A calcium hydroxide lining was placed.

578 Final restoration — Case 3d. The final restoration, with composite filling material.

579

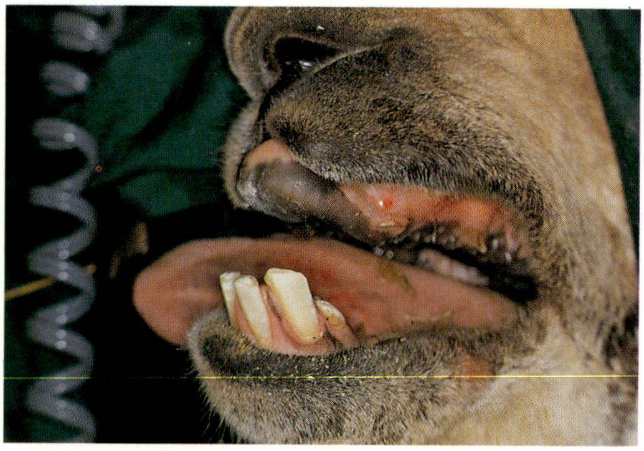

579 Final bite — Case 3e. Postoperative bite is more favourable for the prehension of food. The animal gained weight rapidly after treatment.

580

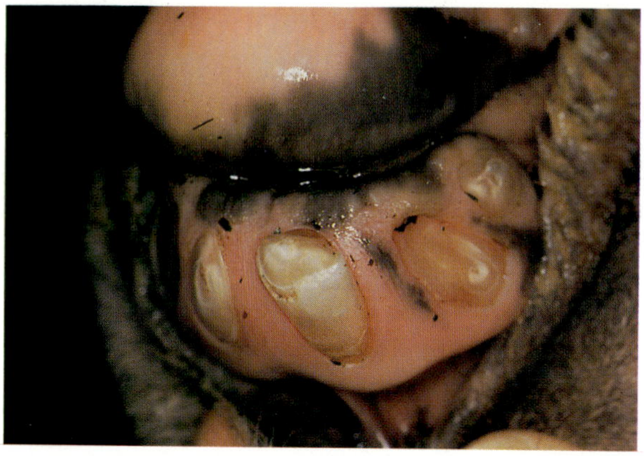

580 Five-year follow-up — Case 3f. No overeruption had taken place as marked abrasion of the incisors was evident. The root canals of the teeth treated had solid secondary dentine and no pulp exposures were present.

581

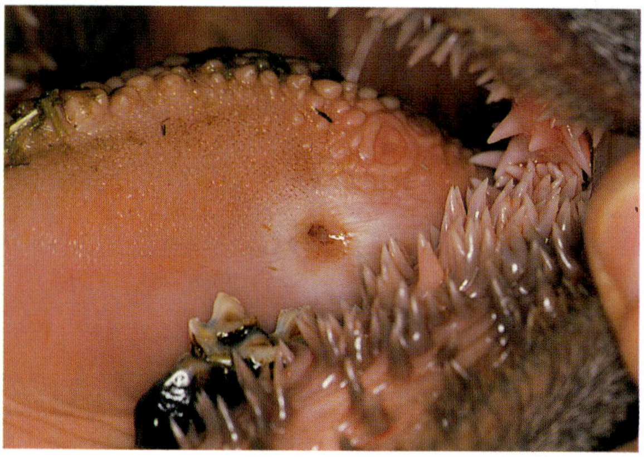

581 Ulcerated tongue. Irregular wear of the cheek teeth can create sharp lingual points that ulcerate the tongue of camelids. The most efficient way to reduce these spurs is with tungsten or diamond burrs in extended industrial die grinders, under sedation or a full general anaesthetic.

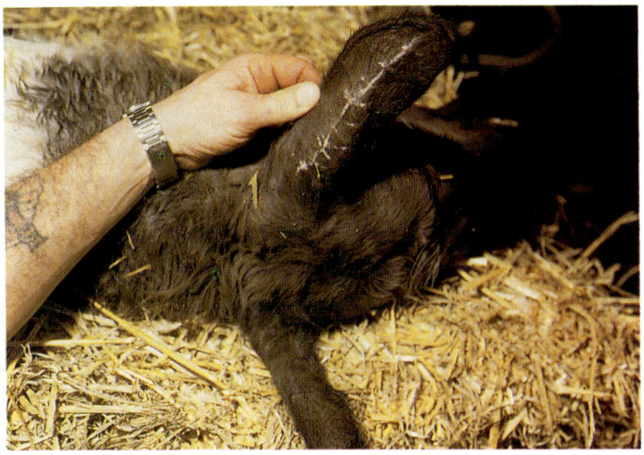

582

582 Split ear — llama. One of the management problems often encountered in the keeping of male camelids is the severe injuries they inflict upon other animals. It is not the author's position to discuss the ethics of disarming but to give guidelines for the most appropriate treatment options in cases where such treatment is to be performed.

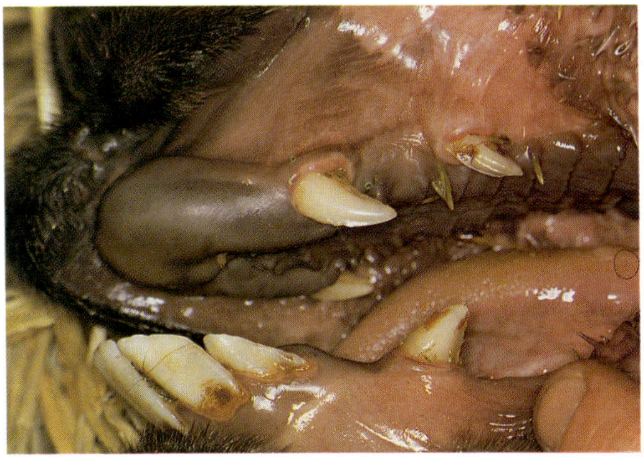

583

583 Canines and upper incisor — Case 4a — llama. The razor-sharp canines and upper incisors are responsible for the trauma. Extraction of these teeth is extremely difficult because of their long bulbous roots and the possibility of mandibular fractures due to the thin body of the mandible in the diastema region.

Amputation of the crowns without following dental principles is unacceptable. Root canal treatment after amputation may be considered, but the morphology of the camelid's apical foramina is a highly complex delta formation which does not lend itself to root canal treatment. It must also be considered that endodontics of six caniform teeth may be an excessively prolonged anaesthetic session. Coronal pulpectomies with calcium hydroxide dressings is another option. The third disarming technique is to amputate the crowns and bury the roots with vital pulp tissue still present apical to the alveolar crest and gingival tissues. The underlying principle is that the exposed pulp tissue will not degenerate, but remain vital if protected from the oral environment, while its blood supply is maintained through the root apex and the overlying periosteum.

584

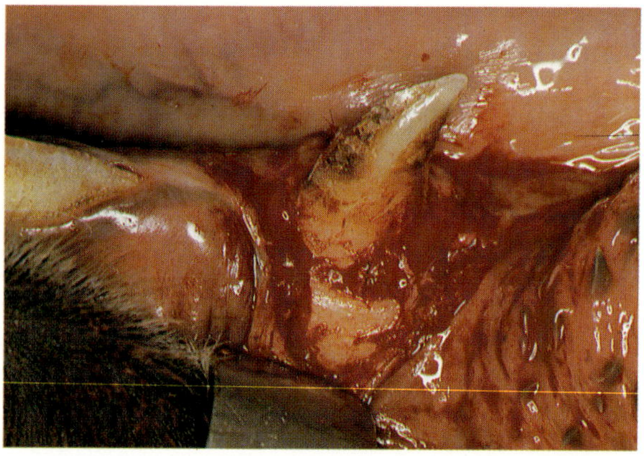

584 Buccal flap reflected — Case 4b. A full-thickness labial mucoperiosteal flap needs to be raised to expose the alveolar bone.

585

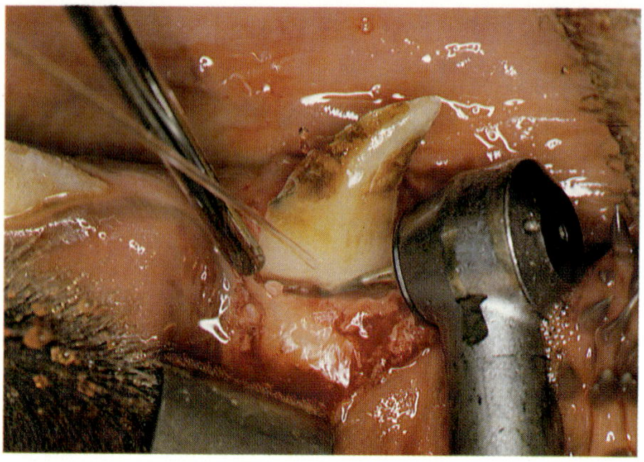

585 Crown being amputated — Case 4c. With an air-rotor and copious irrigation, the crown is amputated apical to the alveolar crest.

586

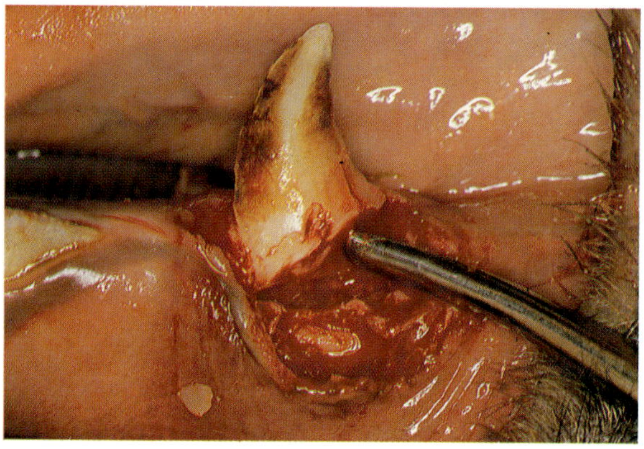

586 Crown being elevated — Case 4d. The amputated crown is dissected away from the alveolar bone and elevated with a Coupland's chisel.

587 Reduction of root — Case 4e. To allow better approximation of the gingival flap and encourage primary healing the root may be reduced further, apical to the alveolar crest. This is best accomplished with a large round burr and profuse irrigation.

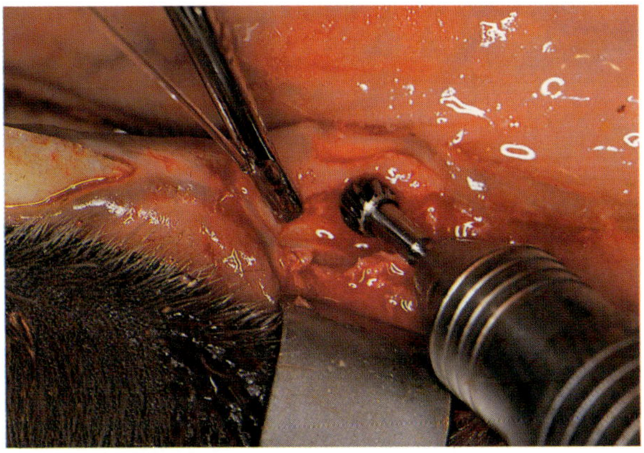
587

588 Sutured flap — Case 4f. The gingival flaps are sutured without tension after having had their margins freshened up. Healing was uneventful.

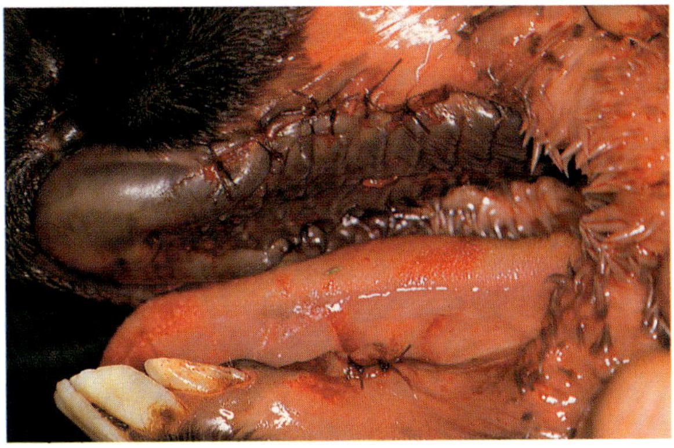
588

589 Buccal sinus tract — llama. A periapical abscess discharging intra-orally. No pulpal exposure was present, but through trauma the apex of the maxillary incisor was fractured horizontally, resulting in pulpal necrosis. The tooth was extracted through a flap procedure.

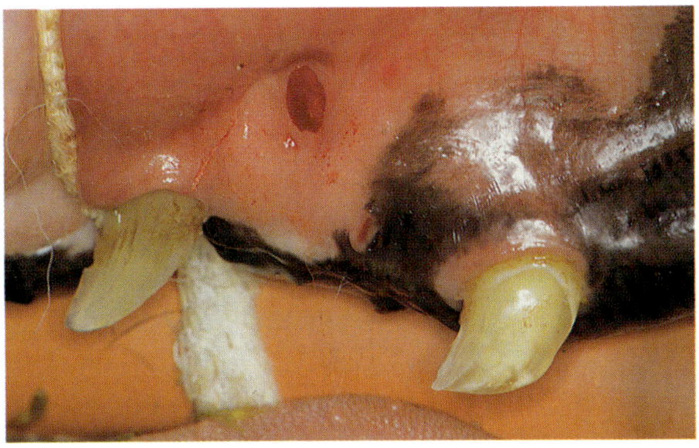
589

Bovidae — sheep family $\frac{0}{3}:\frac{0}{1}:\frac{3}{3}:\frac{3}{3} = 32$

Dental disease of bovids often presents as periodontal disease of the cheek teeth. As with camelids, intra-oral examination is difficult, owing to the limited opening of the mouth, and by the time the disease is diagnosed it is at an advanced and chronic stage. It is doubtful if periodic oral examination and early treatment of periodontal lesions would offer a better prognosis.

590

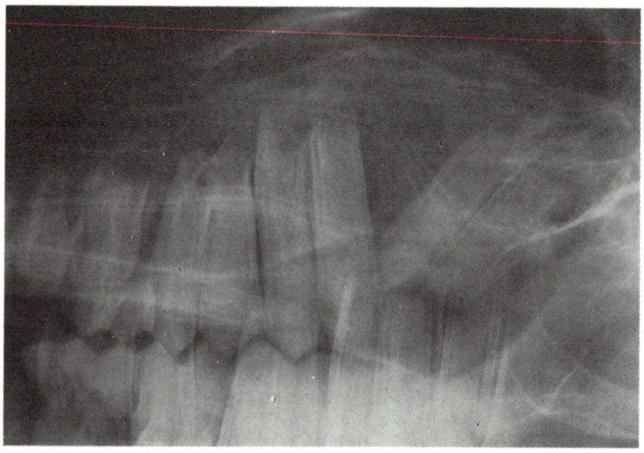

590 Radiograph of an impacted upper third molar — Case 1a — North American bighorn sheep. This two-year-old animal did not exhibit facial swelling or discharge. The only sign of oral pain was a bruxing behaviour. The significance of this phenomenon has not been proven but needs to be noted. Intra-oral endoscopic examination revealed no pathology. Radiographic examination indicated a mesioangularly impacted upper third molar that was fully unerupted.

591

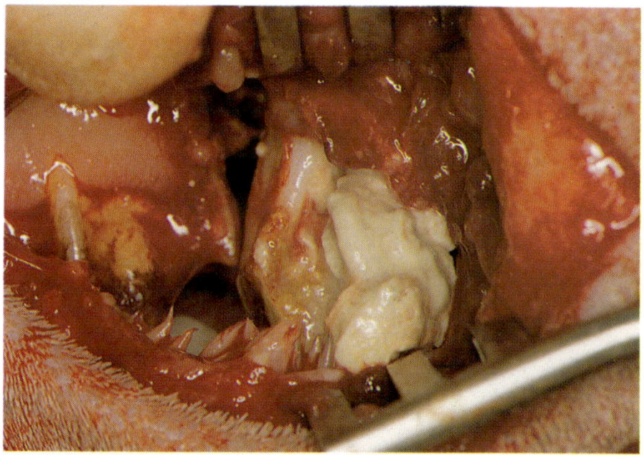

591 The third molar being elevated — Case 1b. Access was through a buccotomy incision. A buccal mucoperiosteal flap was reflected to expose the third molar. Both second and third molars were mobile. Extensive bone destruction was present, with sequestrum formation and frank pus. The teeth involved were extracted. The osseous defect was curetted to healthy bleeding bone. A ribbon gauze pack impregnated with Whitehead's Varnish was placed in the defect to prevent food packing and encourage granulation. The pack was changed at two-week intervals under sedation through a buccostomy. Food packing was controlled and the socket appeared to heal. The stoma was closed one month postoperatively.

592

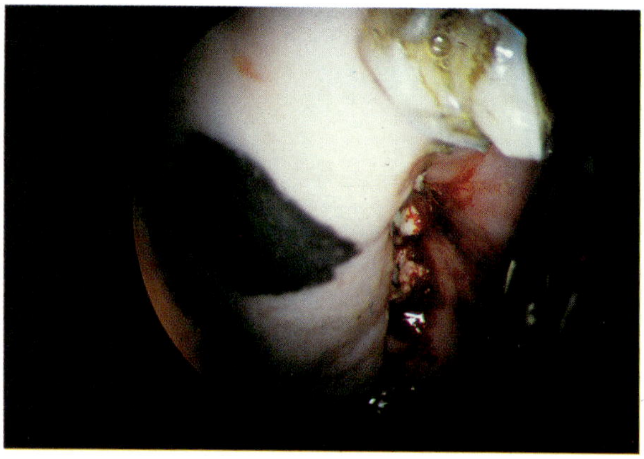

592 Medium-term result — endoscopic view — Case 1c. Two months after removal of the pack, the animal developed a small facial fistula in the infra-orbital region. Intra-oral endoscopic examination revealed a small oro-antral fistula through which food was packing into the maxillary sinus, causing relapse of the osteomyelitis. The animal was euthanised.

593

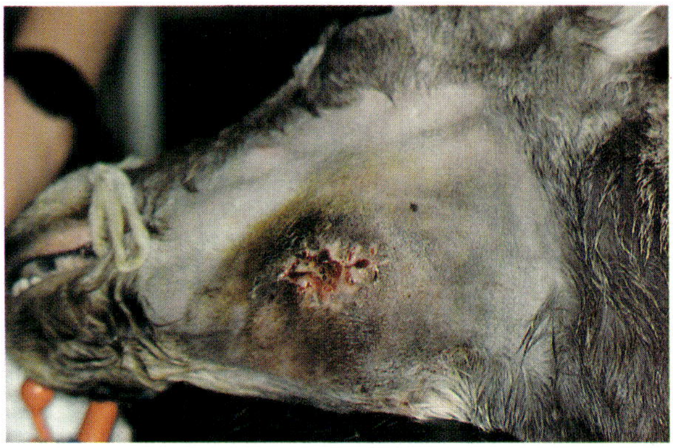

594

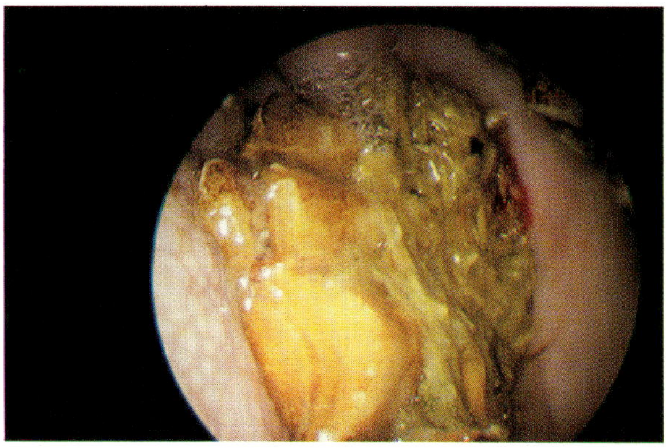

593 Mandibular osteomyelitis — Case 2a — North American bighorn sheep. The animal had a history of intermittent extra-oral swelling and neutrophilia over an eight-month period before a second opinion was requested. Previous radiography revealed no obvious abnormalities. Osteomyelitis, with extra-oral swelling and sinus tract formation, was present on examination.

594 Endoscopic view — Case 2b. Intra-oral examination revealed a periodontally involved lower third molar. Because of the limited opening of the mouth the tooth could not be exfoliated and the food packing and resultant infection became extensive and acute. The animal was suffering with septicaemia.

595

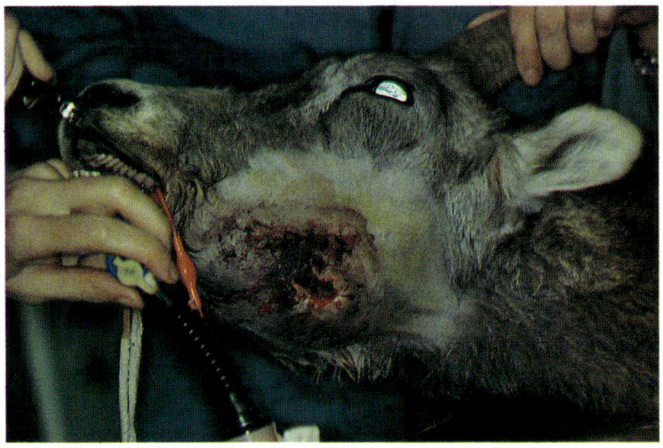

596

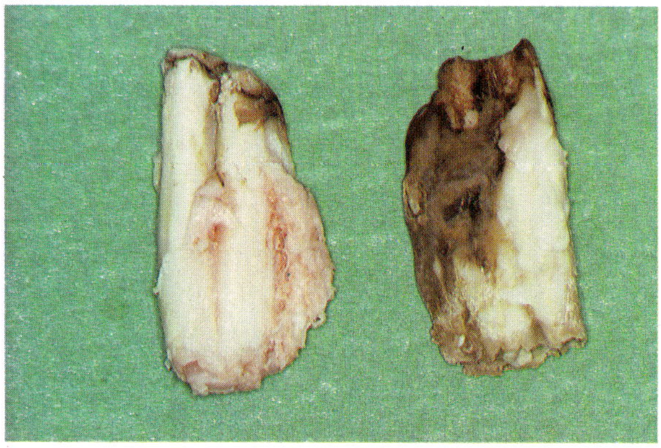

595 Immediate postoperative appearance — Case 2c. Extraction was through a buccotomy, as the lack of space made a labial approach impossible.

596 Extracted teeth — Case 2d. The lower third molar and the opposing upper molar were extracted to minimise the chance of food impaction in the socket. Loss of periodontal ligament and the infected state of the root surface is visible on the lower molar which is on the right hand side of the picture.

597

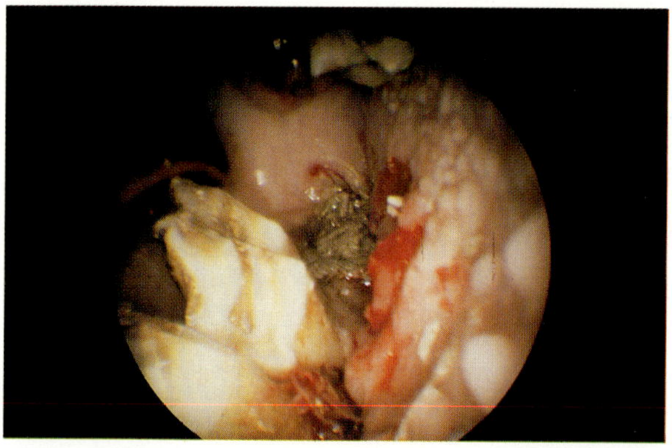

597 Immediate intra-oral postoperative appearance — Case 2e. Defect was curetted and packed as in Case 1. Systemic antibiotics were given for a four-week period.

598

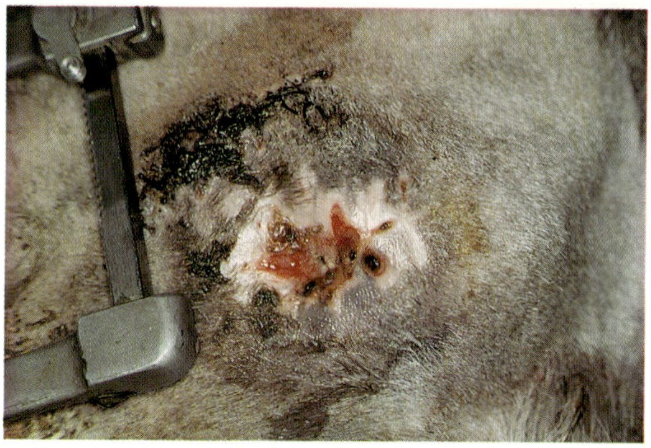

598 One week postoperative condition — Case 2f. The socket was irrigated, the sutures removed and the pack changed. Purulent discharge had ceased by this period. Subsequently, the pack was changed at two-week intervals.

599

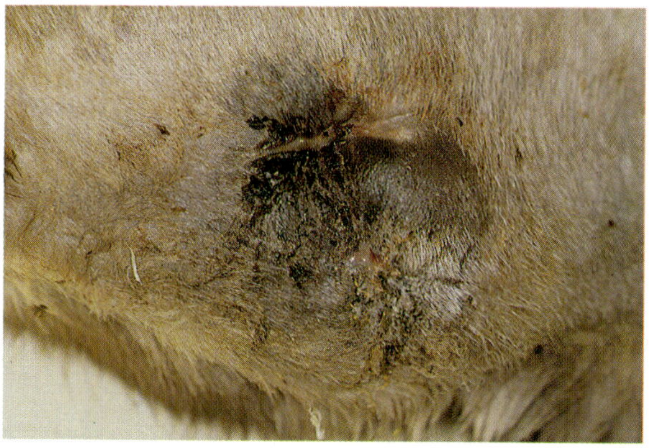

599 Four weeks postoperative condition — Case 2g. Healing was complete in seven weeks and no further infection occurred in a three-year follow-up period.

Anelodonts: brachyodonts

Order Carnivora

Felidae — cat family $\frac{3}{3}:\frac{1}{1}:\frac{3}{2}:\frac{1}{1} = 30$

Developmental defects

600 Malocclusion — Case 1a — Asian lion. This relatively minor occlusal discrepancy of a lower canine traumatising the palatal mucosa, reported by an observant animal keeper, revealed dental abnormalities and periapical infections of developmental origin.

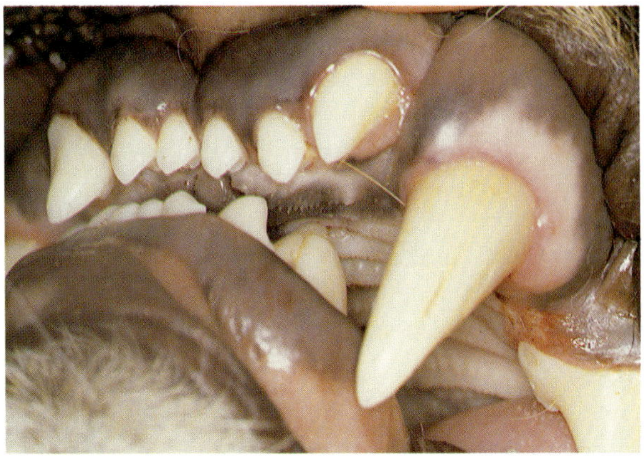

600

601 Malformed crown — Case 1b. Both lower permanent molars had complex enamel invaginations which allowed pulp necrosis to occur. The resultant periapical abscesses were discharging in the buccal sulci.

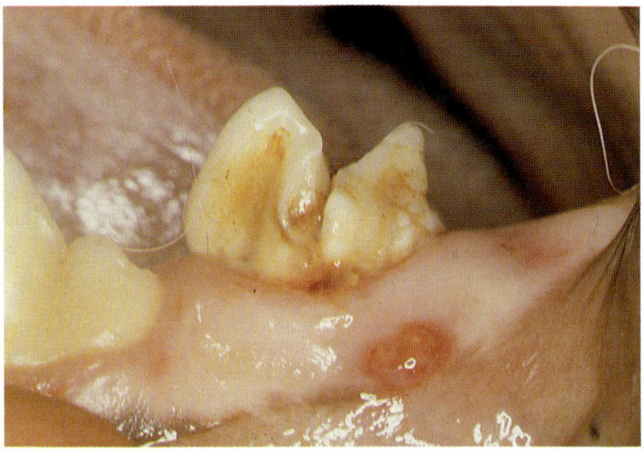

601

602 Radiograph of a molar — Case 1c. The radiographs revealed deformed teeth.

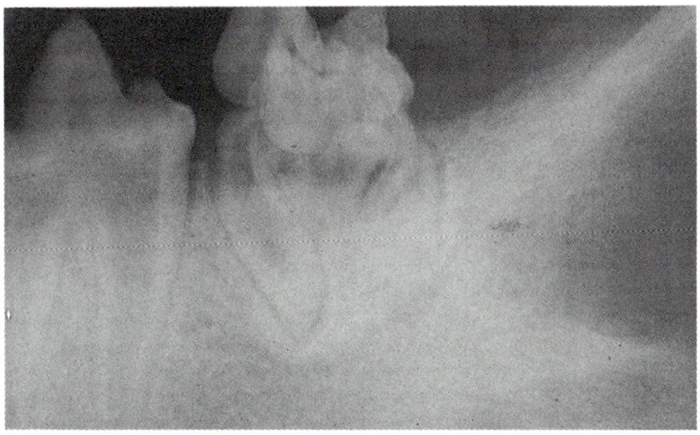

602

603 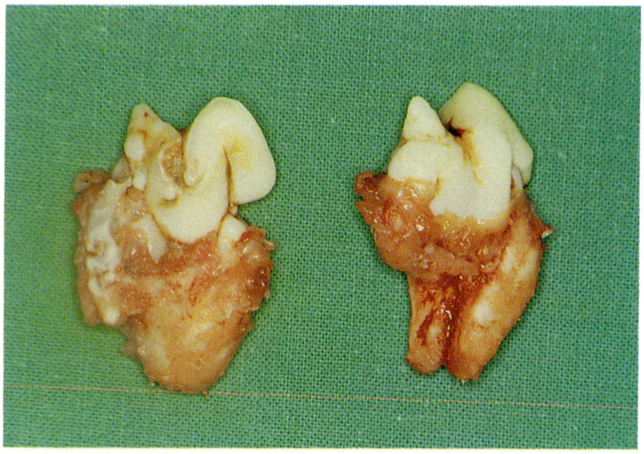

603 Extracted molars — Case 1d. The deformed roots also had developmental perforations into the root canals. Radiographs also revealed abnormalities to the lower canines and upper third incisors, but no treatment was embarked upon as there were no clinical indications for intervention.

604 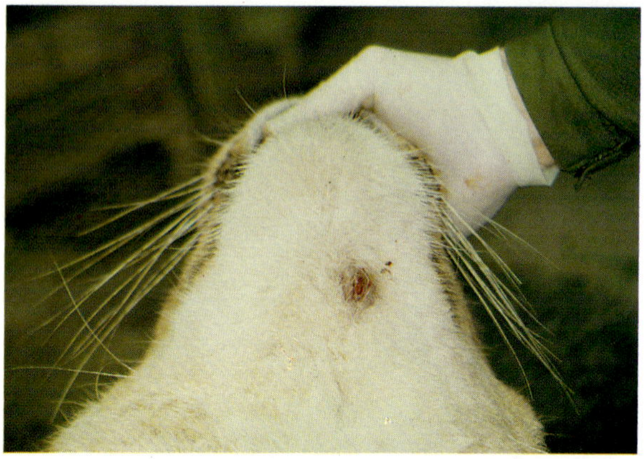

604 Submandibular sinus tract — Case 1e. Nine months after the initial surgery the lower left permanent canine developed submandibular and intra-oral abscesses and associated sinus tracts.

605 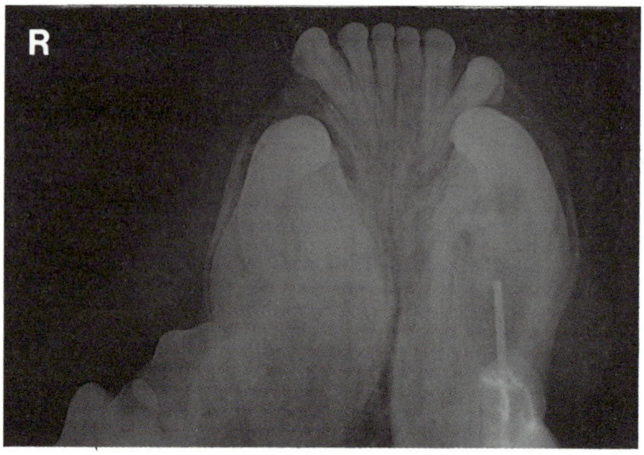

605 Radiograph of deformed lower canines — Case 1f. A metal probe on the radiograph indicates the path of the sinus tract. The tooth was extracted (see **636–639**). The extracted permanent canine had the same complex invaginated pattern with developmental pulp exposures, as that seen on the lower molars.

Discussion: Radiographic examination of the long bones and the ribs of the above animal suggested a developmental disease possibly associated with a dietary deficiency due to hand-rearing.

606 Upper premolar — resorption cavity — Case 2a — leopard. The gingival appearance and subgingival probing indicated a typical feline 'cervical resorption lesion'. In North American zoos, where carnivores are often fed a soft commercially prepared diet, these cavities are common. In Europe, where almost universally the diet of large carnivores is composed of large pieces of fibrous meat, these defects are rare. The lesions are extremely painful for the animal and extraction is the only predictable long-term treatment.

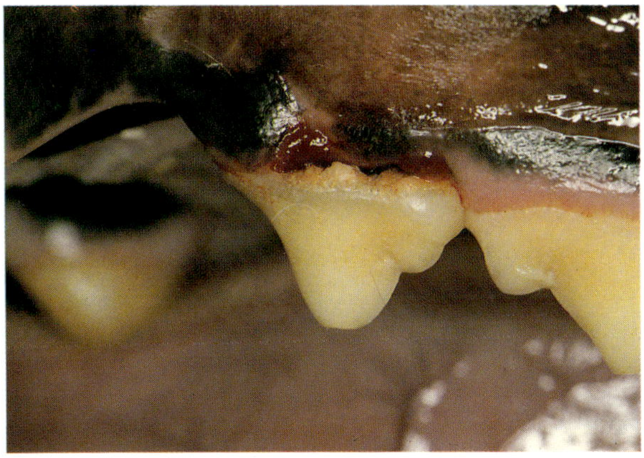

606

607 Radiograph of the tooth shown in 606 — Case 2b. A large radiolucent area at the cervical region of the tooth confirms the extensive subgingival cavity.

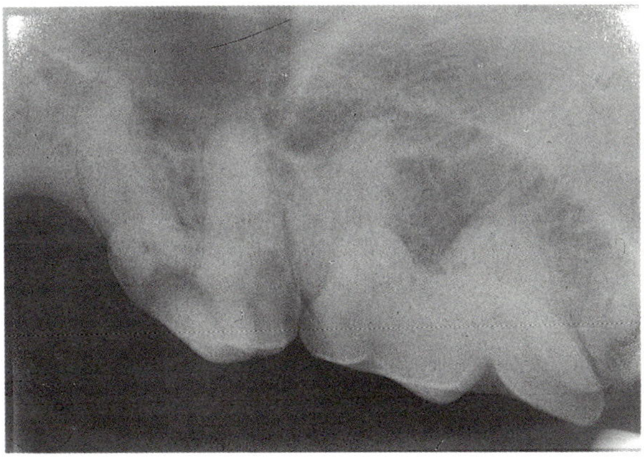

607

608 Buccal flap reflected — Case 2c. Some workers have reported alveolar bone destruction associated with resorption cavities that has lead to sinus and nasal involvement, subsequently necessitating euthanasia. In this case some osteoclastic activity is already evident at the alveolar crest.

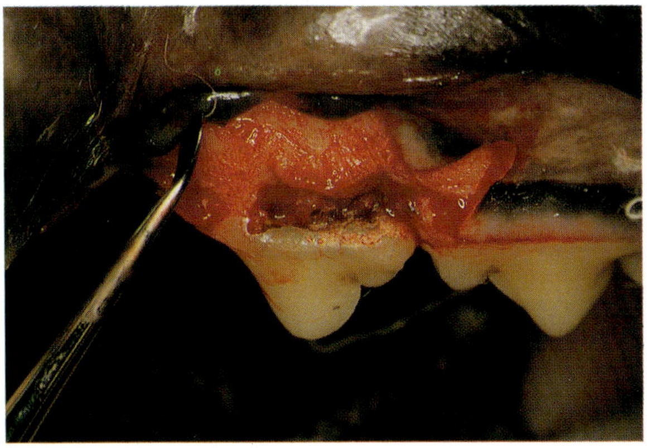

608

609

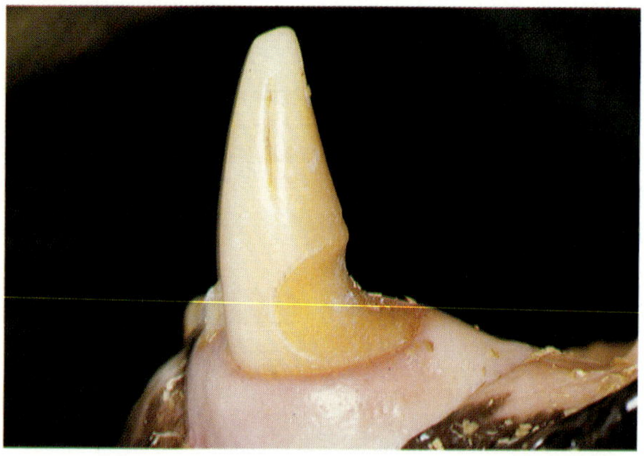

609 Crown abrasion. Bar chewing can contribute to severe abrasion grooves of the canine teeth. The weakened crowns eventually fracture, exposing the pulp. The restoration of such grooves is a futile exercise. No dental material or restorative technique can resist the forces that are inflicted by the animals on their teeth. Failures will occur rapidly.

610

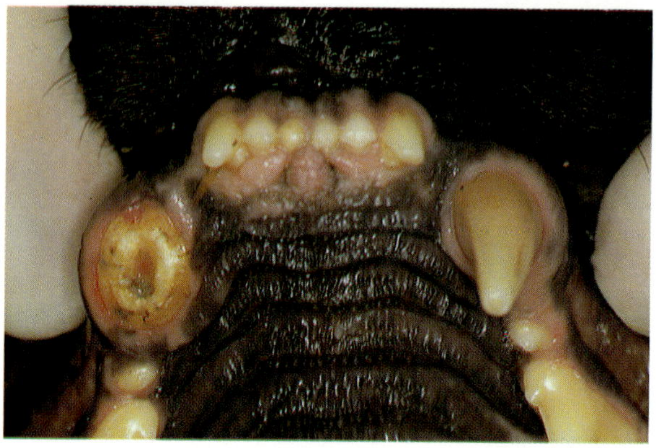

610 Fractured canine — leopard. The fracture of canines among zoo felids is common. At first the pulp will appear pink, while its vitality is maintained.

611

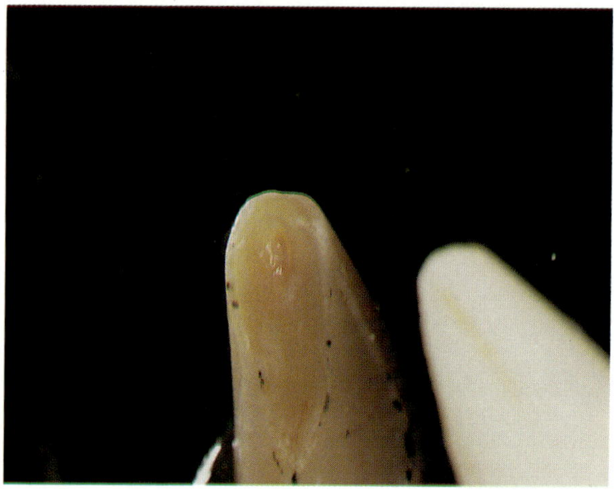

611 Tip fracture — Case 3a — tiger (mirror image). Often, only the tips of the teeth are damaged, presenting very small exposures that are easily overlooked at a cursory examination. The smaller the exposure, the more rapidly pulpitis and consequent pulpal necrosis may occur. This is due to the ease by which the exposure is occluded by debris, and the build-up of inflammatory exudate results in pressure necrosis of the pulp. In the case of this animal the lingually angulated fracture could not be seen until she was anaesthetised.

612

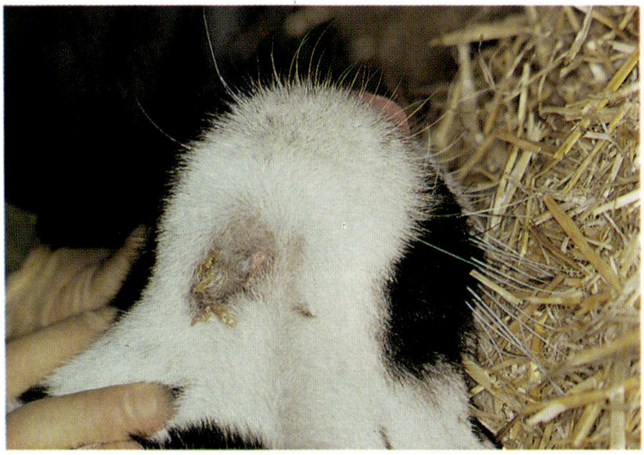

613

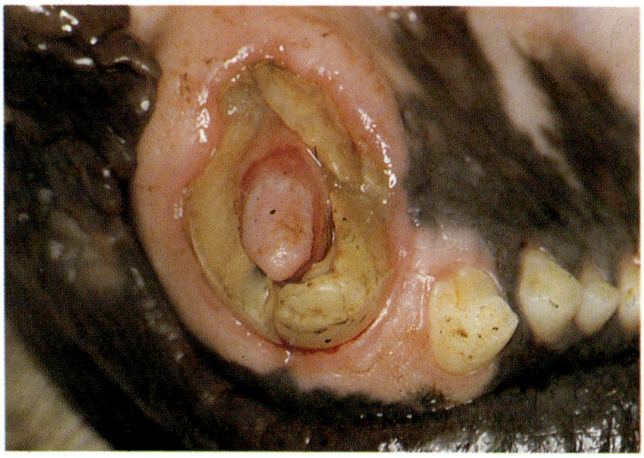

612 Chronic submandibular discharge — Case 3b. Submandibular or infra-orbital sinus tracts in the *Felidae* are usually indicative of periapical abscesses of the canine teeth. The periapical infection in this case developed into a Ludwig's angina, which was controlled with antibiotics before ortho- and retrograde endodontics were carried out on the infected root canal.

613 Pulp polyp — lion. This rare condition may occur in cases of a large pulp exposure when the blood supply to the pulp is still excellent, as in the case of immature teeth with dilated root apices. The hyperplastic pulp tissue becomes epithelialised over and granulates out of the canal. The condition is unstable and irreversible. Endodontics is the treatment of choice.

614

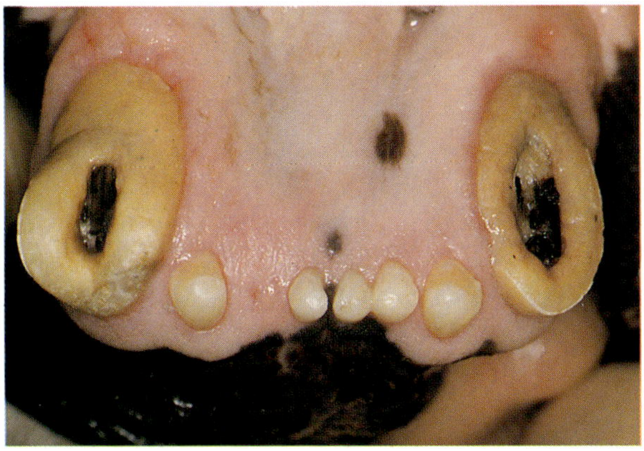

615

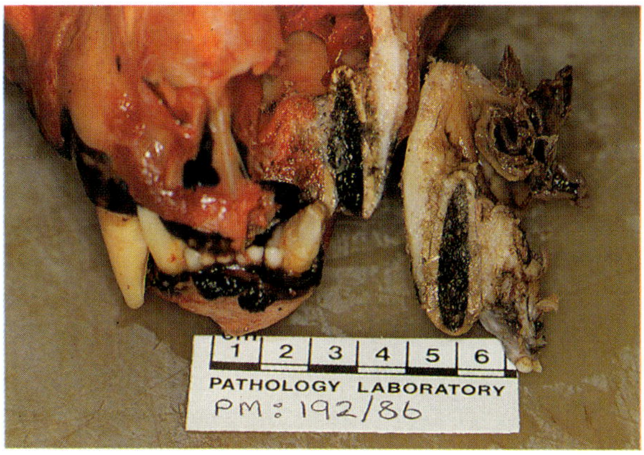

614 Canals filled with debris — lion. The normal sequel of pulp necrosis. The canals filled with putrid material, be it necrotic pulp tissue or food.

615 Postmortem section — cheetah. Clinical signs of dental pain or extra-oral pathology are not always present in cases of dental trauma. Nevertheless, chronic infection of the teeth invariably occurs with the resultant local and systemic consequences. This postmortem case demonstrates the quantity of necrotic material and periapical osteolysis present in a previously undiagnosed fractured canine.

616
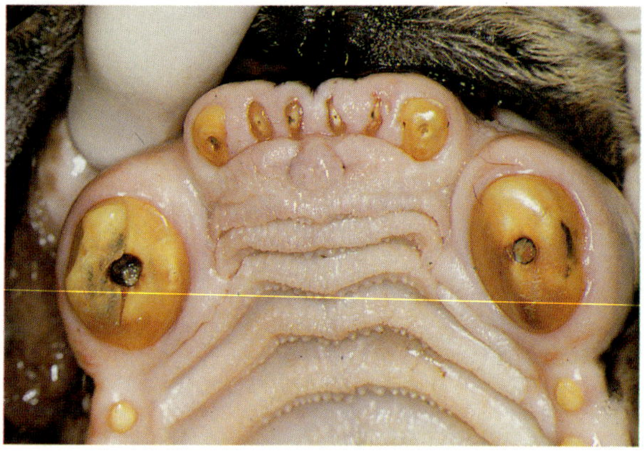

617
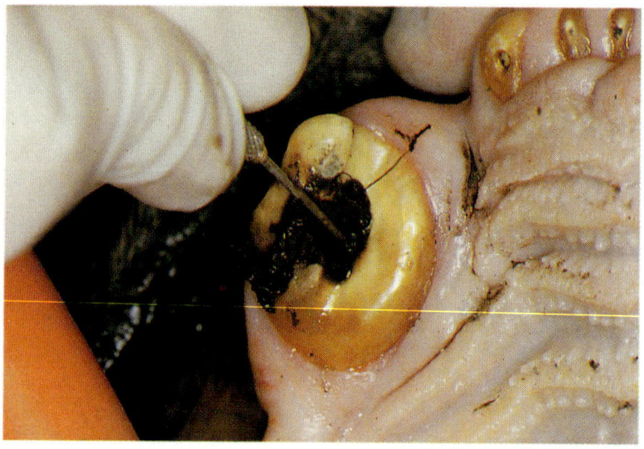

616 Infected root canals — Case 4a — tiger. Root canal exposures, whether the pulp is vital or necrotic, should not be ignored. They should be treated the least traumatic way that will give a predictable result. This usually entails endodontic treatment to a high standard.

617 Root debridement — Case 4b. The principles of endodontic treatment on zoo carnivores are the same as for other animals. The dimensions encountered can make the treatment more difficult and time consuming. Unless one is fully prepared and equipped for such obstacles the results of the treatment will be poor.

618
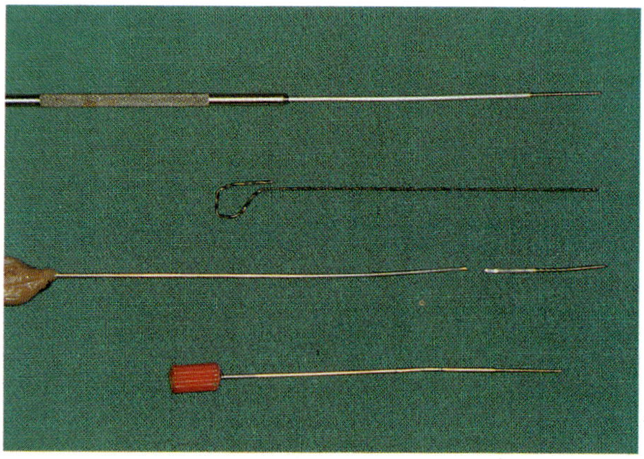

618 Selection of long endodontic instruments. Factory-made files of the required length (at the top of the picture), are far more desirable than instruments of normal length extended by soldering on to home-made handles, which are liable to break. Fractured tips in the canals may not only contribute to failure of the procedure, but extended or repeated general anaesthetics and invasive surgery may be necessary to complete the treatment. Coping saw blades can be used to serve as large-diameter barbed broaches.

619
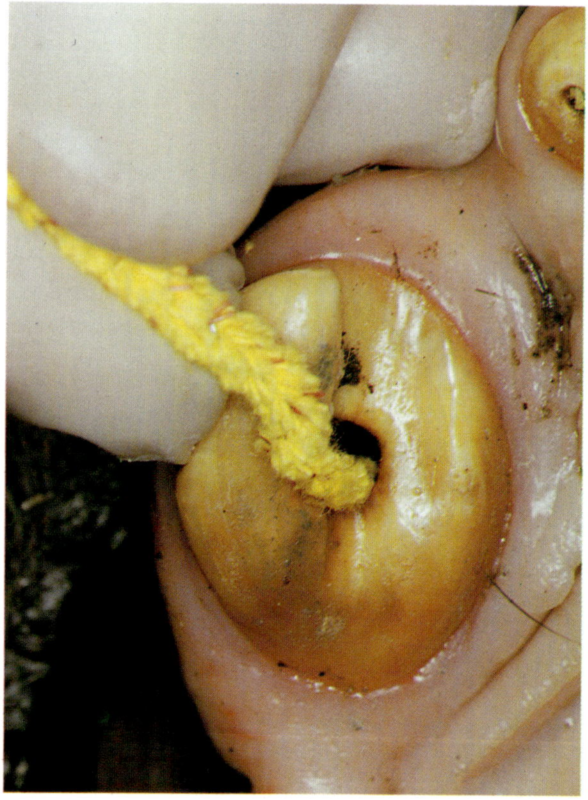

619 Drying the root canal — Case 4c. Pipe cleaners may be used to dry out the root canals after irrigation; ribbon gauze is used in cases of extremely wide canals.

620

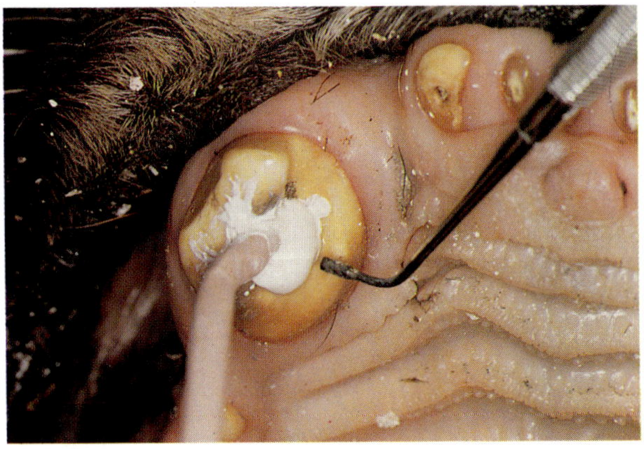

621

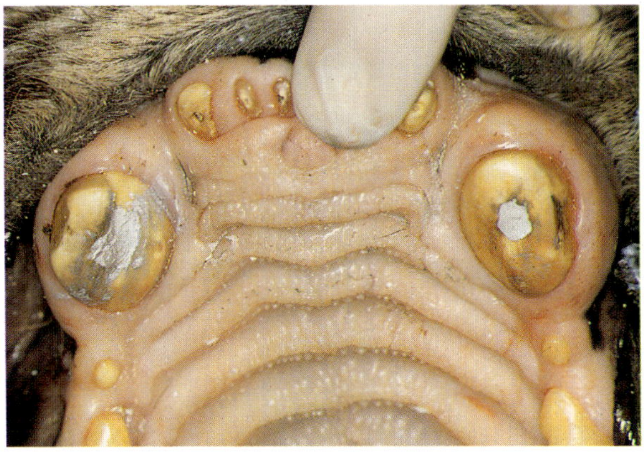

620 Filling the canal — Case 4d. Root canal sealers on their own are not satisfactory as root-filling materials. They may be resorbed through the apical foramina. Gutta percha points in a commercial form do not fulfil the required sizes encountered in large animal endodontics. Prefabricated custom-rolled points are required in a selection of sizes. These may be further customised by careful warming in a water bath and shaping to the contours of the canals once debridement has been completed (*see* **272, 273**).

621 Final amalgam restorations — Case 4e. Amalgam offers the most durable seal for the access cavities. Any further build-up of the teeth to restore function or aesthetics in the form of crown prosthodontics should not be attempted as captive animals do not need to catch or kill their prey. Such unnecessary procedures are not in the best interest of the animal's welfare and prolonging or repeating the treatment session carry increased anaesthetic risks. Restorations will almost universally result in failure due to the same factors that caused the original injury.

622

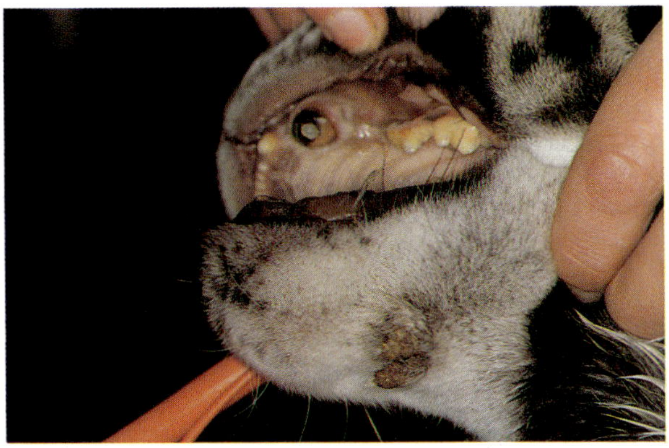

622 Submandibular sinus tract — Case 5a — clouded leopard. Chronic submandibular sinus tracts are often an indication of infection related to primary dental disease. This recently acquired animal to the collection already had endodontic treatment to the lower canines.

623

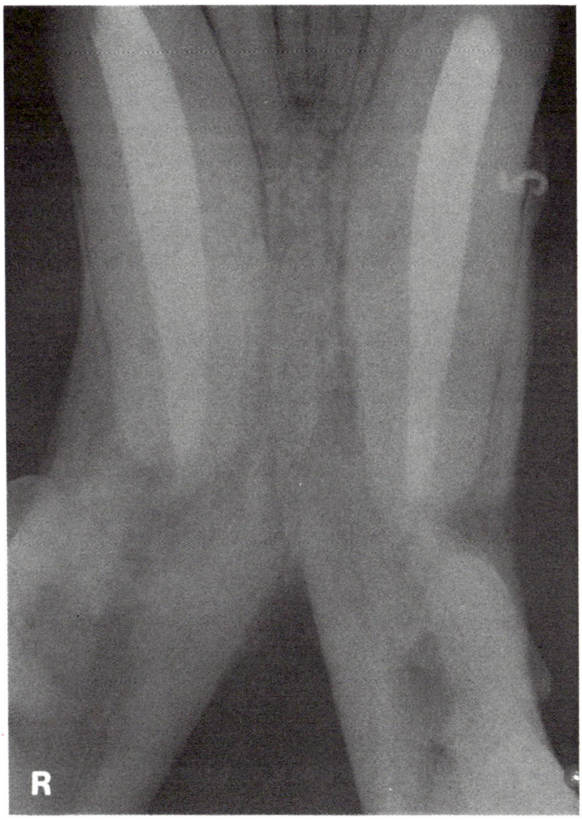

623 Occlusal radiograph — Case 5b. Although reasonable root filling were indicated on the radiograph, a radiolucent area is visible at the periapical region of the animal's lower left canine.

624

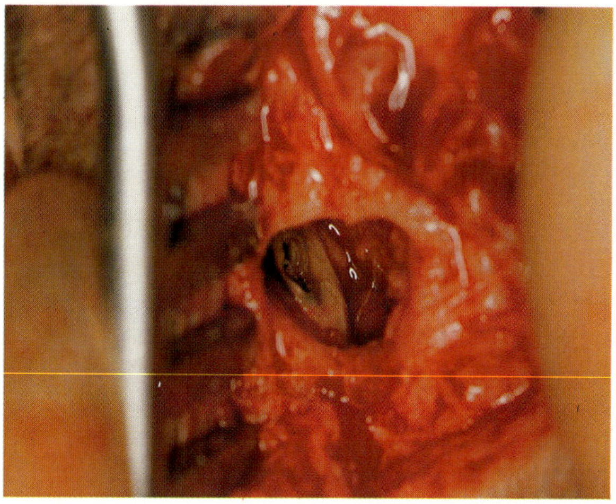

624 Apicectomy — Case 5c. A midline ventral extra-oral approach is required to perform an apicectomy on the lower canines of carnivores in order to avoid the rostral mental foramen and its contents. Once the apex was exposed and resected, an empty root canal was found. The root canal sealer had been resorbed. This case also demonstrates how misleading radiographs can be.

625

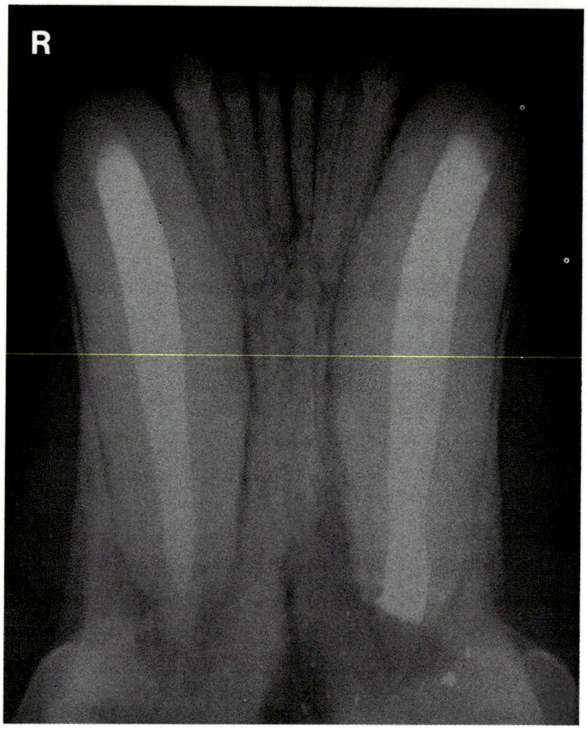

625 Postoperative radiograph — Case 5d. A retrograde amalgam filling was placed in the apical preparation. The submandibular sinus tract healed within 10 days without recurrence.

626

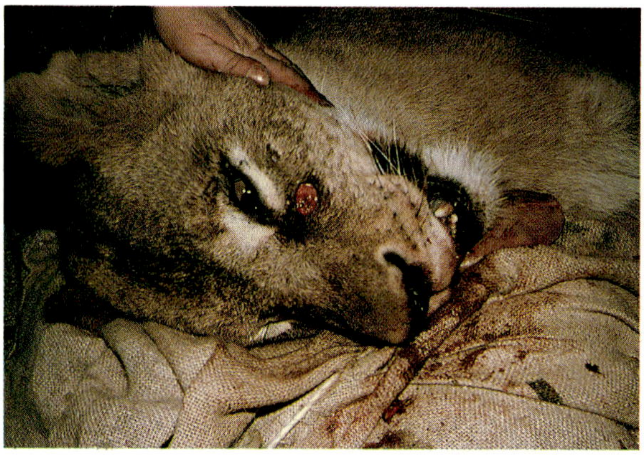

626 Infra-orbital sinus. Chronic periapical abscesses associated with the upper canine teeth of the *Felidae* can give rise to infra-orbital sinus tracts. If the retention of the tooth is clinically indicated, an apicectomy is necessary to eliminate the periapical infection and allow for osseous healing.

62'

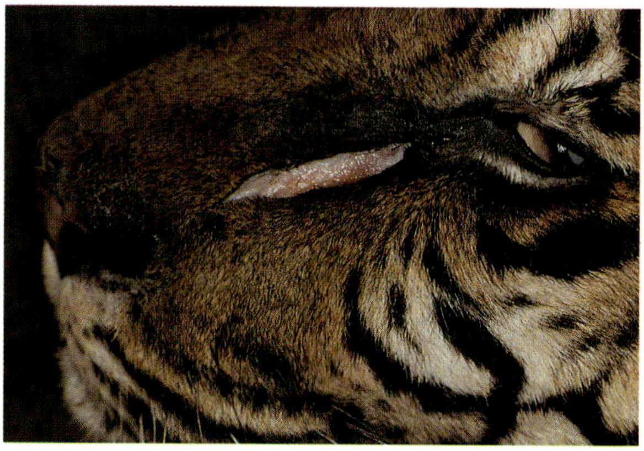

627 Apicectomy approach — Case 6a — tiger cadaver. In the *Felidae* an intra-oral approach to the apex of the upper canine teeth is time-consuming and traumatic. A very large mucoperisteal flap needs to be raised and retraction of the soft tissues, visibility and access to the apex are less than ideal. A far more elegant and practical route is an extra-oral approach through an incision made in a line between the medial canthus of the eye and the nostril.

628

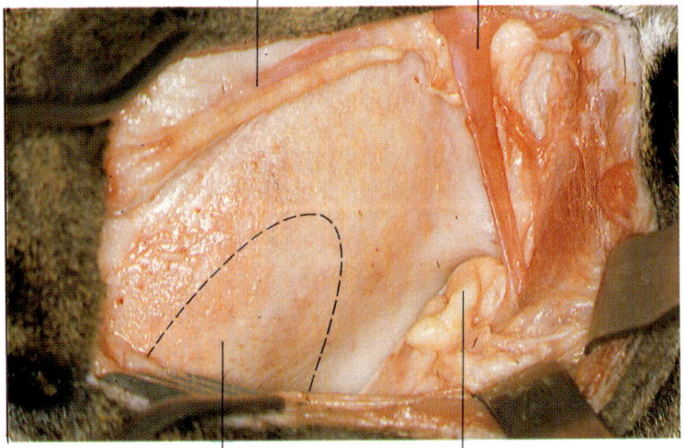

628 Regional anatomy — Case 6b. Once the skin and the periosteum have been raised, the apex of the canine lies almost exactly at the centre of the incision line. The dissection illustrates the regional anatomy and the relative position of the canine tooth. Such an extensive exposure is not necessary to perform the surgery, but vital structures such as the infra-orbital neurovascular bundle should be identified and protected from rotary instruments.

629

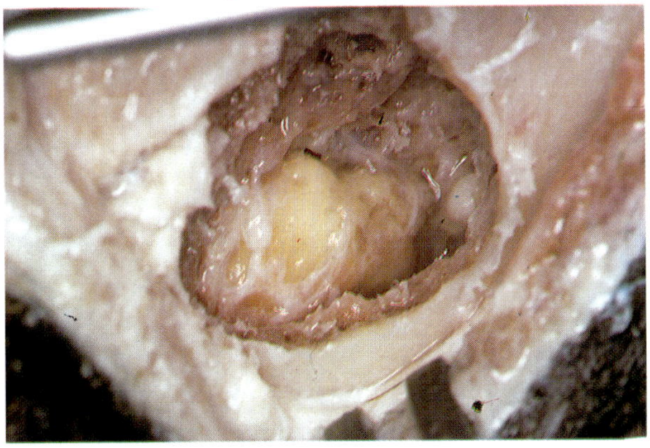

629 Apex exposed — Case 6c. In cases of chronic intra-oral sinus tracts the apex of the canine root requires minimal dissection for exposure.

630

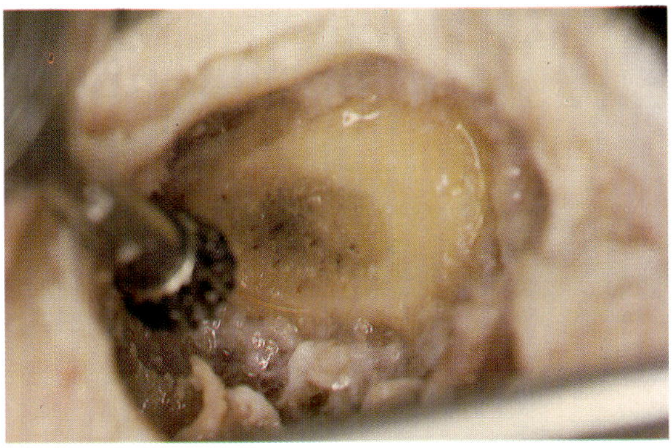

630 Apical delta visible — Case 6d. As the apex of the tooth is resected, the infected apical delta is clearly visible.

631

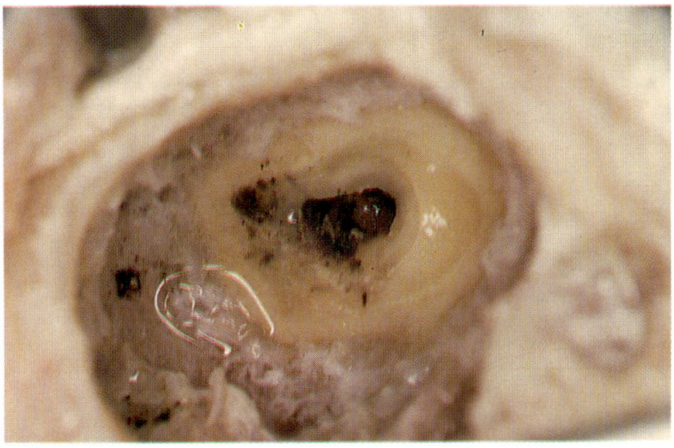

631 Root canal visible — Case 6e. Because of its complex delta formation, resection is advisable in conjunction with an orthograde root filling. If a satisfactory condensation of the gutta percha cannot be achieved it should be complemented with a retrograde amalgam filling.

632

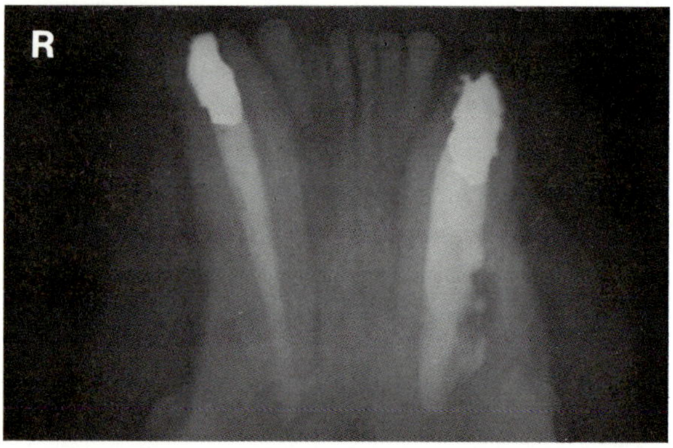

632 Radiograph of a resorption cavity. An attempt was made to root fill these lower canines, which had chronic periapical infections, with extra- and intra-oral fistulas present. This postoperative radiograph demonstrates a perforating internal resorption cavity on the lower left canine that allowed the root canal sealant to escape into the lateral abscess. The tooth was subsequently extracted as the sinus tracts did not heal.

633

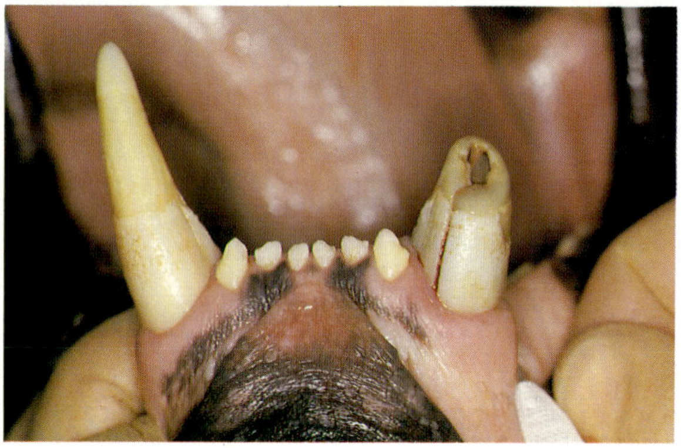

633 Longitudinal fracture of the root — Case 7a. Teeth with longitudinal fractures are unsavable and must be extracted.

634

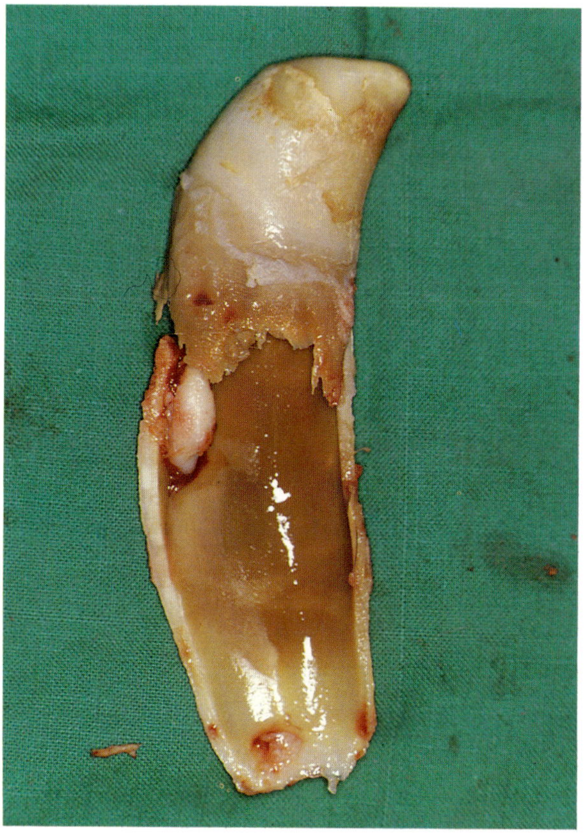

634 Extracted root — Case 7a. The thickness of the dentine walls of the root and the incomplete apical formation indicate that the fracture and pulp necrosis occurred at a young age.

635 Mandibular mucoperiosteal flap — same animal as in 600–605 — Case 8a — lion. To facilitate extraction, a large full-thickness mucoperiosteal flap is reflected. The relieving incision is made at the symphysis region to aid in the exposure of an adequate length of alveolar bone without resorting to a caudal relieving incision in the region of the mental foramen. Care needs to be exercised apical to the canine and first premolar region not to damage the mental nerve. It is best to identify the mental foramen and its contents so they may be protected with retractors.

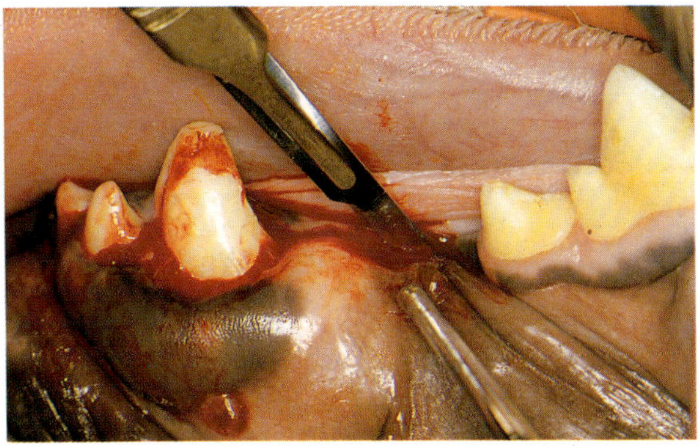
635

636 Root elevation — Case 8b. On large animals, bone removal is best achieved with the use of large-diameter tungsten burrs. Copious irrigation during drilling is mandatory. To minimise vertical bone reduction, which results in increased weakening of the mandible, the alveolar bone is guttered with long surgical fissure burrs to facilitate elevation. Large roots occasionally require large elevators. Coupland chisels with blades up to 9.5 mm wide, are extremely useful in large animal work. Because of the leverages and power possible, especially with the cross-handle versions, great care is required in their use to avoid fracturing the jaw.

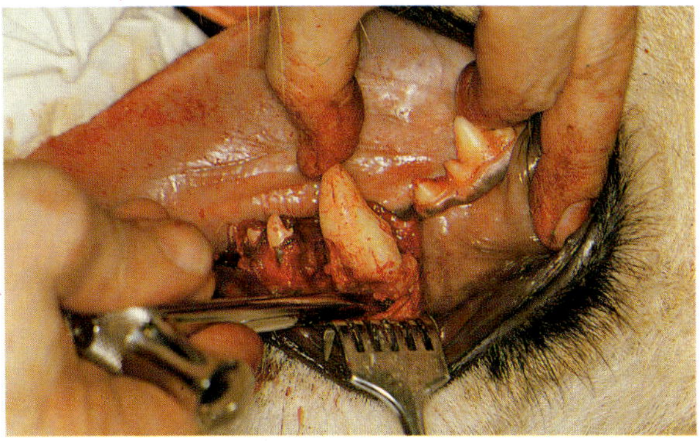
636

637 Postoperative defect — Case 8c. A large osseous defect remains after the extraction. Packing is contraindicated if good apposition of the mucoperiosteal flap can be accomplished.

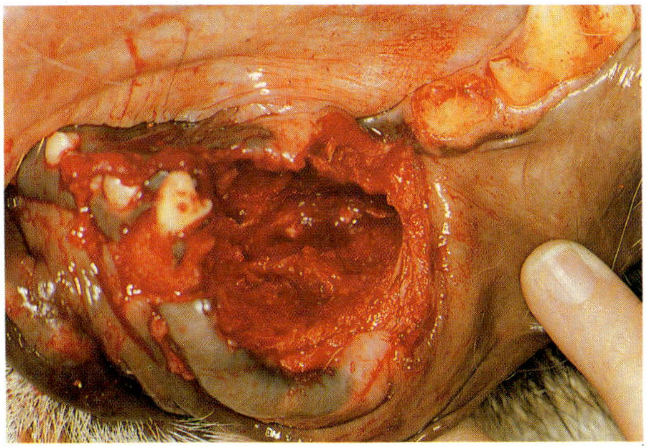
637

638

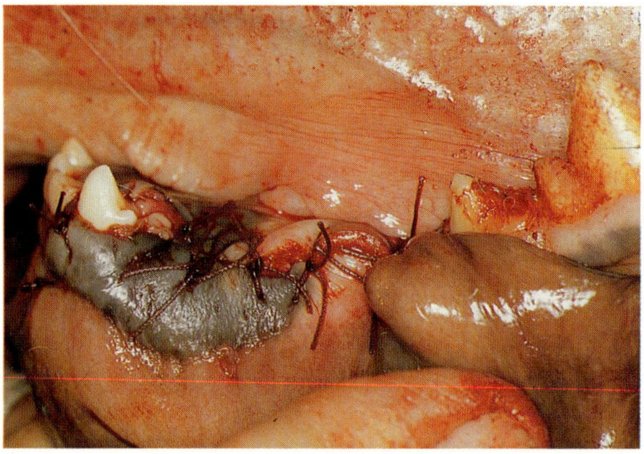

638 Flap closed — Case 8d. Thoughtful flap design allows for good gingival approximation that minimises the danger of food packing and encourages the closure of large defects through primary healing.

Ailuropodidae — panda family $\frac{3}{3}:\frac{1}{1}:\frac{2-3}{3}:\frac{3}{3} = 38-40$

639

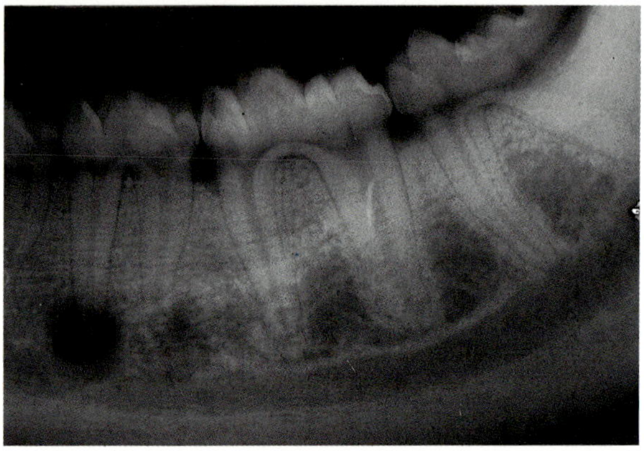

64

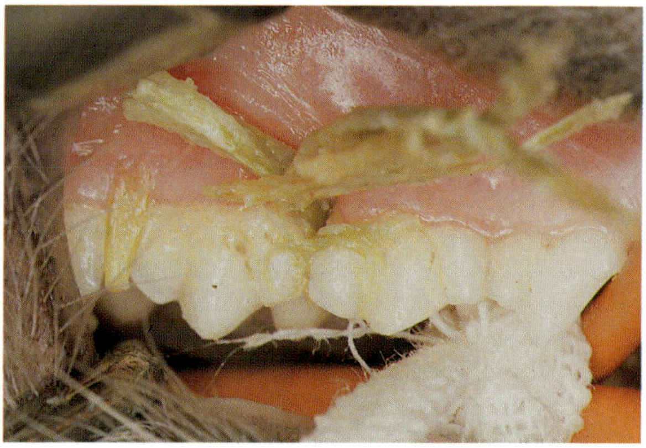

639 Radiograph associated with a chronic facial abscess — red panda. Intra-oral examination did not reveal any oral or dental abnormalities. Radiography of the mandible revealed a periapical abscess of the lower third permanent premolar. The aetiology was unknown. It may have been an undisplaced fracture of the crown through the pulp chamber as a result of occlusal trauma or pulp necrosis through excessive occlusal force. Note the extremely long roots. The tooth was extracted through a planned flap and vertical sectioning procedure. Healing was uneventful.

640 Food packing — red panda. This animal was suffering with a facial abscess. Oral examination revealed food packing between the upper second and third premolars that was perforating the cheek. The third premolar was extracted to eliminate the food-trap area. Healing was uneventful and the condition did not reoccur.

Order Primates

Pongidae — Great apes
Cercopithecidae — Old World monkeys

$$\frac{2}{2}:\frac{1}{1}:\frac{2}{2}:\frac{3}{3} = 32$$

Cebidae — New World monkeys

$$\frac{2}{2}:\frac{1}{1}:\frac{3}{3}:\frac{3}{3} = 36$$

641

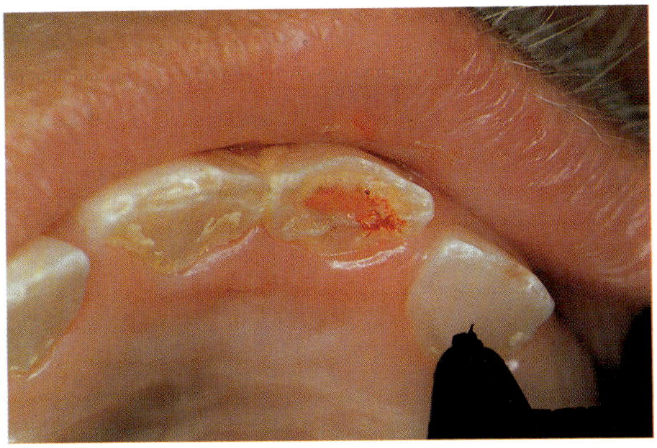

642

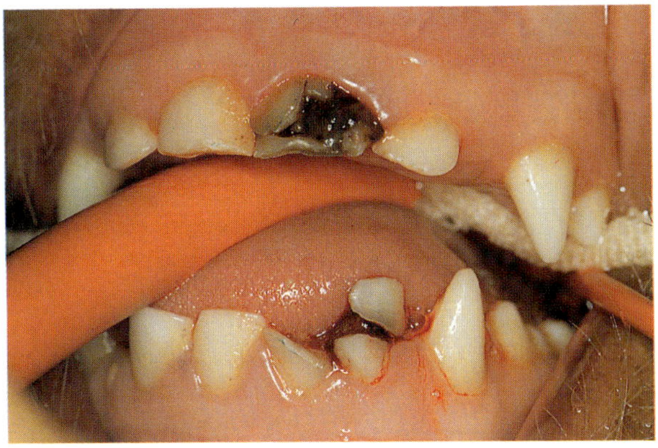

641 Fractured primary incisor — chimpanzee. Exposed pulp; the animal demonstrated pain and anorexia. Total coronal pulpectomy, five minute application of formol cresol moistened cotton pledget to the pulp surface and a restoration lined with a sedative dressing alleviated the symptoms. The tooth was exfoliated at its normal time.

642 Compound fractures of primary incisors — chimpanzee. With the hard floor surface it is inevitable that the anterior teeth, especially those of young active animals, receive injuries. Unless a predictable prognosis can be forecast the damaged teeth should be extracted. This three-year-old chimpanzee was showing oral pain. All the affected teeth had longitudinal fractures and were extracted.

643

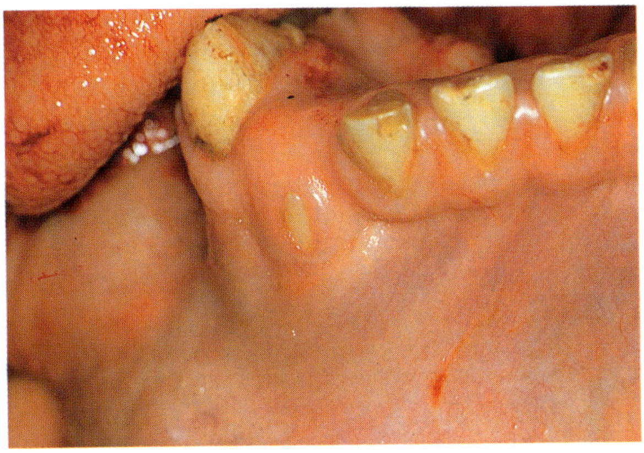

644

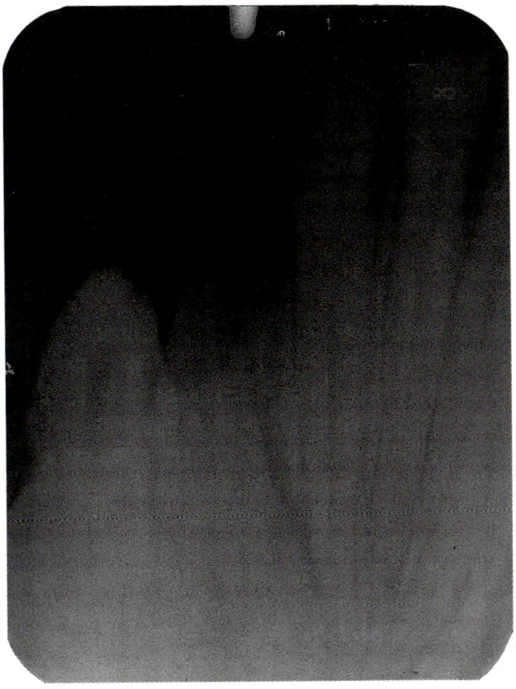

643, 644 Unerupted permanent canines — lowland gorilla. Developmental abnormalities in apes and monkeys are not as common as in man or domestic small animals. These unerupted lower canines were an incidental finding during treatment. The desirability of active treatment of such symptomless conditions must be carefully assessed. Considerable surgical trauma and anaesthetic time would be required for the removal of such canine teeth.

645

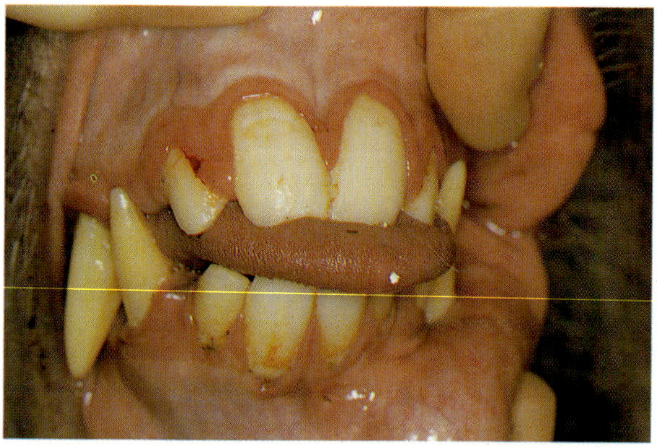

645 **Marginal gingivitis — baboon.** Many primates in the wild and captivity suffer with varying degrees of periodontal disease.

646

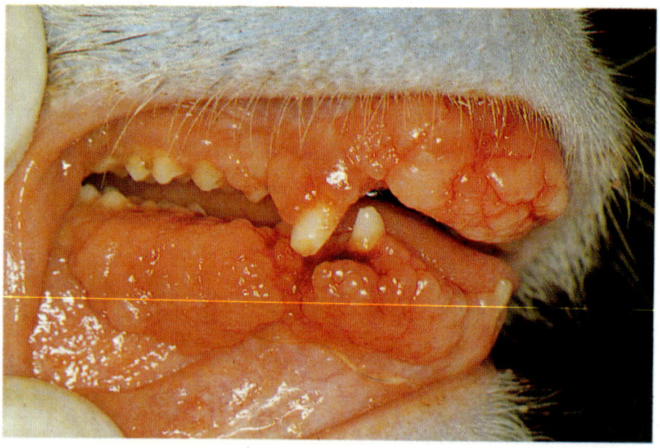

646 **Severe hyperplastic gingivitis — Case 1a — DeBrazza's monkey.** This type of hyperplastic gingivitis, where the tissues are frail and resemble a 'grape bunch' in appearance, is not uncommon among some species of monkeys. Electron microscopic investigations have not been able to demonstrate a viral aetiology.

647

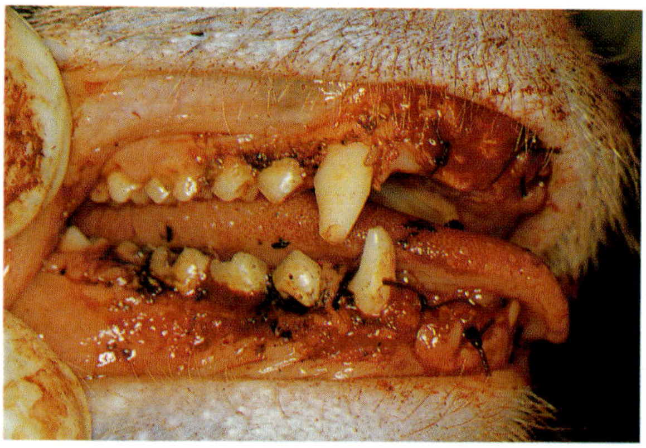

647 **After gingivectomy — Case 1b.** If osseous support to the teeth is good and only false pockets exist, a gingivectomy will eliminate the hyperplastic tissues. Recurrences are common.

648

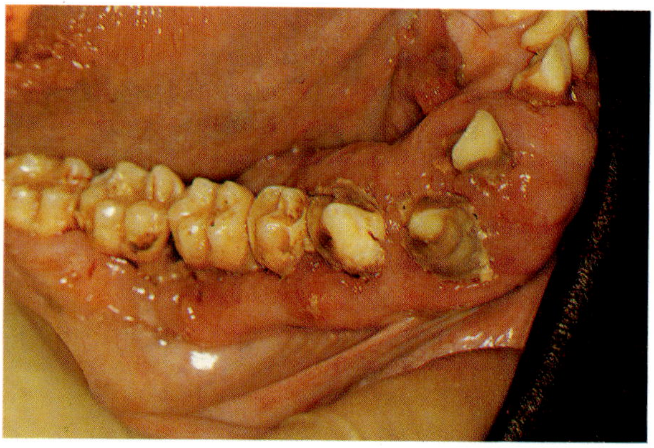

648 **Advanced periodontitis — lowland gorilla.** Hyperplastic gingival proliferation may be present in advanced cases of periodontal disease among the great apes.

649 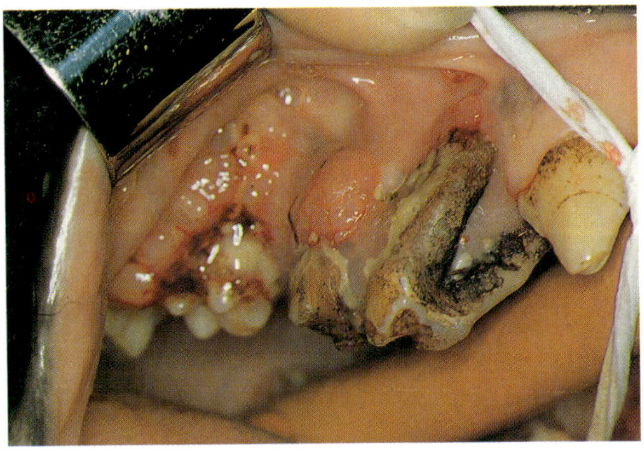

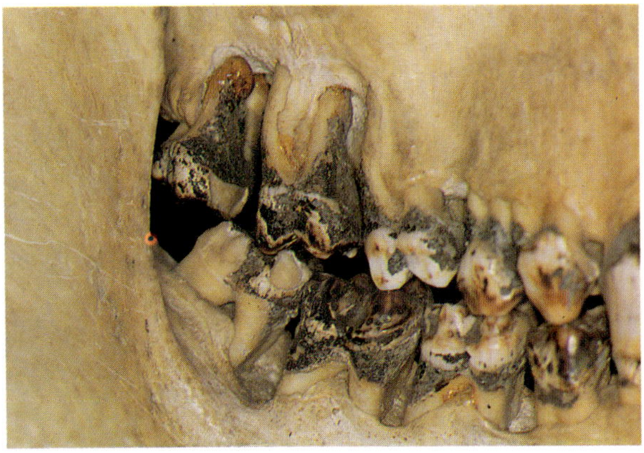 650

649 Advanced periodontal disease — lowland gorilla. The excellent bone support and relatively high root/crown ratio mean that extreme mobility is only demonstrated at the terminal stages of periodontal disease. Because of the long, fine, divergent roots it is often advisable to section posterior teeth prior to extractions, even when periodontally involved, to minimise the fractures of root apices.

650 Periodontal condition — lowland gorilla. Periodontal disease is not confined to captive primates. Gorillas in the wild, as shown in the skull above, also demonstrate alveolar bone loss associated with periodontal disease.

651 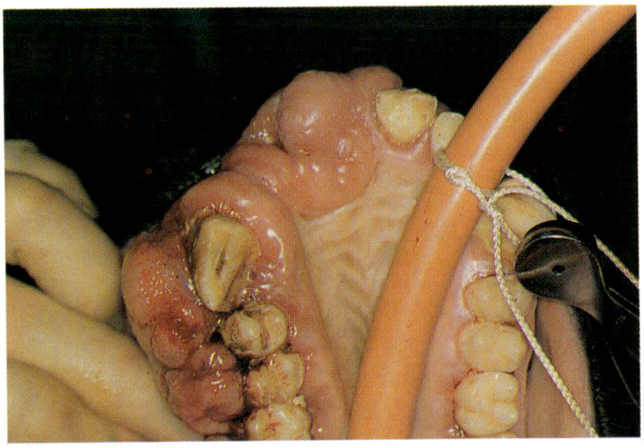

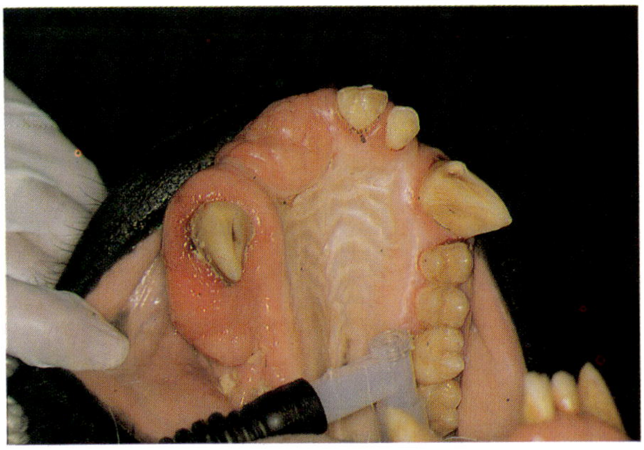 652

651 Advanced periodontal disease — Case 2a — lowland gorilla. Hyperplastic inflammatory gingiva was present, even at previous extraction sites. It is advisable to resect such tissues during extractions as it allows for a better postoperative healing of the sockets.

652 One year postoperative appearance — Case 2b. The edentulous area showed good healing and generally there was a lower level of inflammation of the soft tissues.

653

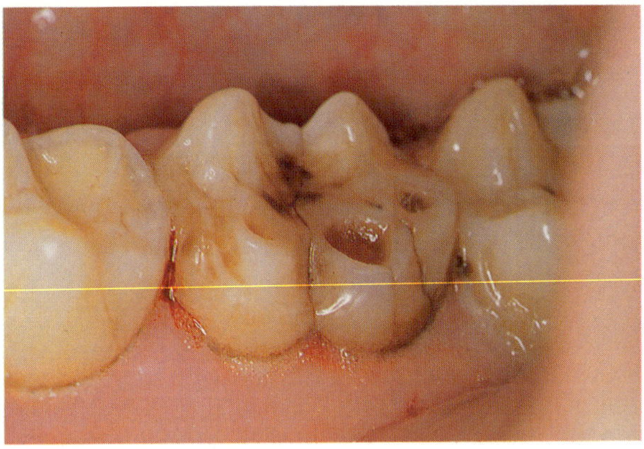

653 Caries — Case 3a — lowland gorilla. Gorillas suffering with dental disease often show signs of pain. This animal held its jaw and avoided hard and cold food. In a captive situation caries is not uncommon if the animals are fed refined carbohydrates. The colour of the crown indicated an abnormality, although the clinical appearance of the tooth was atypical of caries and no soft dentine or sticky fissures could be elicited.

654

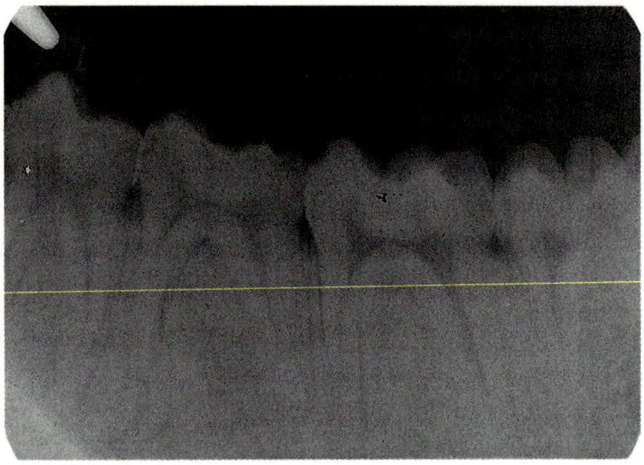

654 Radiographic view — Case 3b. Radiography did not indicate any occlusal caries because of the extensive buccolingual dimension of the crown. It did, however, illustrate the exaggerated crown/root ratio and the fine, divergent root formation. Root canal treatment was thought to be inappropriate due to the prolonged anaesthetic time that would have been required for the treatment of four long fine root canals.

655

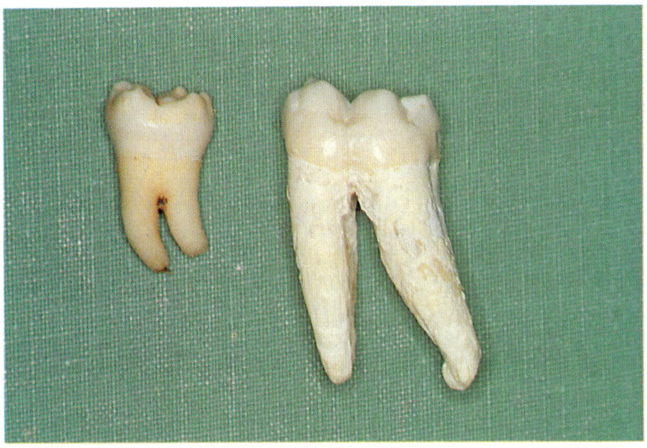

655 Comparison between human and gorilla molars. Extraction of these teeth has to be an open flap procedure. The crown was divided longitudinally into four sections according to the position of the roots, and buccal bone was removed. In the maxilla it is wise to design the buccal flap with care because of the close proximity of the maxillary sinus. Oro-antral fistulas can be created during molar extractions and immediate repairs are mandatory to prevent chronic fistulas and sinusitis.

656

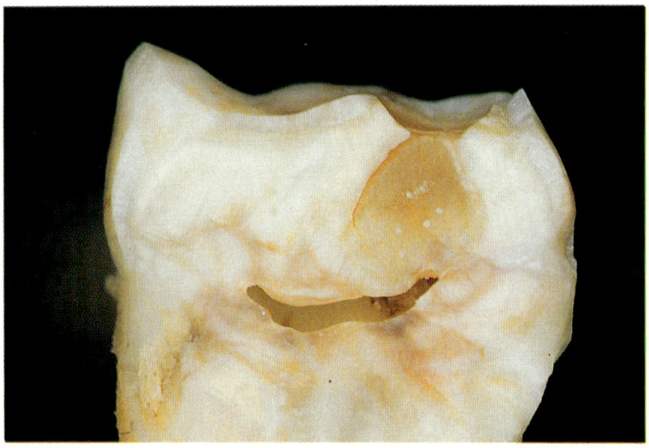

656 Cross-section of extracted crown — Case 3c. The depth of the occlusal caries is visible. The caries was hard in consistency. The red staining of the dentine surrounding the pulp chamber is most likely to have been caused by breakdown products and internal haemorrhage due to episodes of acute pulpitis.

657

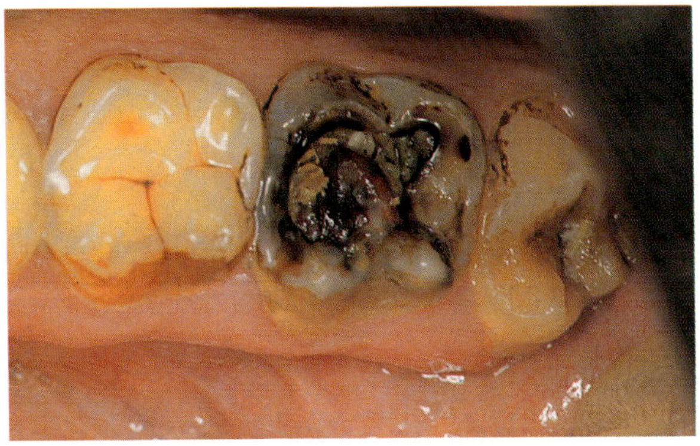

658

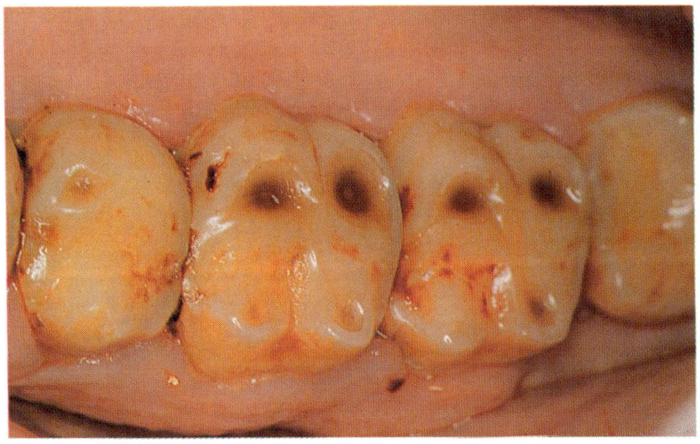

657 Extensive caries — lowland gorilla. Even such large carious lesions did not have the typical soft, leathery consistency of human caries. When assessing a treatment plan for animals it is vital to consider the anaesthetic implications and the long-term prognosis of restorative treatment. Carious molars in primates should only be conserved if the cavities are small and there is substantial sound tooth substance surrounding the lesions to assure a high level of predictability of the restorations.

658 Occlusal attrition — lowland gorilla. It is important to differentiate between caries and stained dentine of occlusal attrition.

Dental trauma

659

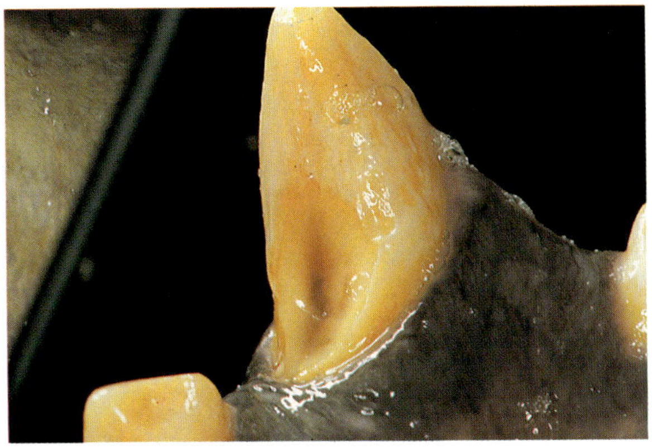

660

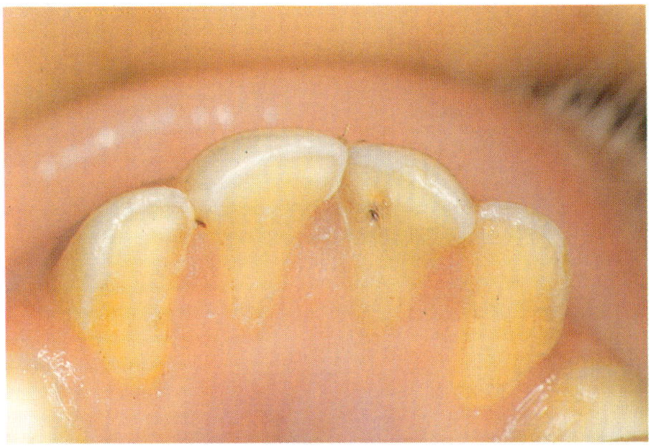

659 Canine attrition — orang-utan (mirror image). Bar-chewing will result in tooth abrasion. The discoloured area is indicative of secondary dentine. The animal had a poor appetite and avoided using the lower canines for a period of months. Radiography did not show any apical infection. The animal's appetite did not improve with the empirical use of antibiotics. Endodontic treatment was the final resort. The pulp was vital and showed no histological abnormalities. Normal appetite returned two weeks postoperatively.

660 Small exposure — baboon. Infected pulpal exposure on the palatal aspect of an upper incisor.

661

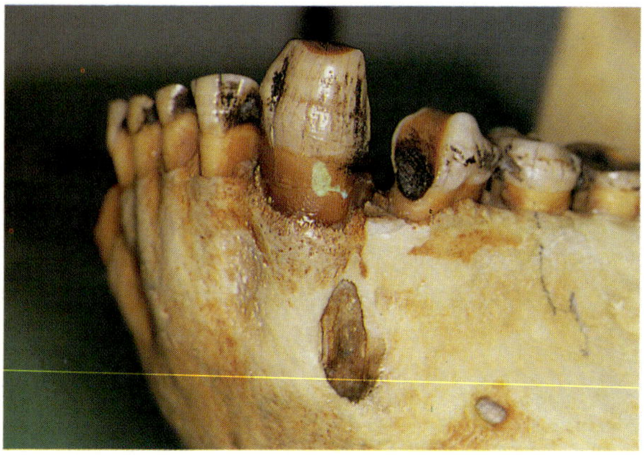

661 Mandibular abscess — lowland gorilla. The osseous destruction that can occur through periapical infection as a result of a fractured and infected lower canine tooth is evident on a dry specimen.

662

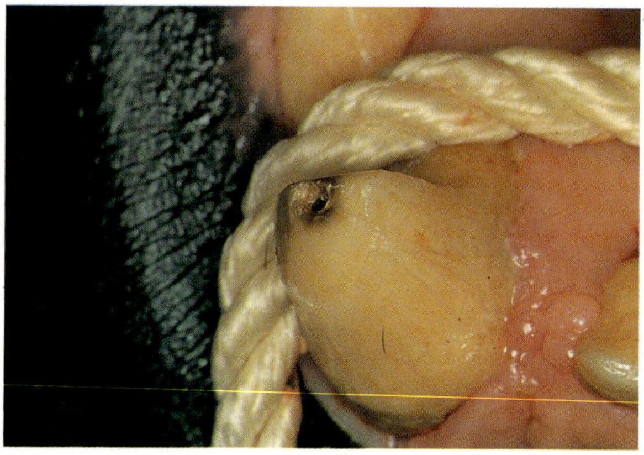

662 Dental trauma — Case 4a — lowland gorilla. The animal had a poor appetite and would not follow his normal habit of eating regurgitated food. A fractured and infected lower canine was diagnosed on oral examination. Root canal treatment of these long single-rooted teeth is a predictable and fast procedure and is far less traumatic for the animal than a surgical extraction.

663

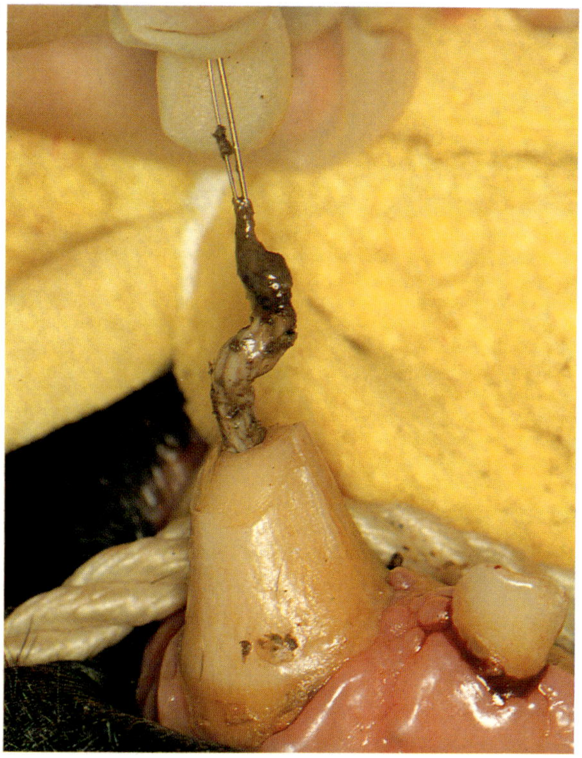

663 Pulp being extirpated — Case 4b. Intact necrotic pulp was removed with two long barbed broaches after a large enough coronal access cavity was prepared.

664

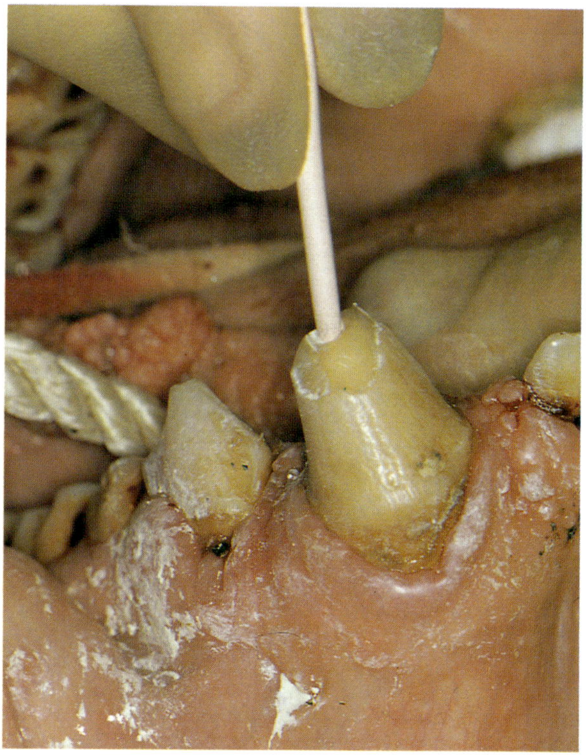

664 Buccal sinus tract — Case 4c. Root canal sealer extruded from a buccal sinus tract originating from the apical abscess. Apicectomy was contraindicated, as an unacceptable increase in anaesthetic time would have been required. Normal appetite returned within days postoperatively, and the animal has not exhibited oral pain over a follow-up period of two and a half years.

665

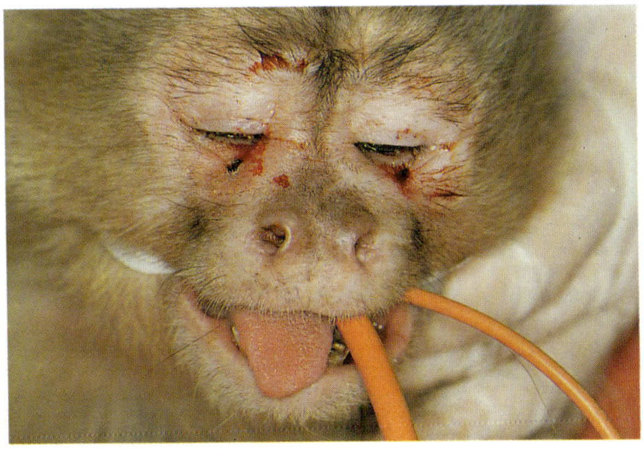

666

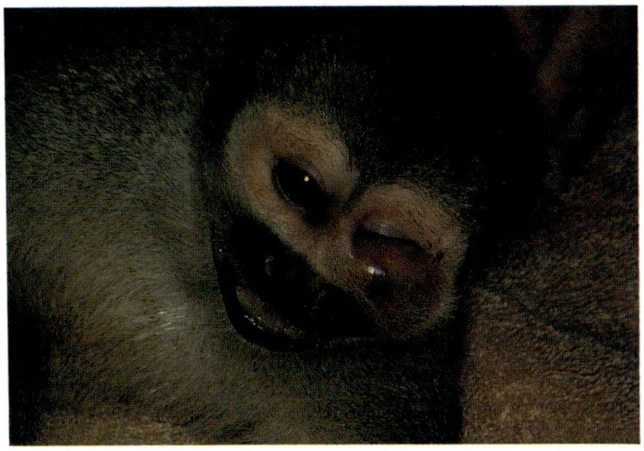

665 Infra-orbital sinus tracts — capuchin monkey. In primates the apices of the upper canines are often close to the infra-orbital region. Chronic sinus tracts associated with pulp necrosis can often be seen in animals that have been disarmed by having had their canine teeth cut off at the gingival margins. This is a cruel procedure that is unfortunately still practised in some countries. When chronic extra-oral sinuses are present, associated with the teeth of these small animals, extractions should be considered as opposed to endodontic treatment.

666 Infra-orbital cellulitis — squirrel monkey. Acute facial cellulitis associated with a fractured canine tooth illustrates how dental disease can become a life-threatening condition.

Order Hyracoidea

Procaviidae — hyrax $\frac{1}{2}:\frac{0}{0}:\frac{4}{3-4}:\frac{3}{3} = 32 - 34$

667

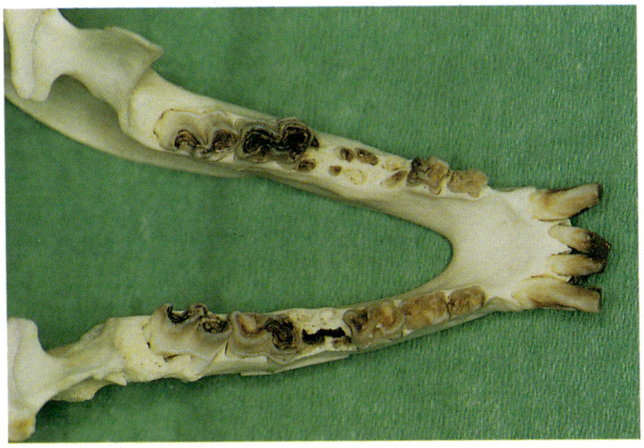

668

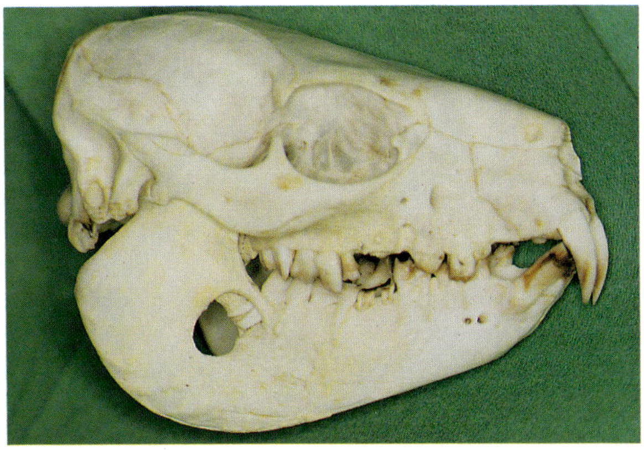

667 Dental caries — Case 1a — rock hyrax. Large carious lesions were present in the cheek teeth, indicating a dietary aetiology.

668 Periapical abscesses — Case 1b. The large periapical osseous defects were the result of caries-induced pulp necrosis. The cause of death was amyloidosis of the major organs, a condition often associated with chronic suppurative disease.

Sequentially erupting teeth

Order Proboscidea

Elephantidae — elephants $\frac{1}{0}:\frac{0}{0}:\frac{0}{0}:\frac{6}{6} = 26$

Molars

669

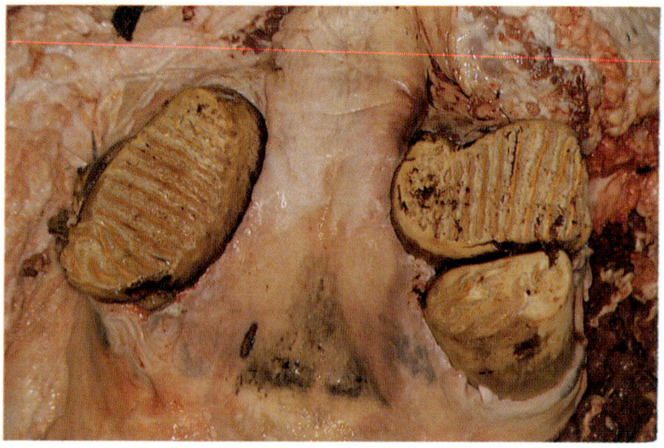

670

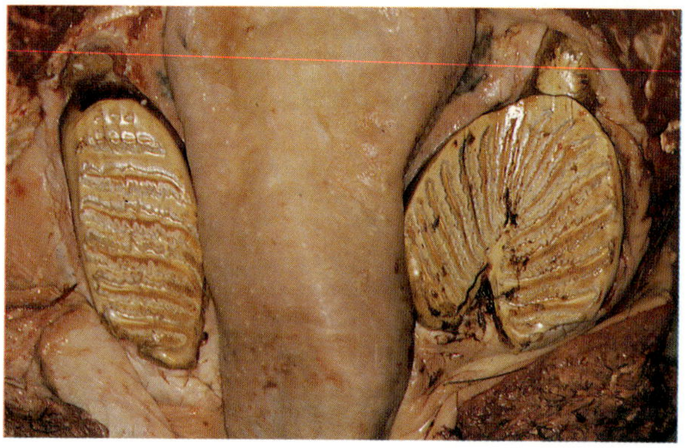

669 Maxilla — postmortem - Case 1a — Asian elephant. Molar malocclusions and eruption-related pathology are occasionally seen in captive elephants. These may be related to the consistency of a soft diet, where normal attrition and eruption patterns do not progress naturally, or a dietary problem, where the nutritional requirements are not met and the complex calcification/resorption associated with the elephant molar eruption sequence is disturbed.

670 Mandible — Case 1b. Malocclusion can lead to rotation of the teeth, which in turn may contribute to food packing and periodontal complications.

671

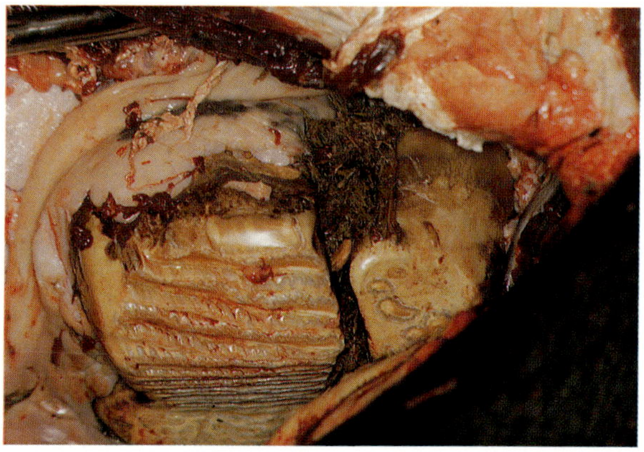

67

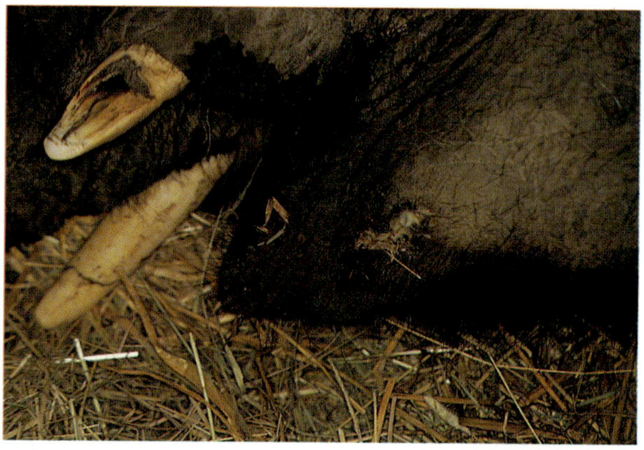

671 Food packing — Case 1c. Close-up view of a 100-mm deep periodontal pocket between the deformed molars, which were packed with necrotic food. The condition may have been clinically relevant and contributed to referred pain. The animal constantly rubbed her tusk of the same side; this finally resulted in its fracture subgingivally, causing a chronic tusk sheath infection. The animal died of an unrelated cause.

672 Mandibular abscess — Case 2a — African elephant. This 7-year-old female was suffering with a periapical abscess discharging at the ventral border of the mandible.

673

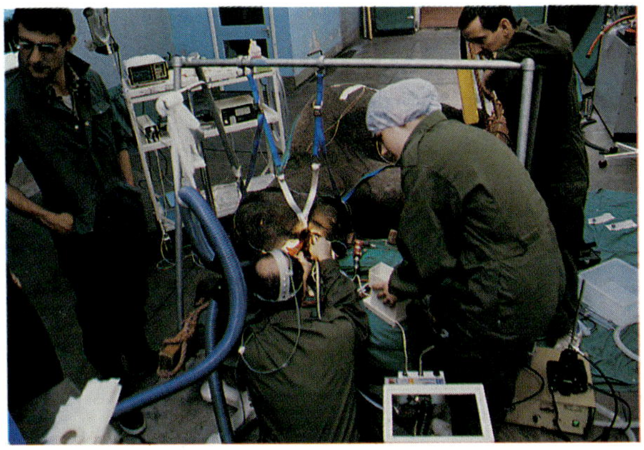

674

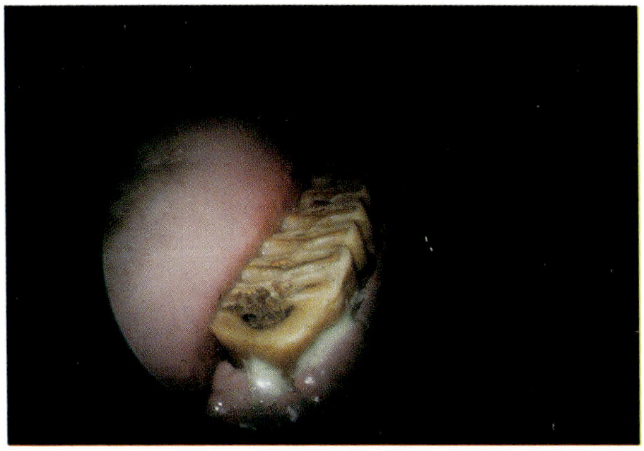

673 Buccal retraction — Case 2b. Access to elephant molars presents a logistic problem, because of the restricted opening of the mouth and the considerable obstruction caused by the cheek and the tongue. Multiple cheek retractors, supported by a custom-made adjustable scaffolding, offer excellent retraction and intra-oral access. Injectable anaesthetics do not provide the necessary muscle relaxation in elephants for extensive intra-oral work and gaseous maintenance is usually required. The mouth is opened with a selection of hardwood wedges, which should have cords attached for safety. The airway is protected with large sponges, which also have cords attached.

674 Endoscopic view of a lower molar — Case 2c. Endoscopic view of a perforation in the occlusal table of the lower third molar, with food debris packed into the pulp chamber. Such perforations of the pulp chambers and associated periapical infections have been reported in wild and captive elephants. The aetiology has been blamed on diets containing abrasive contaminants such as silica.

675

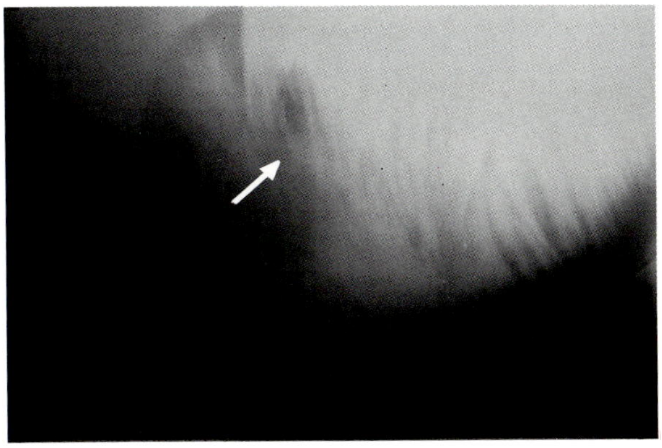

676

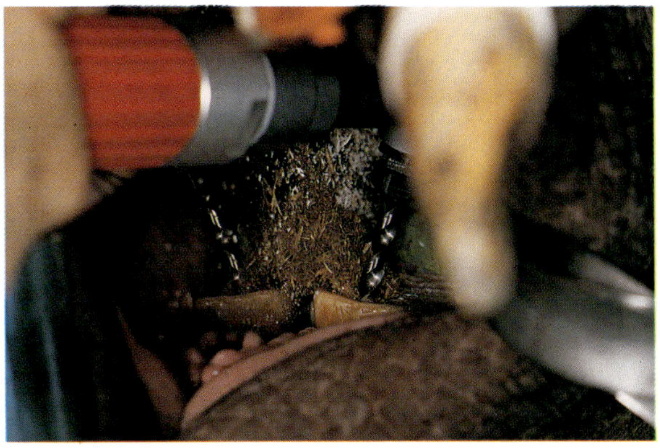

675 Radiograph of mandible — Case 2d. A periapical abscess associated with the perforation is confirmed, with the radiolucent area visible around the mesial root on this lateral oblique radiograph.

676 Removing necrotic material — Case 2e. Basic principles of endodontics were closely followed. Twist drills and extra-long endodontic files were used to debride the canals, followed by thorough irrigation.

677

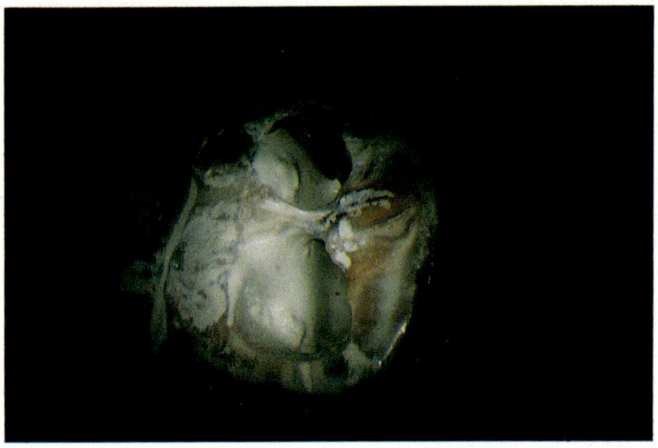

678

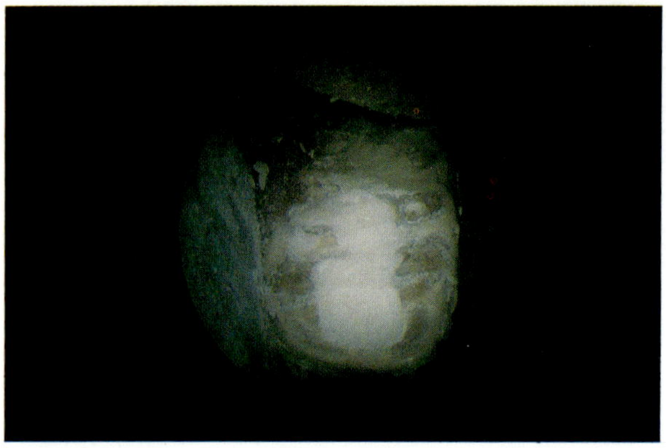

677 Canal filled with cement — Case 2f. The root apices of elephant molars are often dilated. A cellulose gauze saturated in calcium hydroxide-based cement was placed at the apex to minimise the danger of overfilling the canal. The canal was filled with a non-oil of clove-based sealer, as elephants have been reported to react unfavourably if eugenol-based material escapes into the periapical space.

678 Occlusal restoration — Case 2g. Access cavities of the exposed lamellae were restored with 10 ml of self-curing methyl methacrylate.

679

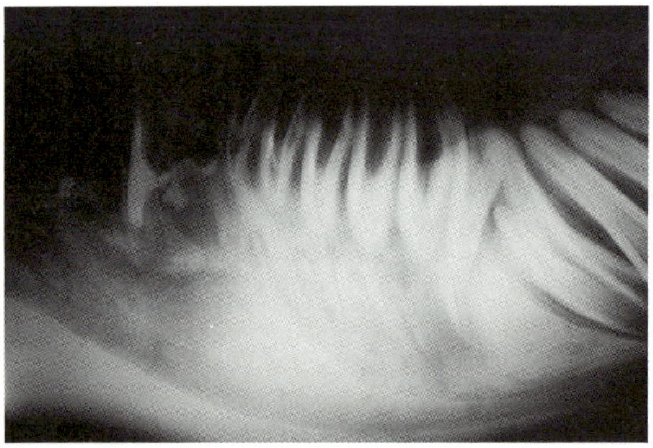

680

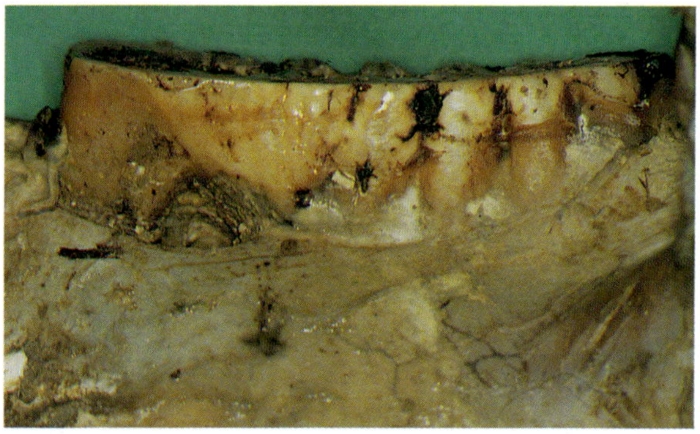

679 Postmortem radiograph — Case 2g. The animal died of an unknown cause 10 months postoperatively. A satisfactory root filling is visible on the radiograph, although some radiolucency is apparent in the mesial periapical region and the bifurcation. This feature may be consistent with natural resorption of the mesial aspect of elephant molars before exfoliation.

680 Postmortem view of hemimandible — Case 2h. A postmortem examination found complete resolution of the gingival and extra-oral sinus tracts. The occlusal restorations survived moderately well, but amalgam would have been preferable. The body of the mandible was somewhat thickened when compared with the opposite side, but no osseous destruction was present, except in the region of the bifurcation.

Discussion: The treatment was a qualified success, but with the benefit of hindsight, sectioning at the bifurcation and extracting the infected mesial piece would have offered a better result, with a considerable reduction in anaesthetic time.

Order Marsupialia

Macropodidae — kangaroos and wallabies $\frac{3}{1}:\frac{0-1}{0}:\frac{2}{2}:\frac{4}{4}=32-34$

'Lumpy jaw' is a vague, inaccurate term used to describe chronic alveolar abscesses or facial exostosis in herbivores and occasionally in other animals, whatever the aetiology of the conditions. The expression is often used to describe facial necrobacillosis in macropods, while in classical veterinary medicine it is confined exclusively to the condition in cattle that is caused by *Actinomyces bovis.*

Aetiology

Necrobacillosis of captive macropods represents a serious management problem. *Fusobacterium necrophorum,* which is found in the gut contents of some herbivores, has been identified as the principal organism associated with the disease. *F. necrophorum* does not readily penetrate healthy, intact skin or mucous membrane and macropods, although frequently affected, are not abnormally susceptible to the organism. It is strongly suggested that this organism is an opportunist that may be excreted in the faeces and invade injuries in the mouth caused by sharp cereal awns and periodontal defects. Experiments suggest that, in pure culture, very large doses of the organism are required to initiate infection, but the presence of faecal and other bacteria, such as *Escherichia coli* and *Corynebacterium (Actinomyces) pyogenes,* greatly increases the infectivity of *F. necrophorum.* Necrobacillosis can also affect the feet and limbs, the lining of the stomach and the liver, lungs and tail of the animal. Poor sanitation and overcrowding, especially in the feeding areas, are important factors in outbreaks of the disease.

Prevention and treatment

Because the main virulent factors of *F. necrophorum* are weakly antigenic, vaccine development has proved unsuccessful. It has been found that less than 10% of wallabies excrete *F. necrophorum* in the faeces and further research on factors that influence such excretion may help in the control of this fatal disease in captive macropods. At present, prevention through minimising faecal contamination and injuries to the oral mucosa offers the best hope of control. Treatment of infections with antibiotics and surgery is moderately successful, but only in early lesions.

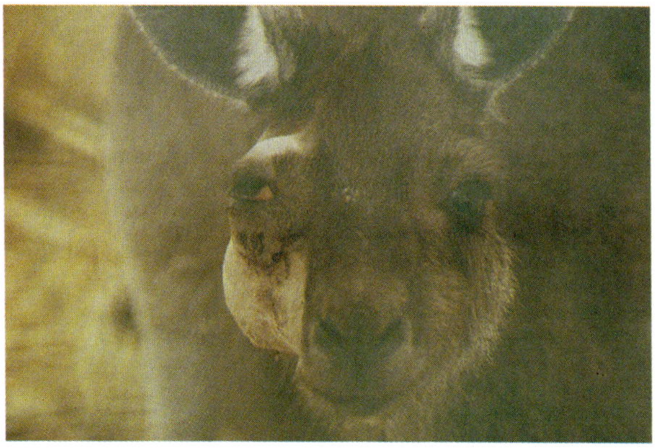

681

681 Facial necrobacillosis — red kangaroo. Poor appetite and weight loss are usually the first signs of the disease. Facial swellings associated with maxillary infections can cause retrobulbar abscesses that give rise to exophthalmus.

682

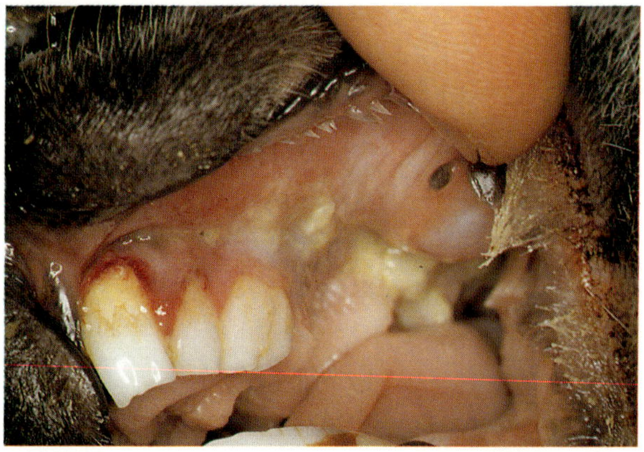

682 Intra-oral view of infection — Case 1a — Bennett's wallaby. Purulent discharge through the oral mucosa often indicates an extensive lesion of the deeper structures.

683

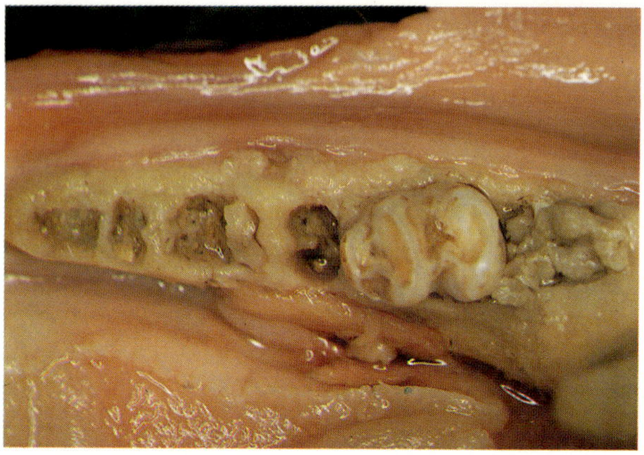

683 Dental condition — post mortem — Case 1b. This intra-oral view confirms a generalised osteomyelitis. Many of the teeth have been lost or only roots have been retained. There is a prolific, fetid, purulent discharge from the soft tissues.

684

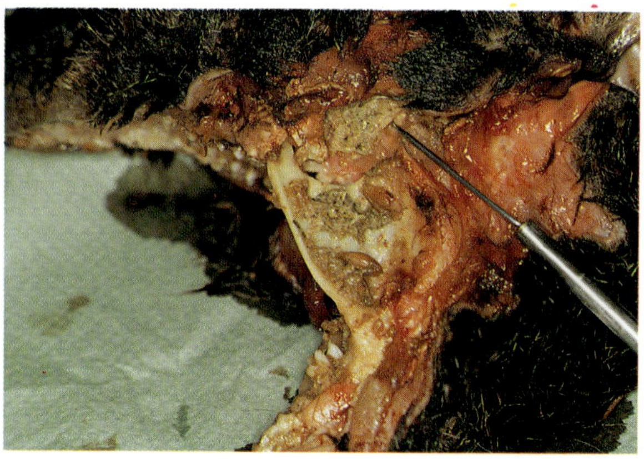

684 Food packing — post mortem — Case 1c. Food contamination of the muscle layers may be present in advanced cases of facial necrobacillosis. In this specimen, grass awns can be seen at the lateral border of the mandibular ramus, and further food debris in the pterygoid region.

685 Necrobacillosis of a mandible — Bennett's wallaby. This radiograph of a mandible illustrates osseous destruction, reactive bone at the ventral aspect of the mandible and sequestrum formation associated with necrobacillosis.

685

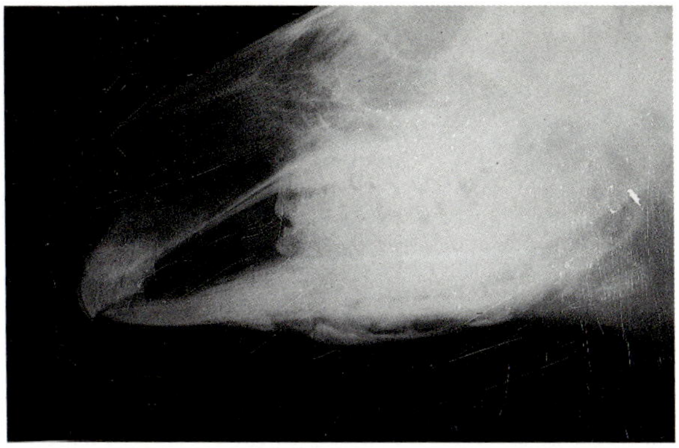

686 Dry mandible — Bennett's wallaby. Osseous destruction can lead to pathological fracture of the mandible.

686

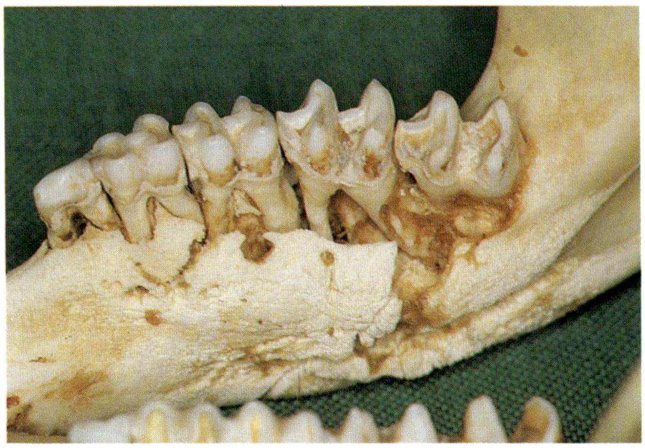

Treatment

The treatment of oral/facial necrobacillosis has proved disappointing in its long-term prognosis. Careful assessment of the condition must be made in the light of experience and advanced cases should be euthanised. If the condition is diagnosed and treated early, a slightly better prognosis may be expected. The most successful treatment is a radical regime in which all the involved teeth are extracted and the diseased bone is thoroughly curetted from the lesion. Occasionally, this procedure cannot be performed through a labial approach, because of the limited access to the posterior teeth. In such cases a buccotomy has proved useful. Postoperatively, the defect is treated on the lines of a localised osteitis. Dressing sockets with a firm zinc oxide/oil of cloves (eugenol) pack affords the necessary protection from immediate food contamination and encourages granulation-tissue formation. The pack may be changed after two to three weeks and the second allowed to be lost naturally. Larger defects are more usefully treated postoperatively with ribbon gauze and Whitehead's Varnish packs. Systemic antibiotic therapy should be used to complement the surgical treatment.

687

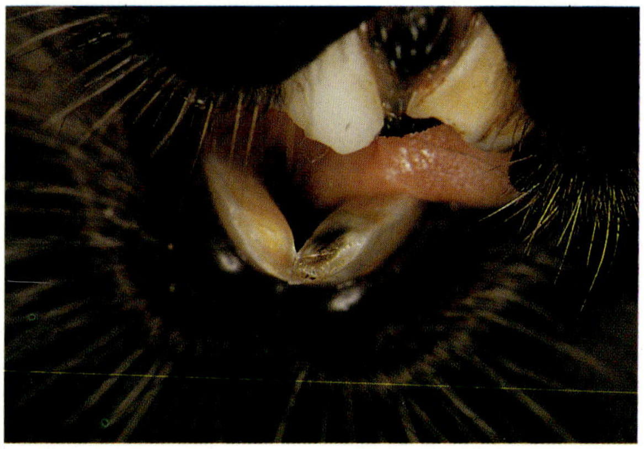

687 Fractured lower incisor — Case 2a — Bennett's wallaby. The lower incisors of wallabies are anelodonts and root canal exposures will lead to pulp necrosis and periapical infection. In this case the typical black spot at the site of exposure is evident. These confined lesions can be confused with necrobacillosis as reactive osseous tissue at the ventral border of the mandible would be palpable.

688

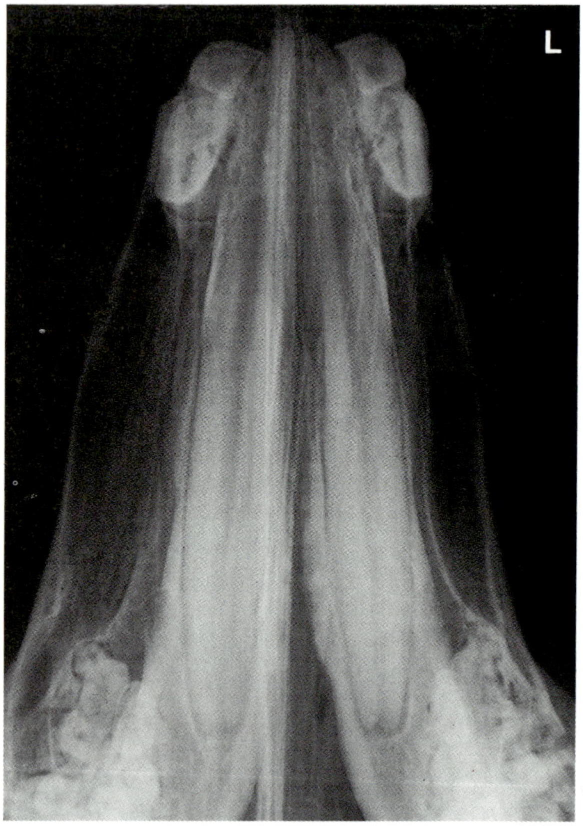

688 Dorsoventral radiograph — Case 2b. A radiolucent periapical lesion of the lower left incisor is visible on the radiograph. Root canal treatment of the fractured incisors is complicated by the fine, long, parallel canals.

689

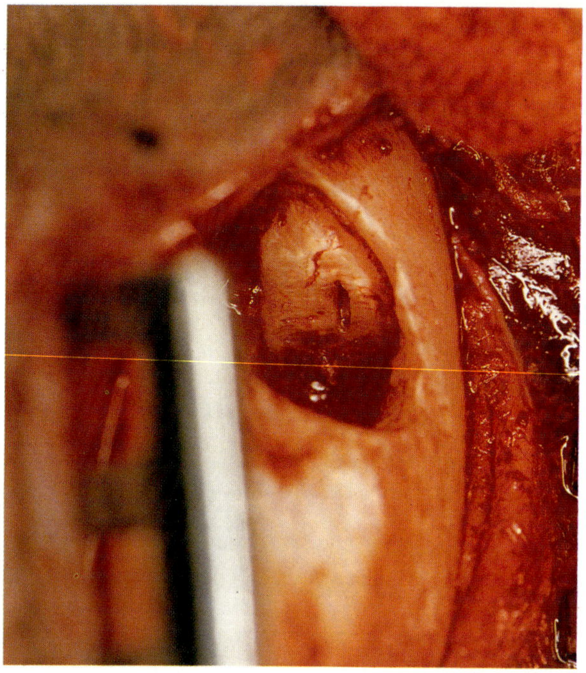

689 Exposure of root apex and periapical defect — Case 2c. An apicectomy and retrograde amalgam seal is advisable to complement the orthograde root filling, which is difficult to condense under the circumstances. A ventral, extra-oral approach is mandatory to access the periapical region.

690

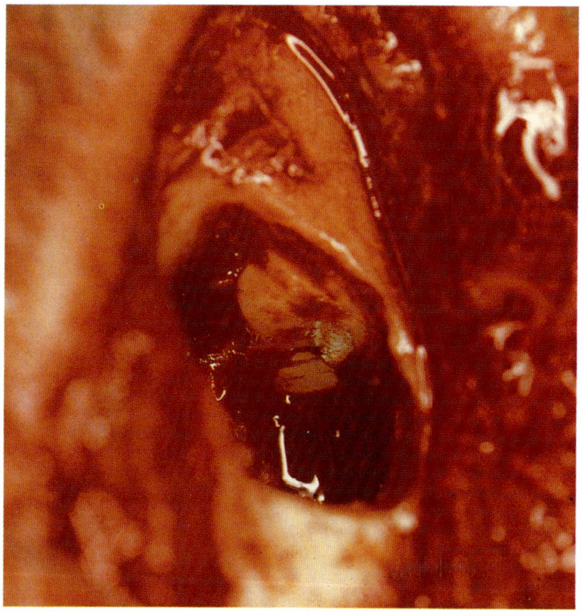

690 Retrograde amalgam — Case 2d.

691 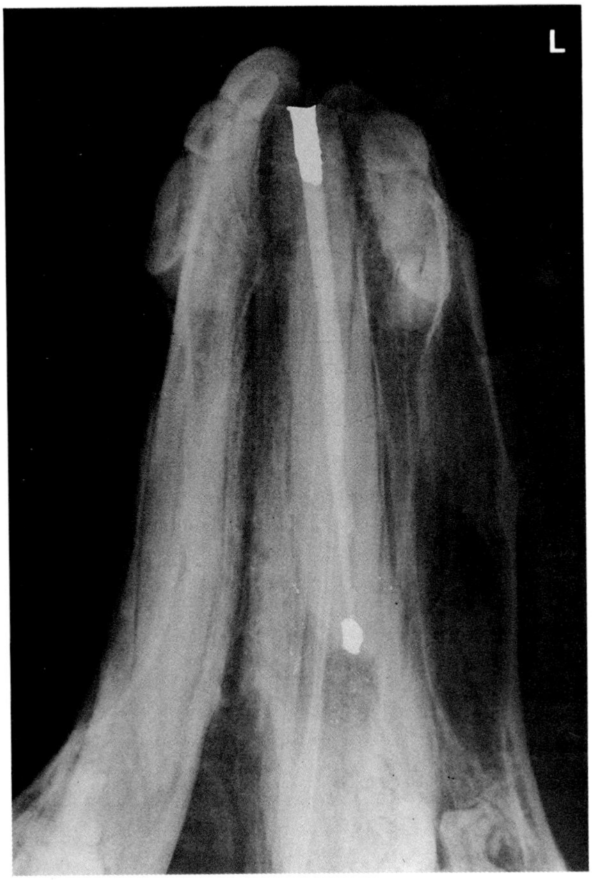

692 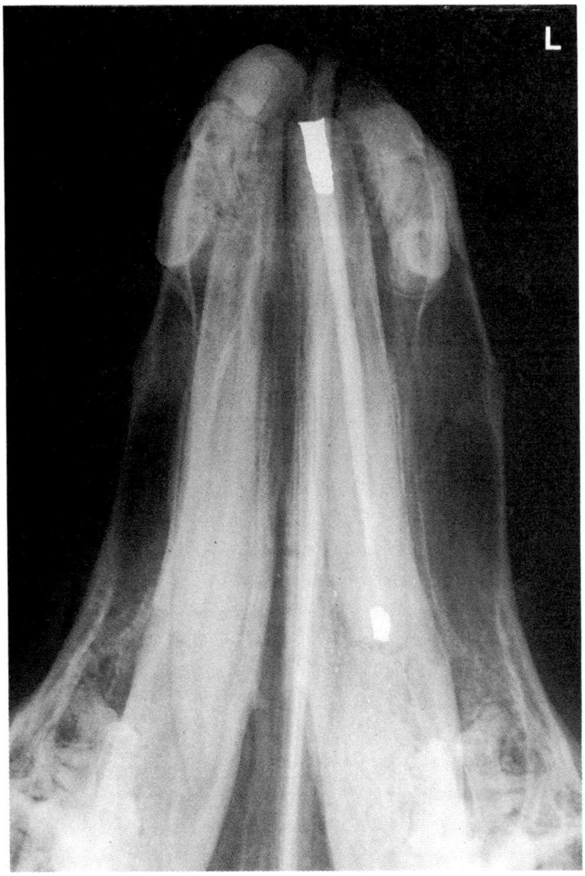

691 Immediate postoperative radiograph — Case 2e. A periapical defect and retrograde amalgam are visible.

692 Follow-up radiograph — Case 2f. Three months postoperatively almost complete healing of the periapical area was evident. The infection did not reoccur in a follow up period of two years.

Miscellaneous

Birds

Guidelines for beak repairs

Lay and professional publications often illustrate prostheses fitted to traumatised beaks. Little in the way of long-term follow-up is available for many of these cases, although most operators admit that the repairs fail within a short period of time. It must also be appreciated that prosthesis and beak surgery often cause more damage than the original trauma. Most birds learn to manage well, despite their injuries. In fact, domestic poultry often have their upper beaks amputated at a very early age to prevent injuries in a battery environment.

It is difficult for most operators to resist the temptation of surgical intervention and the inevitable pressure from some owners for active treatment, rather than to allow the bird to learn to manage with its disability. Certain guidelines must be outlined for the invasive treatment and prosthetic repair of traumatised beaks so as to prevent unnecessary stress and surgery to many birds.

After beak injury a reasonable length of learning time of say two weeks should be allowed, which would involve hand- and possibly force-feeding. No invasive treatment should be embarked upon unless the bird is unable to manage on a modified diet at the end of this period and its life is threatened.

Techniques have also been put forward to correct prognathic beak malocclusions, which are either traumatic or hereditary in origin. Some workers have reported varying degrees of success with oblique bite planes attached to the opposing beak; others have experimented with sliding mandibular osteotomies, where the beak is wired up postoperatively and a pharyngostomy tube is placed throughout the healing phase. There are controversies regarding the ethics of such procedures and readers should study the relevant papers (*see* Bibliography) and draw their own conclusions.

The next section demonstrates, with follow-up photographs, a variety of beak injuries that illustrate the healing potential, the level of regeneration often seen and the results of prosthetic treatment.

693 Toco toucan. The bird suffered a fractured upper beak after a long-standing fungal infection that had undermined and weakened it. Within two days the bird had learned to turn his head on its side and lift the food with the fractured beak.

693

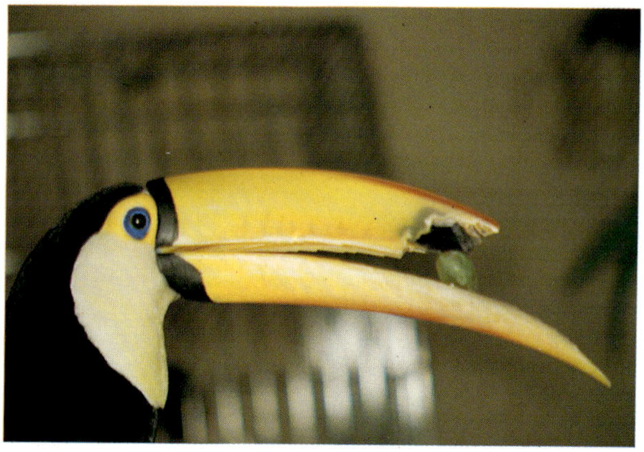

694

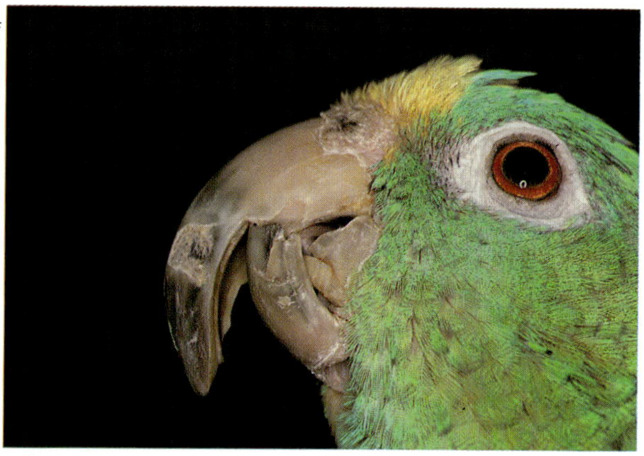

694 Split beak — Case 1a — Yellow-crowned Amazon. A 25-year-old bird with multiple splits of its beak is shown. The bird was managing well and no invasive treatment was given.

695

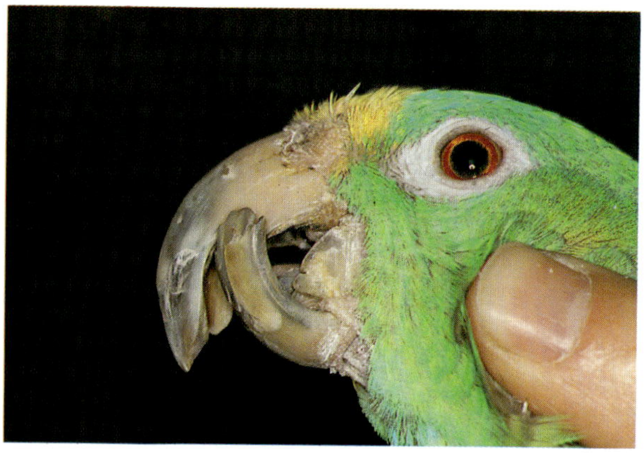

695 Five years later — Case 1b. No healing or growing-out of the cracks took place, but the bird was still eating well. Occasional trimming of the irregular growth and malocclusion was required.

696 Fractured beak — Case 2a — budgerigar. This young bird lost almost the full length of its upper beak through trauma.

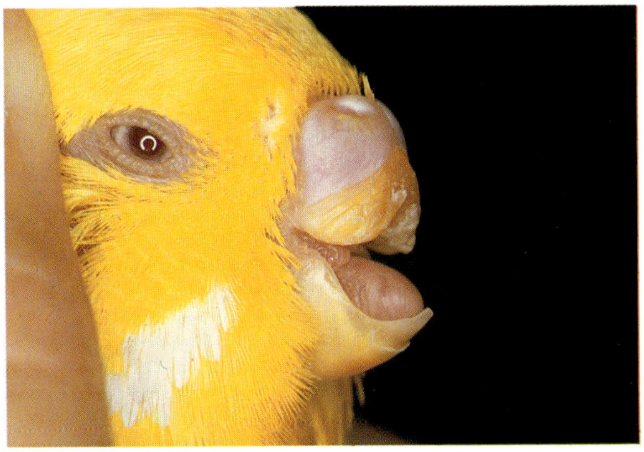

696

697 Close-up of a lost beak — Case 2b. The referring veterinary surgeon anaesthetised the bird seven times in an attempt to replace the lost beak and, subsequently, used an acrylic prosthesis. Repairs failed within one to seven days. The bird was managing on a modified diet. On referral, the bird was placed on a dietary mineral supplement and no prosthesis was placed.

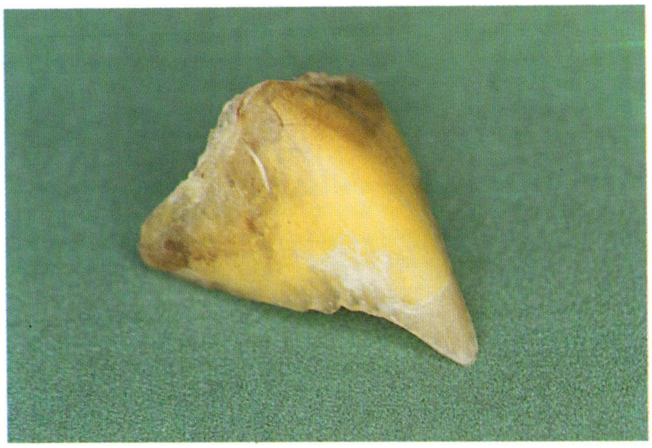

697

698 Five years later — Case 2c. 2.5 mm of new growth has taken place. The bird was feeding well on a normal diet and was able to crack seeds.

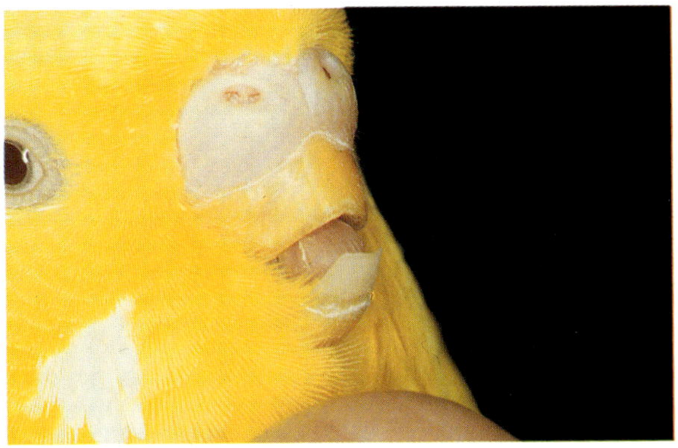

698

699 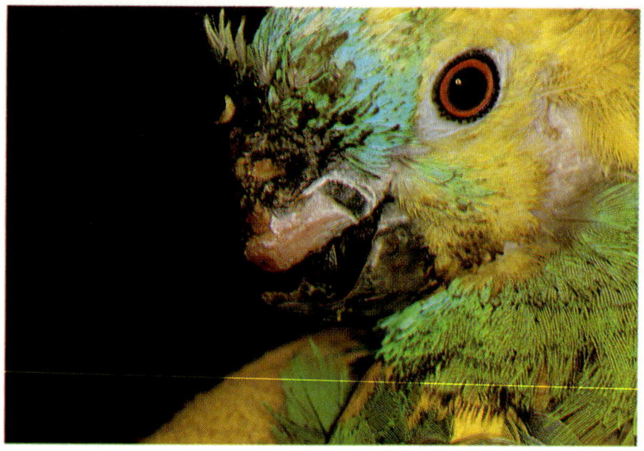

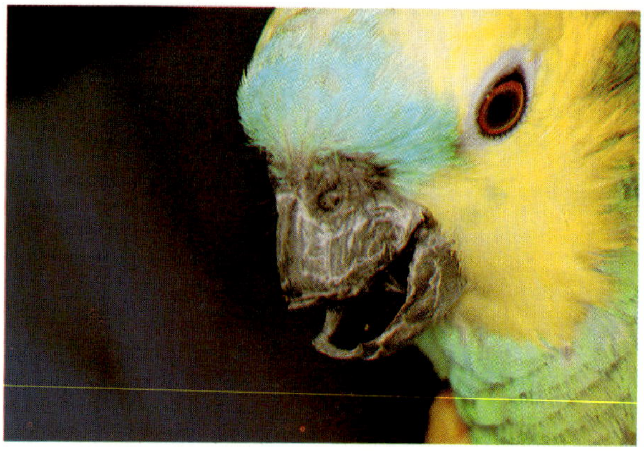 700

699 Recent beak fracture — Case 3a — Bolivian blue-fronted Amazon. The upper beak was fractured traumatically. The bird was managing on a modified diet after learning to use its lower beak in a scooping fashion. No prosthesis was attempted.

700 Five-year follow-up — Case 3b. The length of the beak has not increased appreciably but has thickened and keratinised over well. The bird managed to crack shells with its short beak without difficulty.

701 Deformed beak — cockatiel. This young bird's beak was crushed by a parent. He was unable to eat with the deformity and died.

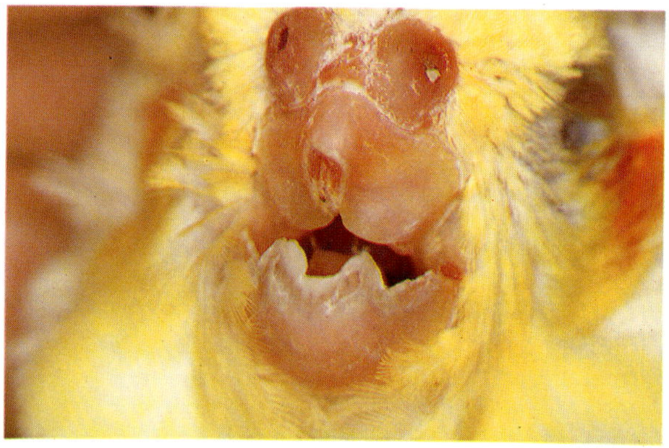 701

702

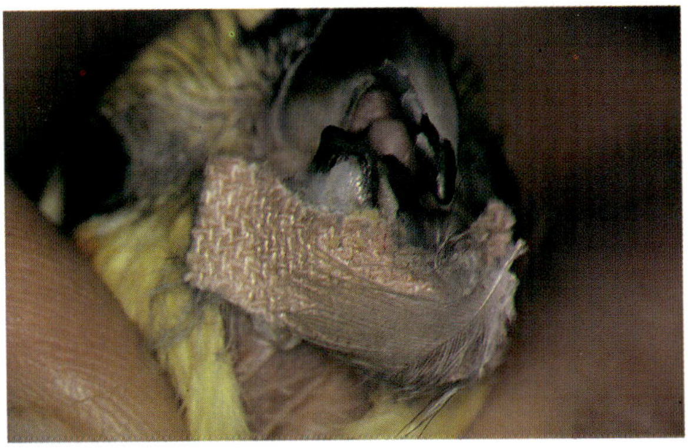

702 Recently split beak — Case 4a — cockatiel. On presentation, adhesive plaster was holding the split beak together. The bird was anorexic and had lost weight rapidly. Intervention was considered necessary.

703

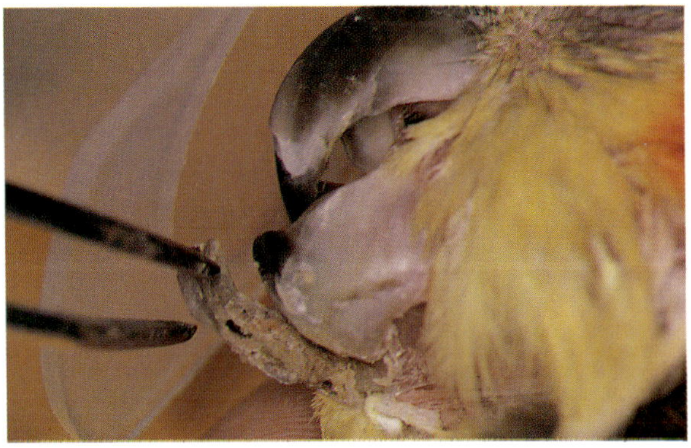

703 Extent of the fracture — Case 4b. The two segments were completely separate, with extensive mobility of the right one.

704

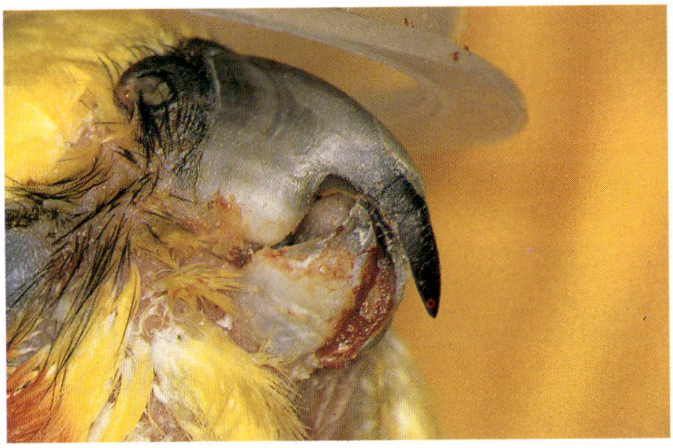

704 Segments approximated. — Case 4c The objective of the treatment was to stabilise the segments and allow the bird to become accustomed to a modified diet and gain weight. The edges of the segments were freshened up to allow healing.

705

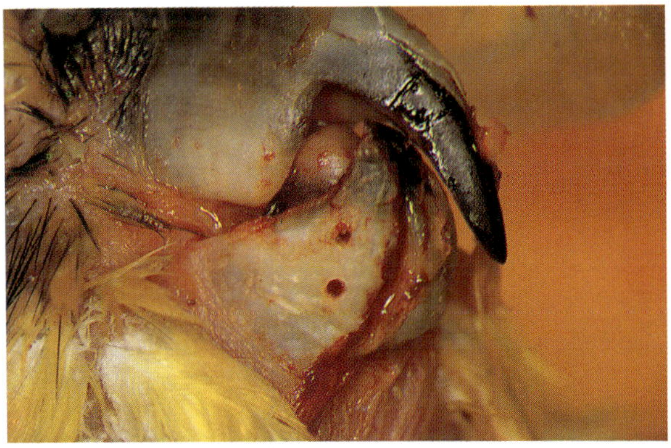

705 Holes drilled — Case 4d. Very fine holes were drilled through the segments to immobilise them with wires.

706

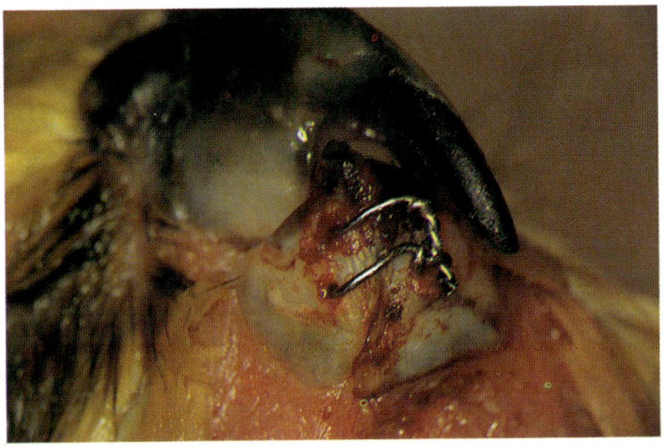

706 Segments wired — Case 4e. Wire ligatures were used to tie the segments together.

707

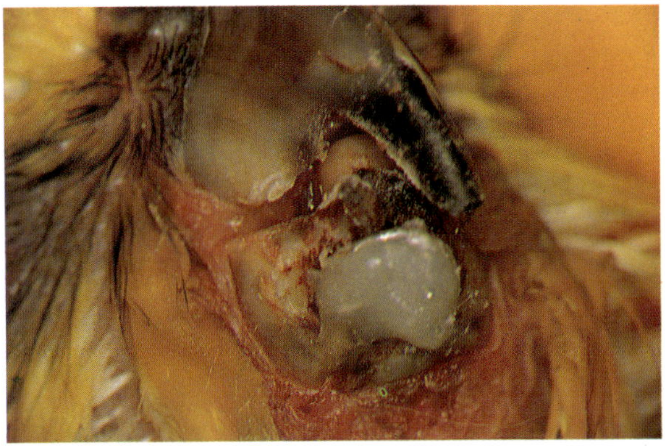

707 Acrylic cover — Case 4f. The wire ligatures had a self-curing acrylic coating placed over them to protect the animal from the sharp ends.

708 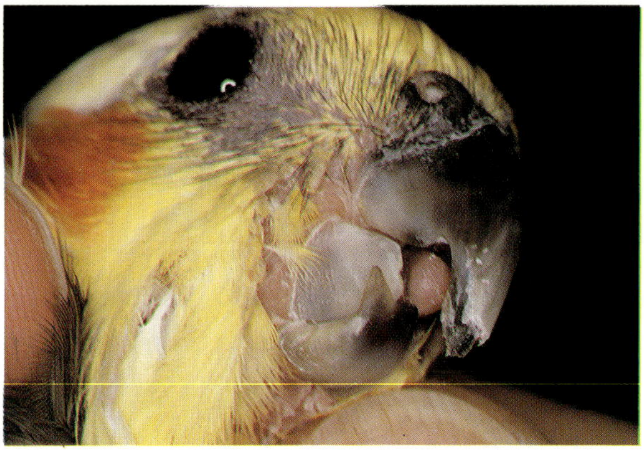

708 Six weeks postoperatively — Case 4g. No healing of the segments occurred. By the time the ligatures were lost through beak growth and abrasion, the bird had recovered in all respects. The beak segments were stable, but not joined, and she was managing well on a modified diet.

Crane/stork bill injuries

The repair of elongated bills has a very high failure rate. A more invasive, but acceptable, treatment alternative, if the bird is unable to feed in a competitive and natural environment, is the amputation of the opposing bill to match the length of the injury. Haemorrhage of the amputation site sometimes needs to be controlled and the length of the tongue occasionally needs to be reduced. It is important to note that among aggressive birds amputated bills mean no defence and the deformed individual may be killed by members of the community within minutes of reintroduction.

709 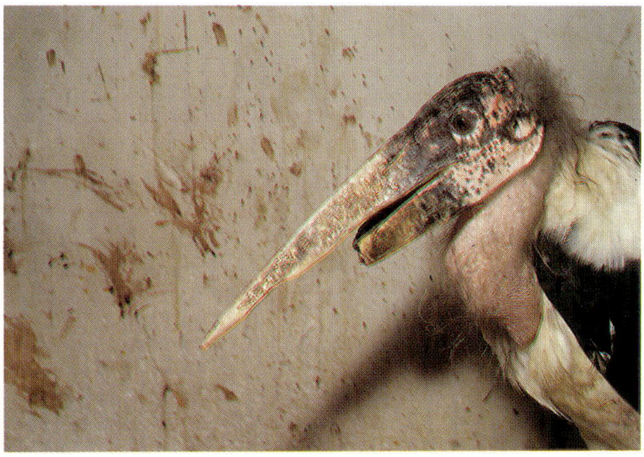

709 Marabou stork — Case 5a. Middle-aged bird was coping well with a fractured lower bill as long as food was supplied deep enough in a container or he was hand fed. The establishment rejected amputation of the upper bill to match the length of the lower. A practitioner attempted to bolt a prosthesis onto the remaining lower bill, which failed within weeks and as a consequence further tissue was lost.

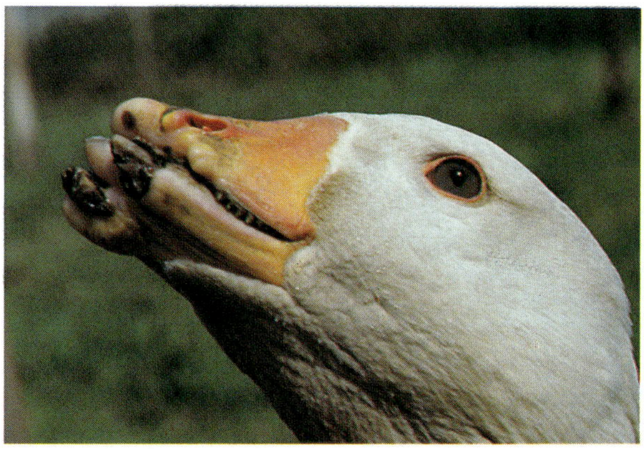 710

710 Fractured bills — goose. Two year old male lost over half the length of its upper bill through trauma. Request from owners for a prosthetic replacement was rejected as the animal, after an initial period of hand feeding, was eating and grazing normally by having learned to turn its head to the side. Three months later the lower bill was also damaged while protecting the eggs of its mate, which resulted in the bird managing to feed more easily with matching lengths of stumps. The animal appears to have also adapted to his disability by holding the tongue further back in the mouth.

Tortoises

It may be surprising that tortoises are included in an atlas on veterinary dentistry, as they do not possess teeth. The aspects covered are the principles of shell repair and the handling procedures of the materials that are in everyday use in dentistry, as much damage and injury can be created through their incorrect use.

In addition to its use in attempts to repair bird beaks, self-curing polymethyl methacrylate (acrylic) is often used in the repair of tortoise shell fractures and defects. The material has many advantages in rapidly creating a hard, inert acrylic mass; however it has some undesirable properties. It is often erroneously assumed that polymethyl methacrylates are adhesives: any bonding to other materials is only through mechanical means and for a true bond a suitable adhesive should also be used.

Self-curing acrylic comprises a monomer, which is the liquid, and a polymer powder. The two have to be combined in the correct proportions for a paste-consistency compound to be obtained. The liquid monomer is highly irritant and so is the paste while it is in an uncured state. Care should be taken to avoid contacting delicate tissues, as chemical burns may result. Although the material used is also called 'cold cured', this only means that no external heat is required for polymerisation to take place, as opposed to 'heat cured' materials. In fact, many of the self-curing products generate enough heat for thermal burns to be created. The reader is strongly urged to protect living tissues from the material while it is in an uncured state and not allow it to set in close proximity until the initial shape has been created. The thicker the material, the more heat will be generated.

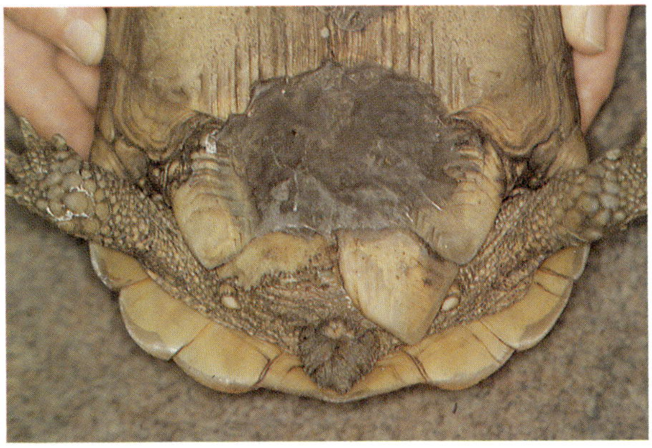

711

711 Abdominal repair — Case 1a — tortoise. A tortoise with two abdominal defects, which were previously repaired by placing liquid self-curing acrylic directly onto the shell and the injury. The operator was not aware of the dangers of the material.

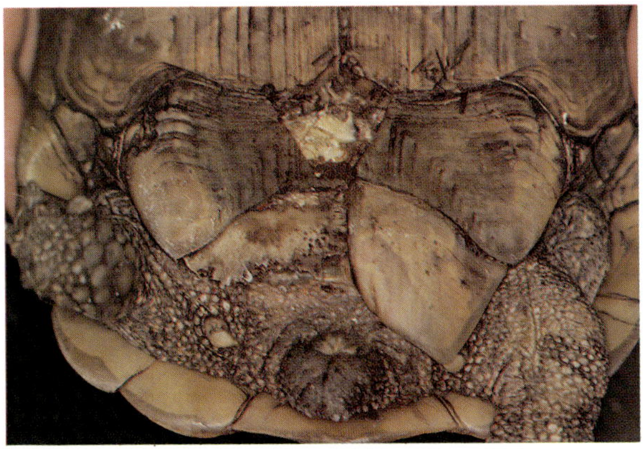

712

712 Necrotic bone — Case 1b. Once the loose piece of acrylic had been removed, necrotic bone was apparent around the repair.

713

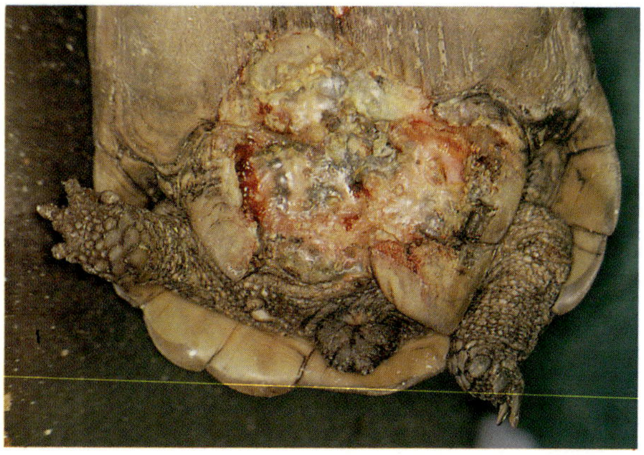

714

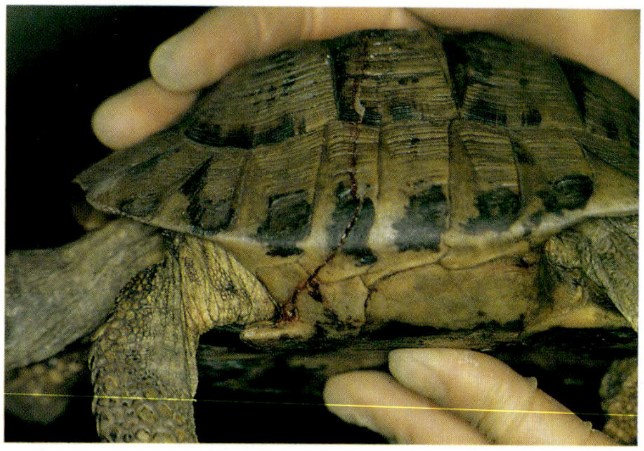

713 Full extent of destruction — Case 1c. The osteomyelitis had spread under the apparently healthy shell and hardly any vital tissue remained in the ventral aspect. Euthanasia was considered the most humane option.

714 Fractured shell — Case 2a — tortoise. Traumatic injuries to tortoise shells are common. As the shell is composed of bone, with a thin keratinised external layer, healing of the fractures takes place from an internal direction. If shell fractures are neglected, bacterial invasion can result in osteomyelitis.

715

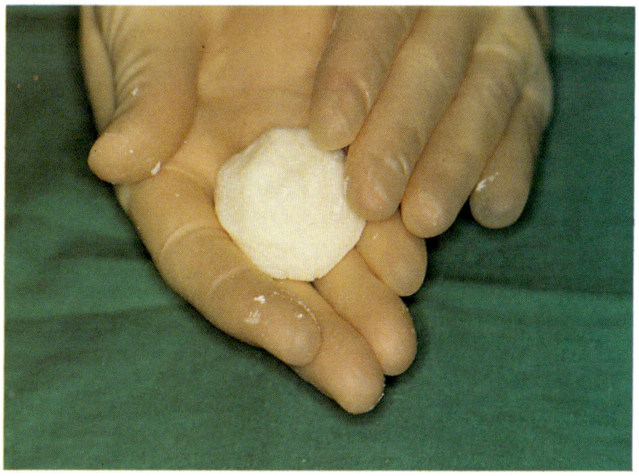

716

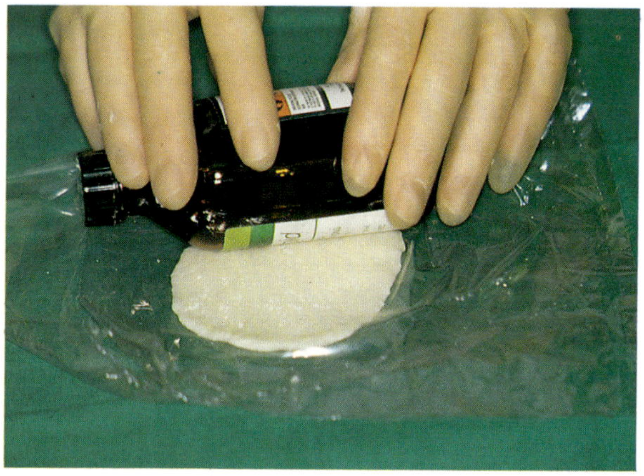

715 Acrylic ball — Case 2b. Methyl methacrylate is an irritant material. Mixing is best carried out in a disposable cup. The manufacturer's recommended liquid to powder ratio must be adhered to or the physical properties and the setting time will be seriously altered. The material will go through specific phases: liquid, tacky, dough, then solid. Once it has reached a doughy stage it is rolled into a ball with gloved hands.

716 Flattened acrylic — Case 2c. The ball is quickly placed into a thin plastic bag and pressed and rolled on a flat surface to an even thickness.

717 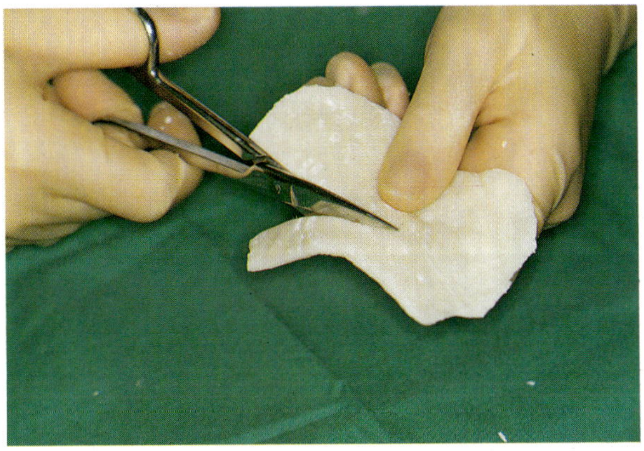

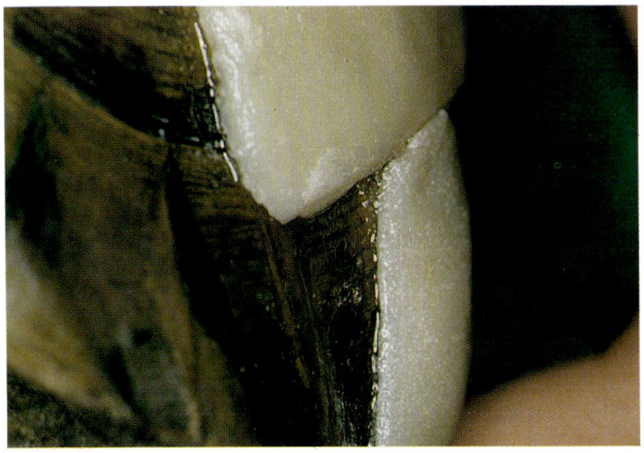 718

717 **Cutting the strip — Case 2d.** The acrylic is removed from the plastic bag and cut into the shape required with a pair of scissors. Before the doughy material is applied to the body, the shell and the injury is covered with kitchen foil or 'cling film' so the material can be easily applied and removed repeatedly to give the acrylic the required shape and prevent the tissues of the animal becoming irritated or overheated. Self-curing acrylic distorts during setting. Once it is fully cured it may be necesary to reline the fitting surface with more material to obtain the accuracy of fit necessary for maximum adhesion. The separating material is kept in position during the relining stage.

718 **The strap is bonded into place — Case 2e.** The glaze from the surface of the shell can be carefully roughened to improve the bonding of the adhesive. The relined strap shows the close adaptation of the material. The ideal adhesive is a cyanoacrylate gel, which improves the bond strength up to a gap of 0.5 mm. Cyanoacrylates are usually self-curing and set rapidly under the anaerobic, humid conditions that exist at the surface interface of joints. The material is applied to the acrylic and the shell surface, and setting takes place under pressure within 30 seconds at room temperature. Excess uncured material from the margins of the straps can be removed with gauze.

719 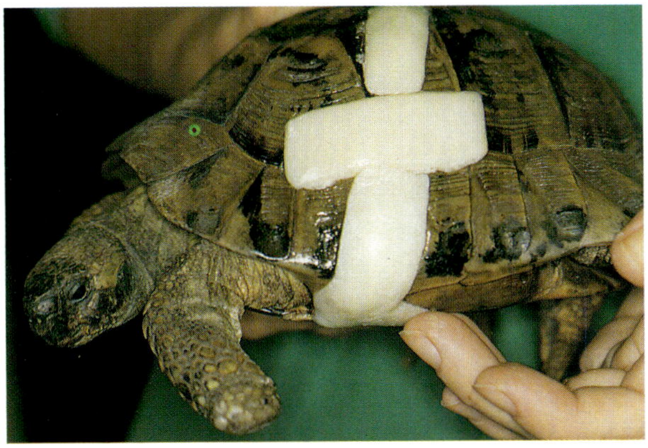

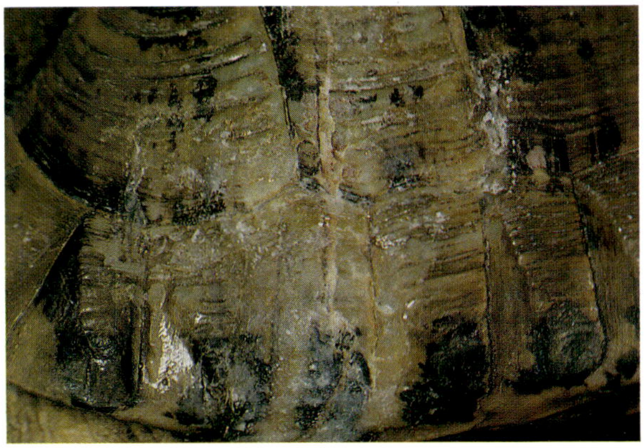 720

719 **Final result — Case 2f.** The cross-straps enhance the stabilisation of the segments. As cyanoacrylate is hydrophilic, the exposed adhesive joints were varnished with a moisture-resistant material.

720 **Two years postoperative — Case 2g.** The acrylic straps were totally intact two years after the injury and completely attached to the shell. The removal was achieved through thinning the material with a tungsten burr and the final remains with a scalpel. Chemical solvents are strongly contraindicated. The callus in the fracture line is clearly visible. Care must be exercised in the removal of the acrylic as the thin keratinised layer is easily damaged.

Bibliography

History of the oral and dental treatment of animals

Bartlett, E. (1899). *Wild Animals in Captivity*. Chapman & Hall, London.

Brightwell, L.R. (1952). *The Zoo Story*. Museum Press, London.

Merillat, L.A. (1914). *Animal Dentistry and Diseases of the Mouth*. Alexander Eger, Chicago.

Swartz, K. (1979). Tierqualerische chirurgische Eingriffe am Maul und an den Backen des Pferdes in der Stallmeisterzeit (Inhumane surgical operations on the mouth and cheeks of the horse in the period of the Masters of the Horse). Inaugural dissertation, Ludwig-Maximillians Universität, München.

Yu, Benjuan and Yu, Benheng (1979). *Yuan Heng Liao Ma Niu Tuo Jing Quanji (Complete Collection of Yuan's and Heng's Treatment for the Horse, Cattle and Camel)*. Nongye Chubanshe, Beijing.

Dental anatomy and comparative odontology

Bland-Sutton, J. (1884). Comparative dental pathology. *Transactions of the Odontological Society of Great Britain* new series, **16**, 88–145.

Miles, A.E.W. & Grigson, C. (1990). *Colyer's Variation and Diseases of the Teeth of Animals*, (revised edn). Cambridge University Press, Cambridge.

Peyer, B. (1968). *Comparative Odontology*. The University of Chicago Press, Chicago.

Scott, J.H. & Symons, N.R.B. (1982). *Introduction to Dental Anatomy*, 9th edn. Livingstone, Edinburgh and London.

Tomes, C.S. (1904). *A Manual of Dental Anatomy*. J.& A. Churchill, London.

Widdowson, T.W. (1939). *Special or Dental Anatomy and Physiology and Dental Histology, Human and Comparative*. John Bale, Sons & Curnow, London.

Periodontal disease

Allen, D.L., McFall, W.T., Jr & Hunter, G.C. (1986). *Periodontics for the Dental Hygienist*, 4th edn. Lea & Feibiger, Philadelphia.

Grant, D.A., Stern, I.B. & Lisgarten, M.A. (1988). *Periodontics*, 6th edn. C.V. Mosby, St. Louis.

Macphee, T. & Cowling, G. (1981). *Essentials of Periodontology and Periodontics*, 3rd edn. Blackwell Scientific Publications, Oxford.

Diseases of the calcified dental tissues and conservative dentistry

Cawson, R.A. (1991). *Essentials of Dental Surgery and Pathology*, 5th edn. J. & A. Churchill, London.

Shafer, W.G., Hine, M.K., & Levy, B.M. (1983). *A Textbook of Oral Pathology*, 4th edn. W.B. Saunders, Philadelphia.

Dental trauma and endodontics

Messing, J.J. & Stock, C.J.R. (1988). *A Colour Atlas of Endodontics*. Wolfe Medical Publications, London.

Oral surgery: extractions

Howe, G.L. (1985). *Minor Oral Surgery*, 3rd edn. John Wright & Sons, Bristol.

Dental diseases and their treatment in captive wild animals

Clipsham, R. (1989). Surgical beak restoration and correction. *Proceedings of the Association of Avian Veterinarians*, pp. 164–76.

Hess, R.E. Jr. & Collins, R. (1987). The correction of a beak deformity in a Southern bald eagle. *Proceedings of the First International Conference on Zoological and Avian Medicine*, pp. 323–4.

Howard, P.E. (1989). Management of beak fractures in cranes. *Proceedings of the 1989 Exotic Animal Dentistry Conference, Philadelphia*, pp. 24–31.

Appendix

Photographic technical information for Chapters 1–10 and 14

Equipment used

Nikon F bodies. Cameras were hand-held for all the clinical photographs. The lens used was a Medical-Nikkor 120 mm/f4. Some of the photographs of the domestic cat were taken with a Medical-Nikkor 200 mm/f4. Radiographs were photographed with the camera mounted on a tripod, with a Micro-Nikkor 55 mm/f3.5.

Film used for colour photographs

Kodak Ektachrome Professional 64 ASA; flash was set at 45 ASA for intra-oral close-ups (× *0.5* and × 2), and at 55 ASA for extra-oral photographs (× *0.04* to × *0.9)* and light-toned close-up subjects. The film speed was set at 25 ASA for mirror-reflected images. Films were processed at normal speed.

Endoscopic photographs

Olympus OM2 body and Zuiko 100 mm/f2.8lens. For some photographs, close-up rings were also used. The laparoscopes were 10 mm in diameter with 50° or 0° angulation. Light sources were Wolf continuous source model No. 5105 or flash source model No. 5005. Film used was Fujichrome 1600, exposed and processed at 1600 ASA.

Radiographs

Small specimens were radiographed on Kodak Industrex AX, and then photographed onto Agfa Dia Direct 12 ASA.

Glossary

This atlas will be read by professionals of diverse specialities — practising and student veterinary and dental surgeons, veterinary and dental auxiliaries, zoologists, zoo curators and keepers and laboratory workers. Since the readers will have different training and technical vocabularies, the inclusion of a glossary is considered vital. The glossary is a comprehensive guide to the vocabulary the reader may encounter in the study, discussion and treatment of animal dentitions. Classical definitions in dentistry are traditionally based on human teeth, hence some important modifications have been made so they are applicable to the whole range of dentitions. Some entries contain encyclopaedic details to enrich the reader's insight into the subject.

- American variations in terminology are indicated *N. Amer.*
- A subject field, e.g. *Biology, Dentistry,* is given when the meaning of the entry varies, or the area of use is not clear in the explanation. Note that *Medicine* includes surgical terms.
- The etymology of many of the entries is given in [square brackets].
- Words in SMALL CAPITALS indicate a separate main entry in the glossary.
- Prefixes and suffixes used frequently in the etymologies are given as main entries in order not to repeat information.

The convention used in this atlas for hyphenation is as follows:

- Hyphens are used if two consecutive vowels are present and there is a danger of a diphthong being created, e.g. oro-antral, pre-operative, or when two or more words are used as a single adjective, e.g. root-filling material, tooth-like structure.
- Hyphens are not used if a connecting vowel is employed in the construction of a term, e.g. oronasal, dorsoventral, or where the joint usage of the words has become so common that they are considered a single expression, e.g. postoperative, postmortem.

abrasion: tooth wear caused by frictional contact of a tooth with non-dental material. [from L. *abradere* to scrape away] Compare ATTRITION and EROSION.

abscess: localised collection of pus, generally as a result of an infection. [from L. *abscedere* to go away]

acid etching: the microscopic roughening of the enamel surface with a dilute acid to increase its mechanically retentive property to restorative materials. Usually the procedure preferentially removes the enamel prism cores and leaves the prism peripheries intact.

acrodont: tooth that is attached to the crest of the jaw through ankylosis and lacks a root formation. [from Gr. *akros* at the top + -ODONT]

acrylic: referring to synthetic compounds that contain acrylic acid, which is formed by the oxidisation of acrolein. See METHYL METHACRYLATE, COLD-CURED, HEAT-CURED, MONOMER and POLYMER..

acute necrotising/ulcerative gingivitis: see VINCENT'S INFECTION.

air rotor or **air turbine:** *Dentistry.* compressed-air-operated turbine that drives friction grip miniature burrs, usually at speeds between 200,000 to 500,000 rpm.

alginate: a commercial mixture containing powdered alginate obtained from brown seaweed, diatomaceous earth filler and calcium sulphate which are mixed with water to produce a PLASTIC (1), irreversible, colloid type elastic impression material. [from L. *alga* seaweed]

alveolar: of or pertaining to the sockets of the teeth. See ALVEOLUS.

alveolar bone: bone that constitutes the alveolar processes.

alveolar crest: the most coronal point of the bone that surrounds the teeth.

alveolar mucosa: loosely attached mucous membrane covering bone that contains the teeth.

alveolar process: the part of the maxilla or mandible that contains the sockets of erupted teeth or the crypts of developing unerupted teeth. See ALVEOLUS.

alveolus: the sockets in the jaw that retain the teeth. [L. a diminutive of *alveus;* small cavity, socket, sac-like dilation]

amalgam: an alloy of mercury with one or more other metals. [possibly from Gr. *malagma* a soft mass]

amelo-: (prefix) indicating enamel or tissues of epithelial odontogenic origin. [from Old Fr. *amail* enamel]

ameloblast: germ cell originating from epithelium from which the enamel is formed. [from AMELO- + -BLAST]

amelogenesis: the process of enamel formation. [from AMELO- + Gr. *genesis* (suffix) development, generation]

amelogenesis imperfecta: disturbance in the formation of enamel.

amyloid: *Pathology.* abnormal, complex, insoluble glycoprotein-like substance, the aetiology of which has been connected with immunoglobins. [from L. *amylum* starch, the substance it was originally thought to be related to]

amyloidosis: a degenerative condition where amyloid is deposited in the parenchymal organs (e.g. kidneys, liver and spleen) rendering the cells nonfunctional. The condition often follows a chronic suppurative focus in the body, when it is termed *secondary* or *reactive* amyloidosis.

anatomical crown: that part of the tooth where enamel constitutes a portion of its external or internal structure. Compare CLINICAL CROWN.

anatomical root: that part of the tooth where enamel does not constitute a portion of its external or internal structure and is covered with cementum.

anelodont: *New term.* type of tooth that has a limited period of growth. [from Gr. *an-* (prefix) not + *elo-* (prefix) an abbreviation of L. *elongare* to lengthen + -ODONT] Compare ELODONT.

anisognathic: having jaws of unequal width. Usually implies an upper jaw that is significantly wider than the opposing mandible. [from Gr. *an-* *(prefix)* not + *isos* equal + -GNATHIC]

ankylosis: the joining together of bone and bone, or tooth and bone by direct union of the parts, resulting in rigidity. [from Gr. *ankuloun* to crook]

anodontia: the absence of teeth, partial or total and qualified accordingly, usually indicating a failure of tooth development. [from Gr. *an-* (prefix) not + -ODONT + *-ia* (suffix) denoting a condition]

anterior teeth: collective term for the incisors and canines.

antral: relating to an antrum.

antrum:
- an air-filled natural cavity, usually in bone.
- also called a sinus, e.g. *maxillary antrum* = maxillary sinus. [from Gr. *antron* cave]

ANUG: acute necrotising ulcerative gingivitis. See VINCENT'S INFECTION.

apex: the terminal extremity of a tooth root. [L. summit, tip]

apical: pertaining to, towards or located at the root tip of a tooth. [from APEX]

apical delta: a type of foramen at the tip of a tooth root, where the innervation and vascular supply to the pulp is through multiple fine channels. [from a type of river mouth where the main channel divides into multiple distributaries resembling the shape of the Greek letter Δ]

apical foramen: aperture at the apex of a tooth root through which the vascular supply and innervation to the pulp enter the root canal.

apicectomy (*N. Amer.* apicoectomy)**:** endodontic treatment that involves amputation of the root tip [from APEX + -ECTOMY]

apicoectomy: see APICECTOMY.

approximal or **proximal:** *Dentistry.* collective term that refers to surfaces of teeth that face adjoining teeth of the same dental arch. [from L. *approximare* side by side, close together; from *proximus* nearest] Compare PROXIMAL.

arcade: see DENTAL ARCADE.

arch: see DENTAL ARCH.

attached gingiva: see GINGIVA.

attrition: tooth wear caused by tooth-to-tooth frictional contact. [from L. *terere* to rub] Compare ABRASION and EROSION.

AUG: acute ulcerative gingivitis. See VINCENT'S INFECTION.

bacterial plaque or **dental plaque:** soft mass of micro-organisms, cellular material and food debris that adheres to the surfaces of the teeth and/or gingiva.

barbed broach: instrument used in endodontics, with small spikes on the side of its working tip, used for removing pulp tissue.

biopsy: samples of tissue taken from a living body for diagnostic purposes, usually examined with a microscope. [from Gr. *bios* life + *opsis* sight]

bishoping:
- to burn.
- tampering with the appearance of an animal, normally a horse, to make it look younger for fraudulent reasons.
- making an old horse appear younger by burning, or drilling and staining an artificial concavity in the dentine of the incisor tables in an attempt to mimic the infundibulum of a younger animal. [Although the techniques of falsifying the appearance of a horse's age were described in detail in early farrier texts, the term 'Bishoping' first appeared in 1725 as a 'Jockey's term' in *The Family Dictionary* by R. Bradley. There is no evidence to support the theory that the practice was initiated by a person of such a name. As burning with a small iron was the original method used to falsify the infundibula of horses' incisors, the etymology of the term is almost certainly derived from the old expression 'to bishop' which means 'to burn'. William Tyndale (1492–1536) recorded its usage in proverbs from the north of England: 'If the porage be burned to, or the meate ouer roasted we say the bishop hath put his foote in the potte or the bishop has played the cooke, because the bishops burn who they lust and whosoever displeaseth them'. It is ironic that Tyndale himself was burnt at the stake for heresy on the orders of an archbishop.]

-blast: (suffix) *Histology.* embryonic cell or formative layer. [from Gr. *blastos* bud]

body of the mandible: part of the lower jaw that contains the alveolar processes and the teeth; in animals it is often incorrectly termed *horizontal ramus*. [from Old High Ger. *botah* body. The meaning of body employed in this usage: the main or principal part, as distinguished from subordinate parts which are attached to it as appendages.] See RAMUS OF THE MANDIBLE.

bonding, enamel: process used to increase the retentive properties of an etched enamel surface by polymerising within it a matrix of unfilled resin. See ACID ETCHING.

brachy-: (prefix) indicating something short. [from Gr. *brakhus* short]

brachycephalic:
- having a head or muzzle that is abnormally short for the species.
- having a head that is almost as wide as its rostrocaudal/anteroposterior dimension. [from BRACHY- + CEPHALIC] Compare DOLICHOCEPHALIC and MESOCEPHALIC.

brachygnathic: having an abnormally short mandible. [from BRACHY- + -GNATHIC]

brachyodont: teeth which have anatomical crowns that are shorter than their roots. [from BRACHY- + -ODONT] Compare HYPSODONT.

brachytherapy: radiation treatment using an implanted or closely appliead radioactive isotope. [from BRACHY- (used in this context to indicate 'from a short distance') + Gr. *therapeia* attendance]

bridge: prosthesis attached to natural teeth and/or dental implants used for the replacement of missing teeth.

buccal:
- of or pertaining to the cheek.
- surfaces of the posterior teeth and adjacent tissues facing the buccinator muscle of the cheek. [from L. *bucca* cheek]

bucco-: (prefix) signifying buccal, cheek.

bucco-occlusal angle: junction where the buccal and occlusal surfaces of a tooth meet.

buccostomy: the formation of a surgical opening through the side of the face that is kept patent beyond the duration of the operation. [from BUCCO- + L. *os* mouth, entrance to a passage + -TOMY]

buccotomy: surgical incision made through the side of the face, usually performed in herbivores, to accomplish an intra-oral procedure that is inaccessible through a labial approach. [from BUCCO- + -TOMY]

bunodont: teeth that have prominent conical cusps to the occlusal surfaces of their posterior teeth (e.g. pigs, bears). [from Gr. *bunos* mound + -ODONT]

burr or **bur:** rotary cutting instrument used in handpieces for the reduction of tooth, bone or existing dental restorations. [from Danish *burre*]

cachexia: condition of weakness of the body that results from a debilitating chronic disease. [from Gr. *kakos* bad + *hexis* condition]

calcium hydroxide: a white powder that is able to encourage the deposition of secondary dentine under certain clinical situations. It is often used in lining materials and in products used in partial coronal pulpectomy. Also called slaked lime or calcium hydrate.

calculus: an abnormal mineralised deposit found on the teeth through precipitation of calcium and phosphorus salts in the saliva. [from L. *calx* small stone]

cancellous: *Anatomy.* having an open, porous, spongy internal structure. [from L. *cancellus* lattice, cross-bars]

canine tooth: conical and pointed crowned tooth, so named because of its resemblance to that of the dog. When present, the single canine tooth per quadrant lies distal to the incisors and mesial to the premolars. [from L. *canis* dog]

caries: demineralisation of calcified dental tissues through the acid produced by micro-organisms. [L. decay; related to Gr. *ker* death]

carnassial teeth: large, opposing and blade-like teeth, adapted for cutting and slicing meat. Term used to describe the last upper premolars and the first lower molars of 'true carnivores' (e.g. felids and canids, but excludes e.g. bears and pandas which do not have such specialised teeth). [from Fr. *carnassier* meat eating]

caudal: *Veterinary.* at or towards the the tail end of the body or structure. [from L. *cauda* tail] Compare ROSTRAL.

cavitation: the formation and collapse of microscopic bubbles on the liquid covered surface of a structure. This action, after which the first ultrasonic scaler was named, is one of the principles by which ultrasonic instruments function.

Cavitron: trade name of the first ultrasonic scaler marketed in 1955 by the Cavitron Corporation. Often other makes of ultrasonic scalers are erroneously called by this name.

cellulitis: diffuse inflammation, often purulent, of the soft tissues.

cement, dental:
- a PLASTIC (1) material that is used to affix dental restorations.
- a type of filling material.

cemento-enamel junction: a line on the tooth surface where the cementum of the roots meets the enamel of the crown.

cementum: a bone-like connective tissue that covers the outer surface of anatomical tooth roots. Cementum is also found:
- in the infundibula of hypsodont crowns.
- surrounding or lying between the enamel folds or plates of some hypsodont teeth.
- covering the non-occlusal surfaces of some hypsodont crowns. [from L. *caementum* stone]

cephalic: relating to the skull or head. [from Gr. *kephalos* head]

cervical: pertaining to the clinical neck of the tooth adjacent to the gingival margin. Sometimes used to indicate the cemento-enamel junction. [from L. *cervix* neck]

cGy: a centigray, 1/100 of a gray. See GRAY.

cheek teeth: *Veterinary.* usually an equine term to describe all the premolar and molar teeth but sometimes used to describe those teeth of other animals.

chemotherapy: the treatment of disease with chemical agents that affect the pathological parts or organisms.

choking up: *Veterinary.* restriction of the airway.

chuck: part of the handpiece that holds the burr.

clinical crown: that part of a tooth which is
- visible in the mouth.
- not covered with gingiva or embedded in the alveolus. See CROWN. Compare ANATOMICAL CROWN.

closed apex: See CONSTRICTED APEX.

cold-cured: a form of acrylic resin that does not require heat for the hardening process to take place; however, heat is usually generated by the reaction. See EXOTHERMIC. Compare HEAT-CURED.

collagen: a fibrous form of protein that is an important constituent of periodontal ligament, cartilage, bone and connective tissue. [from Gr. *kolla* glue + *-gen* (suffix) producing; from *genes* born. (Tissues that contain collagen yield gelatin on boiling.)]

commissure:
- band of tissue joining two parts or organs together.
- corners of the mouth, where the upper and lower lips join (c. *labialis*). [from L. *commissura* joining together]

composite resin: restorative dental material, usually tooth coloured. Most composite resins are composed of an organic polymer matrix, which is an aromatic diacrylate, and inorganic quartz or silica fillers, which increase hardness and wear-resistance.

concha: any organ of the body that resembles a shell in shape. Nasal turbinate bone. [from Gr. *konkhe* shellfish]

condyle of the mandible: a rounded articular process at the caudal/posterior part of the mandibular ramus which articulates with the temporal bone, forming the temporomandibular joint; a cartilaginous disc is present between the articulate surfaces. [from Gr. *kondulos* knuckle, joint]

congenital: denoting a condition, usually abnormal, present at or before birth, but one that is not necessarily hereditary. [from L. *congenitus* born with] Compare HEREDITARY.

conservative dentistry: collective name for the aspects of dentistry that are concerned with the preservation of injured and diseased teeth.

conservative treatment: *Medicine.* treatment not involving surgery.

constricted apex: *New term.* apical foramen that is narrower in diameter than the adjoining terminal root canal. Found in mature anelodont teeth. Usually inaccurately termed *closed apex.* Compare DILATED APEX.

contra-angle handpiece: instrument in which the burr is at an angle to the body of the instrument. Compare STRAIGHT HANDPIECE.

coral formation: *Veterinary.* metaplastic calcification of conchal cartilage through chronic infection.

corona: crown. [L.]

coronal: relating to or towards the crown part of a tooth.

corono-: combining form of *corona.*

coronoid process: part of the ramus of the mandible on which the temporal muscle is inserted. [from Gr. *korone* a crow, resembling a crow's beak]

cortex: the external layer of an organ or bones; hence, cortical. [L. bark, outer layer]

cortical: see CORTEX.

crown:
- part of a tooth where enamel constitutes a portion of its external or internal structure.
- part of a brachyodont tooth that is covered with enamel.
- part of a tooth that is utilised in mastication.
- a dental prosthesis which restores a fractured or decayed tooth through covering the remaining part. [from CORONA] See ANATOMICAL CROWN and CLINICAL CROWN.

crib-biting: destructive behaviour when horses bite their food container, resulting in an abnormal wear pattern to their incisors and the ingestion of air.

crypt: a cavity in the alveolar process containing the bud of a developing tooth.

cusp: pointed projection usually found on the occlusal surface of posterior teeth. [from L. *cuspis* point]

cyanoacrylate: adhesive material usually self-curing in the presence of moisture in an anaerobic environment.

cyst: membrane-lined cavity containing liquid, gas or granulation tissue. [from Gr. *kustis* bag, bladder]

debridement:
- *Dentistry.* the removal of debris from a cavity in a tooth, extraction socket or root canal.
- *Medicine.* the surgical removal of cellular debris from the surface of a wound. [from Old Fr. *desbrider* removal of bridle]

deciduous teeth: See PRIMARY TEETH.

dehiscence: *Medicine.* the spontaneous breakdown of a surgical wound. [from L. *dehiscere* to split open]

delta formation: See APICAL DELTA.

dens: tooth. [L.]

dental arcade: *Veterinary.* a term for the arrangement of all the cheek teeth and associated tissues in any one of the dental quadrants of the horse. [The term appears to have originated from the meaning of 'arcade': 'a line of shops in a covered passage', as the cheek teeth of the horse are also closely abutting, similar units in a straight line. The phrase is ambiguous, and is often used in error to imply a dental arch as 'arcade' derives etymologically from L. *arcus* bow, arch.] Compare DENTAL ARCH.

dental arch: the arrangement of the complete upper or lower dentition.

dental cap:
- *Colloquial.* crown prosthesis.
- *Veterinary.* the coronal remains of a horse's primary molars once the roots have been resorbed.

dental formula: a system of alphanumeric notation introduced in 1849, used to illustrate the numbers and arrangement of the teeth, usually of the permanent dentition, in the jaws of any mammal. See Chapter 4.

dental notation: a system of shorthand whereby the position of a tooth or teeth in the mouth can be recorded. See PALMER'S DENTAL NOTATION, INTERNATIONAL TWO-DIGIT SYSTEM.

dental plaque: See BACTERIAL PLAQUE.

dental sac: *Veterinary.* term usually used in horses to describe the remains of the dental follicle at the dilated root apices of immature teeth.

dentigerous: containing teeth or tooth-like structures. [from L. *dentiger* tooth-bearing + *-ous* having, characterised by]

dentine: sensitive calcified tissue that constitutes the bulk of the tooth and surrounds the pulp cavity. [from DENS + *-ine* of or pertaining to] See SECONDARY DENTINE.

diastema: wide spacing between teeth that indicates either:
- naturally occurring space in most mammals except man, between adjacent types of teeth in the rostral aspect of the jaws.
- an abnormal space between adjacent teeth in man. [Gr. interval]

diathermy: *Medicine.* the local application of a high frequency electric current through external electrodes, which generates heat in the tissues. In surgery, depending on the wave pattern and current filtration employed, it is utilised for cutting or destruction of tissues, and/or the coagulation of bleeding vessels. [from Gr. *dia* through + *therme* heat + *-y* denoting an action]

dichotomy: division into two parts. [from Gr. *dikho* cut in two]

dilated apex: *New term.* apical foramen that is the same diameter or wider than the adjoining terminal root canal or pulp chamber. Usually found in immature anelodont teeth or throughout the life of elodont teeth. Usually inaccurately termed *open apex*. Compare CONSTRICTED APEX.

diphyodont: animals that develop two sets of teeth, a primary and a permanent dentition. [from Gr. *dis* twice + -PHY + -ODONT] Compare MONOPHYODONT and POLYPHYODONT.

disarming: *Veterinary.* procedure where one or more teeth are either extracted or shortened in order to prevent animals from inflicting injuries.

distal:
- *Dentistry.* tooth surfaces that face away from the centre of the dental arch, where the median plane bisects the jaw between the first incisor teeth. Compare MESIAL.
- *Anatomy.* situated away from the centre of the body, the median plane, or from the point of origin of a limb or organ. [from L. *distare* to be distant] Compare PROXIMAL.

distemper teeth: *Veterinary.* enamel hypoplasia seen in dogs, not necessarily associated with that disease.

dolichocephalic:
- having a head or muzzle that is abnormally long for the species.
- having a head that is much longer in its rostro-caudal/anteroposterior dimension than in its width. [from Gr. *dolikhos* long + CEPHALIC] Compare BRACHYCEPHALIC and MESOCEPHALIC.

dorsal: *Anatomy.*
- pertaining to, or indicating a position situated on, near or towards the back or spine of the body.
- indicating a relative position nearer the spinal side of the body as opposed to one which is nearer the side of the belly. [from L. *dorsum* back] Compare VENTRAL.

dysphagia: difficulty in swallowing. [from Gr. *dus* abnormal + *phagein* eating]

dysplasia: abnormal development of a part or organ. [from Gr. *dus* abnormal, diseased + -PLASIA]

dyspnoea: difficulty in breathing. [from Gr. *dus* abnormal, difficult + *pnein* breathing]

-ectomy: (suffix) *Medicine.* excision of a part. [from Gr. *ek* out + -TOMY]

edentate: *Zoology.*
- animals that are normally devoid of anterior teeth.
- animals that are normally edentulous.

edentulous: devoid of teeth.

elastomers: synthetic, elastic, PLASTIC (1) materials for use in making a permanent, accurate impression.

elevator, dental: hand instrument used in extractions for loosening teeth or roots.

elevator, periosteal: hand instrument used in raising the fibrous membrane that covers the bone.

elodont: *New term.* a type of tooth that increases in its height or length on the pulpal axis throughout life. [from *elo-* (prefix) abbreviation of L. *elongare* to lengthen + -ODONT] Compare ANELODONT.

embolism: the sudden blockage of a blood vessel by a blood clot, fat or air. [from Gr. *embolos* stopper]

empyema: the accumulation of pus in a hollow organ or body cavity. [from Gr. *empuein* to suppurate]

emphysema: the abnormal presence of air in a part of the body. [from Gr. *emphusan* to inflate]

enamel: hard, white, highly calcified prismatic tissue that lacks innervation.
- part of the external or internal structure of the total length of most intra-oral elodont teeth.
- part of the external or internal structure of the anatomical crowns of anelodont teeth.
- the outer cover to the anatomical crowns of all brachyodont teeth. [from Old Fr. *amail* enamel]

enamel hypoplasia: incomplete or partial formation of the enamel. [from Gr. *hypo* less, incomplete + -PLASIA]

enamel points: *Veterinary.* sharp projections occurring at the bucco-occlusal angle of the upper or linguo-occlusal angle of the lower cheek teeth giving rise to ulcerations of the oral mucosa. This term is usually applied to horses but can occur in any hypsodont or elodont dentition where anisognathisism is present.

endo-: (prefix) within. [from Gr. *endon*]

endocarditis: inflammation of the inside lining of the heart and the valves.

endodontic file: hand or mechanically operated steel instrument used in the debridement of root canals.

endodontics: branch of dentistry involved with treating the pulp and root canals of teeth. [from ENDO- + -ODONTICS]

endoscope: instrument used for examining inside hollow organs and the abdominal cavity. [from ENDO- + *skopein* to look at]

endosteitis: inflammation of the endosteum, the vascular lining of the medullary cavities in bone. [from ENDO- + OSTEO- + -ITIS]

endothermic: a chemical reaction or the formation of a compound that occurs with the absorption of heat. Compare EXOTHERMIC.

epistaxis: haemorrhage from the nose. [from Gr. *epistasein* to let fall in drops on the ground]

epithelial attachment: interface at the base of the gingival sulcus or periodontal pocket that unites the gingiva to the tooth.

epithelium: thin cellular layer that covers the external and internal surfaces of the body or organs.

erosion: loss of tooth substance caused by a chemical process without the activity of bacteria. [from L. *erodere* to eat away] Compare ABRASION and ATTRITION.

etching: See ACID ETCHING.

eugenol: oil of cloves, a topical dental analgesic, extracted from the clove *Eugenia caryophyllata.*

exfoliate: to shed. [from Gr. *ex-* (prefix) away from + L. *folium* leaf]

exostosis: local deposition of new bone that projects beyond the normal limits of the skeleton.

exothermic: a chemical reaction that generates heat. Compare ENDOTHERMIC.

exposure: the contents of the root canal becoming open to the oral environment due to the loss of dentine, or infundibular cementum in some herbivores, through developmental abnormality, trauma, caries or resorption.

external fixation: *Medicine.* any method by which fractured bones are supported by means outside the body.

external fixator: *Medicine.* method by which fractured bones are immobilised with percutaneous pins that are joined outside the body.

extirpate: to completely remove or destroy a part or organ. [from L. *extirpare* to root out]

extra-alveolar: outside the bone that surrounds the teeth.

extra-oral: outside the mouth.

extra-oral traction: force applied to the teeth in orthodontics through an anchorage outside the mouth.

facial: *(N. Amer.)* a collective term for the labial and buccal surfaces of the teeth.

false pocket: space between the gingivae and the tooth surface caused by hyperplasia of the gingiva rather than apical migration of the epithelial attachment. Compare POCKET, PERIODONTAL POCKET and TRUE POCKET.

fetid: having a smell of decaying matter. [from L. *fetidus* stinking]

file, endodontic: hand or mechanically operated steel instrument used in the debridement and preparation of root canals.

fissure: fine developmental groove or invagination of the enamel, especially on the occlusal surface of some brachyodont posterior teeth.

fistula:

- epithelial-lined pathological connection between two hollow anatomical structures or an anatomical structure and the outside surface.
- a communication between two mucous membrane surfaces or a mucous membrane and the skin. [L. tube or pipe] Compare SINUS.

flap: portion of mucous membrane or skin separated from the surrounding tissues except for at least one edge.

floating: *Veterinary.* the process of smoothing down the sharp buccal or lingual enamel points on the cheek teeth of horses. [from the similarity of the process to that of making a surface flat or level, as in plastering a ceiling or wall]

follicle: fibrous sac which surrounds the developing tooth germ and by which it is attached to the oral mucosa. [from L. *folliculus* small bag]

foramen: a natural opening or passage, usually through a bone or the apex of a tooth root, through which nerves and vessels pass. [from L. *forare* to pierce]

formol cresol or **formocresol:** antiseptic solution containing *formaldehyde* and *tricresol*, used in endodontics for devitalising and preventing the necrosis of the pulp tissue of primary teeth through fixation. [*formol* indicating formaldehyde in solution]

fraenum or **frenum:** fold of membrane or gingival tissue that limits the movement of an anatomical structure (e.g. lingual or labial fraenum). *Frenulum* is a small fraenum. [L. bridle]

frank: *Medicine.* clinically evident, unmistakable, true. Usually used to describe disease, haemorrhage or pus.

free gingiva: *Obsolete.* that part of the gingiva that is not attached to the tooth and forms the wall of the gingival sulcus. (See Chapter 3, p. 32.)

free gingival crest: See GINGIVAL MARGIN.

friction-grip: type of head used on a dental handpiece where the burr is held in place through a tight fit. Compare LATCH-GRIP.

furcation: being divided into parts. Teeth with multiple roots have bi- or trifurcation, at the point where the roots meet coronally. [from L. *furca* fork]

gag: an instrument to prevent the closure of the mouth during oral examination or surgery.

gemination: the fusion of two tooth buds during their development. The term is used by some to denote the division of a single tooth bud. [from L. *geminare* to be united] Compare DICHOTOMY.

general anaesthesia: controlled, drug-induced unconsciousness, whereby pain, voluntary muscle movement and an effective swallowing reflex are eliminated. [from Gr. *an-* (prefix) not + *aisthesis* feeling] Compare SEDATION.

gray or **Gy:** SI unit of absorbed ionising radiation dose; named after the British physicist Louis Harold Gray (1905–1965).

gingiv- or **gingivo-:** (prefix) denoting the gingiva.

gingiva: keratinised oral mucous membrane that is attached to the teeth and the alveolar bone. [L.]

gingival sulcus or **gingival crevice:** in conditions of periodontal health, a shallow space occurring immediately apical to the gingival margin, between the gingiva and the tooth surface.

gingival margin: the most coronal aspect of the gingiva.

gingivectomy: resection of unattached gingival tissue to eliminate the presence of periodontal pockets. [from GINGIV- + -ECTOMY]

gingivitis: inflammation of the gingivae. [from GINGIV- + -ITIS] Compare PERIODONTITIS.

gingivoplasty: minor surgical recontouring of the shape of the gingival margins, but still leaving their general outline normal. [from GINGIVO- + *-plasty* (suffix) indicating plastic surgery]

glass ionomer: dental material that is made by reacting an aluminosilicoglass base with polyalkenoic acid. The resulting cement adheres to dentine by both mechanical and chemical means.

-gnathic: relating to the jaw, meaning the mandible in modern usage. [from Gr. *gnathos* jaw]

-gnathism: indicating a state or condition of the mandible. [from Gr. *gnathos* jaw + *-ism* (suffix) condition]

gomphosis: attachment of the teeth to the alveolar processes through socketing and root formation. [from Gr. *gomphos* tooth, peg]

granuloma: localised mass of reactive connective tissue associated with an area of chronic suppuration and/or healing.

grouped eruption: where the permanent posterior teeth erupt side by side in a vertical direction and no sequential replacement of tooth loss takes place horizontally from a caudal direction. Compare SEQUENTIAL ERUPTION.

gutta percha: an ionomer of rubber extracted from the bark of certain tropical trees. Thermoplastic material used in endodontics. [from Malay *getah* gum + *percha* the name of the tree producing the latex]

haemostasis: to arrest haemorrhage. [from L. *haemo-* (prefix) blood + Gr. *stasis* standing still]

Haussmann gag: a metal-framed, ratchet-operated device, used to keep the mouth of herbivores, especially horses, open for examination or treatment. [In Great Britain similar appliances have been termed the American, Eclipse or Climax Gag, while in North America they are often referred to as the English or McPherson Mouth Speculum. The origin of the design appears to be from the USA. In their 1900 catalogue Arnold & Sons, of London, named the device as an 'American Pattern'. The instrument was advertised by the Haussmann & Dunn Co. of Chicago c.1902 as their newly patented 'Haussmann Mouth Speculum'.]

heat-cured: a form of acrylic resin where external heat is required for the hardening process to take place. See ENDOTHERMIC. Compare COLD-CURED.

hereditary: inherited condition passed on genetically; may or may not be apparent at birth. [from L. *hereditas* inheritance] Compare CONGENITAL.

heterodont: dentition of an animal having teeth which differ in form. [from Gr. *heteros* different + -ODONT]

homodont: dentition of animals where all the teeth are alike in form. [from Gr. *homos* the same + -ODONT]

host response: a current theory of the aetiology of periodontal disease which states that the individual's resistance or lack of immunity to toxins liberated from the bacterial plaque reflects the level of periodontal inflammation and destruction.

humoral: *Medicine.* ancient theory of physiology and pathology that originated in Greek and Roman medicine. It was based on the belief that the body contained four chief fluids (humors) that determined emotional and physical disposition: black bile (melancholia), blood (sanguis), yellow bile (choler) and sputum (phlegm). According to the hypothesis, when these were in perfect harmony the body was healthy and an imbalance produced ill-health. [from L. *humor* liquid]

hyper-: (prefix) exaggerated, excessive. [from Gr. *huper* over]

hyperplasia: enlargement or overdevelopment of organ or tissue through increased production of cells. [from HYPER- + -PLASIA]

hyperplastic: affected by hyperplasia.

hypso-: (prefix) indicating height. [from Gr. *hupsos* height]

hypsodont: teeth that have anatomical crowns which are greater in height than their roots. [from HYPSO- + -ODONT]

iatrogenic: *Medicine.* condition caused by treatment. [from Gr. *iatros* physician + *genes* born]

idiopathic: *Medicine.* disease of unknown origin. [from Gr. *idios* peculiar, own, personal + *pathos* suffering]

impacted: position of a tooth where full or normal eruption is obstructed by alveolar bone, gingiva or another tooth. [from L. *im-* (prefix) having a causative function + *pangere* to fasten, drive in]

implant:
- *Dentistry.* (intra-osseous), biocompatible structure placed in the alveolar bone which is used as a support in prosthodontics.
- *Medicine.* (orthopaedic), biocompatible structure (stainless steel, titanium, carbon fibre, etc.) used as a graft or internal splint to immobilise bone.

impression: mould taken of the teeth and/or intra-oral contours of the jaw for the preparation of a replica model.

impression material: a PLASTIC (1) substance used in the making of a mould of the teeth and/or the contours of the jaws.

impression tray: receptacle, usually custom-made in veterinary use to fit the jaw being worked on, for carrying the impression material.

incisal: pertaining to the cutting edges or tables of the incisor teeth. [from L. *incedere* to cut]

incisor: cutting tooth, usually chisel-edged, lying in the most anterior, mesial/rostral part of the jaw. [L. cutter, from *incidere* to cut]

inferior: *Anatomy usually Human.* indicating the relative position of a structure that is lower than others specified when the body is in an anatomical position; often with reference to parts or organs of the same or a similar kind. [from L. *inferus* low] Compare SUPERIOR.

infiltration anaesthesia: the injection of a local anaesthetic solution into an area to cause the loss of pain sensation to the tissues in the immediate vicinity of the injection site.

inflammation: reaction of living tissue to infection or injury.

infra-: (prefix) below, underneath.
- *Anatomy.* indicating a position beneath the structure being qualified.
- *Dentistry.* indicating a position apical to the the structure being qualified. [L.] Compare SUPRA-.

infrabony pocket: a periodontal defect that has a base which is apical to the alveolar crest and has one or more bony walls.

infundibulum: invagination on the occlusal surface or incisal tips of many hypsodont teeth, usually containing some cementum. [L. funnel]

innervation: nerve supply to a part or organ.

inter-: (prefix) between. [L.]

interalveolar septum: bony wall between the sockets of two roots.

interdental: indicating a position between the approximal surfaces of adjacent teeth.

interdigitate: the teeth from opposing jaws interlock like the fingers of clasped hands. [from INTER- + *digitus* finger or toe]

internal fixation: *Medicine.* method by which fractured bones are immobilised with implants within the confines of the body.

international two-digit system: a method of tooth charting where the first digit indicates the quadrants of the mouth, numbered 1 to 4 in a clockwise sequence, starting at the upper right. The second digit 1 to 8 indicates individual teeth, starting with the first incisor and 8 indicating the third molar in each quadrant. Compare PALMER'S DENTAL NOTATION.

interstitial: pertaining to or occurring in the space between adjacent teeth. [from L. *interstitium* interval]

intra-oral: indicating inside the mouth.

invagination: *Anatomy.* the infolding of the outer layer of an organ or structure so as to form a pocket.

-itis: (suffix) indicating inflammation of the specified part. [from Gr. *ites*]

ivory: type of dentine that constitutes the tusks of elephants, hippopotami, walruses, narwhals and mammoths (fossil ivory). [from Old Fr. *ivurie*, L. *evoreus* made of ivory]

keratin: *Histology.* insoluble, fibrous protein found in the outer layer of the skin that is a major component of hair, nail, hooves, horns and beaks. [from Gr. *keras* horn]

keratinised: tissues that are covered or impregnated with keratin.

Kirschner wire: a fine pointed metallic pin widely used in orthopaedic surgery.

labial:
- of, or pertaining to the lips.
- surfaces of the incisor and canine teeth and related tissues that face the lips. [from L. *labium* lip]

lacuna: a cavity, a depression. [L. hole]

lamina dura: a thin layer of compact bone with increased radio-opacity that lines the tooth sockets. [from L. *lamina* thin bone + *dura* hard]

lampas: *Veterinary.* physiological swelling of the mucous membrane of the hard palate of a young horse, especially at periods of tooth eruption. Usually the incisive papilla and the rostral rugae close to the incisors are involved. [origin unclear, possibly L. *lampas* lamp; Bavarian expression for something that hangs down; expression used in the Austrian army up to c. 1918 for the raised red piping on the side of trousers]

latch-grip: contra-angle dental handpiece in which burrs are locked in a chuck with a hinge or sliding mechanism. Compare FRICTION-GRIP.

lateral canal or **accessory canal:** fine channel in the root that contains pulp tissue which exits on the side of the root rather than at its apex.

light-cured: *Dentistry.* any material, usually PLASTIC (1+2) restorative, for which a filtered, visible, blue light (460 nm to 500 nm) acts as an initiator in the setting process. Further filtration is used to eliminate ultraviolet radiation.

lingual:
- of, or pertaining to the tongue.
- surfaces of the mandibular teeth and associated tissues that face towards the tongue. [from L. *lingua* tongue]

linguo-occlusal angle: junction where the lingual and occlusal surfaces of a tooth meet.

lining: *Dentistry.* insulating and/or sedative materials, usually rigid in consistency, used in cavities to protect the pulp from thermal and chemical irritation.

lophodont: teeth with occlusal surfaces that have a pattern of ridges, usually transverse (e.g. elephant molars). [from Gr. *lophos* crest + -ODONT]

Ludwig's angina: severe form of submandibular and/or sublingual cellulitis that spreads into the parapharyngeal space. [Wilhelm Friedrich von Ludwig, German surgeon 1790–1865; from Gr. *ankhone* strangling]

lumpy jaw: *Veterinary.*
- a term in classical veterinary medicine confined to a condition in cattle caused by *Actinomyces bovis.*
- a term often used to describe necrobacillosis in macropods.
- a vague and inaccurate term used to describe chronic alveolar abscesses or facial exostoses in herbivores and, occasionally, other animals. See NECROBACILLOSIS.

luxation:
- *Medicine.* the action of dislocation or displacement of bone extremities from their natural position of forming a joint.
- *Dentistry.* the displacement of a tooth from its socket. If a tooth is displaced from its natural position, but retained in the socket it is termed *subluxation.* [from L. *luxare* to displace]

lyssa or **lytta:** *Veterinary.*
- a thin, rod-like encapsulated structure (*septum linguae*), found in the tongue of dogs. Composed of adipose tissue and muscle, it is situated in the ventral aspect of the free end of the tongue, between the fraenum and the rostral tip, and is believed to act as a stretch receptor. It was believed from classical Greek times that the *septum linguae* was a 'worm' that caused rabies.
- *Obsolete.* a term for rabies, hydrophobia, fear of water.
- *Obsolete.* a term for the pustules that are sometimes found on the sublingual mucosa in cases of rabies. [from Gr. *lussa* madness, rage, fury]

malar: relating to the zygoma, cheek bone. [from L. *mala* cheek]

malocclusion: a condition where opposing teeth or jaws meet in a way that is abnormal for the type of animal, species or breed.

mandible:
- the lower jaw of vertebrates. A single bone often fused at the symphysis, or which has a fibrous joint.
- *Ornithology.* the lower part of the beak; the use of the term to describe both the upper or lower part of the beak is becoming less common. [from L. *mandere* to chew]

matrix: *Histology.* intercellular substance.

maxilla: the bone comprising half the upper jaw of vertebrates. [L. jaw]

meatus: *Anatomy.* a naturally occurring canal or channel. [L. passage]

median plane: *Anatomy.* an imaginary vertical plane running through the centre of the body from rostral to caudal or front to back, dividing it into left and right halves.

mental: relating to the chin. [from L. *mentum* chin]

mental foramen: anatomical opening(s) on the lateral surface of the mandible in the canine/premolar region, through which the mental neurovascular bundle emerges to supply the chin and the lower lip.

mesial:
- *Dentistry.* tooth surfaces that face towards the centre of the dental arch, where the median plane bisects the jaw between the first incisor teeth.
- *Anatomy.* pertaining to, situated in or directed towards the middle of the body. [from Gr. *misos* middle] Compare DISTAL.

mesocephalic:
- having a head or muzzle of normal length for the species.
- having a head that is between the brachycephalic and mesocephalic width to rostrocaudal/anteroposterior dimension ratio. [from Gr. *misos* middle + CEPHALIC] Compare BRACHYCEPHALIC and DOLICHOCEPHALIC.

metaplasia: *Pathology.* the transformation of one type of tissue into another. [from Gr. *meta* after, indicating change + -PLASIA]

metastasis: the spreading of disease, especially a malignant tumour, from one part of the body (primary) to another distant site (secondary). [Gr. transition]

methyl methacrylate: liquid monomer used in the manufacture of acrylic resins by mixing it with a powder polymer. See ACRYLIC, COLD CURED, HEAT CURED, MONOMER and POLYMER.

molar:
- tooth at the posterior/caudal aspect of the mouth, usually used for grinding, except in the case of true carnivores, where lateral excursion movements of the mandible are prohibited by the carnassial and canine teeth as well as the shape of the condyles of the mandible. In these instances the molars only slice or crush.

- *Veterinary.* general term for all the cheek teeth of the horse, including premolars and molars, with the exception of the wolf tooth. [from L. *mola* millstone]

monomer: liquid component of acrylic resin composed of simple molecules. Compare POLYMER.

monophyodont: an animal in which the permanent dentition does not have a primary precursor or a successor (e.g. dolphins). [from Gr. *mono* one + -PHY + -ODONT] Compare DIPHYODONT and POLYPHYODONT.

morphology: *Biology.* study of the form and structure of an organism or part of it. [from Gr. *morphe* form, shape + *-logy* (suffix) the science of, from Gr. *logos* word]

mucoperiosteum: periosteum that has a mucous membrane covering.

mummification: in endodontics the use of mummification in permanent teeth is controversial. It is claimed that the chemically fixed pulp tissue in the root canals can act as an effective root filling. [from Arabic *mum* wax (used in embalming bodies)]

necrobacillosis: *Pathology.* disease caused by *Fusobacterium necrophorum,* an anaerobe found in the gut contents of some herbivores. Pathogenecity of organisms is strongly enhanced by other faecal contaminants. The aetiology of oral lesions is connected with wounds of the mucous membrane, possibly caused by dietary trauma through sharp cereal awns, which allow the opportunist organisms to enter.

necrosis: the death of organic tissue; hence, *necrotic.* [from Gr. *nekros* corpse]

neoplasm: benign or malignant tumor, morbid mass of tissue growing at an abnormal rate. [from Gr. *neos* new + *-plasm* (suffix) indicating a material forming cell]

non-vital: *Dentistry.* tooth or pulp tissue that has lost its innervation and vascular supply.

occlusal: relating to:
- the closing of the mouth.
- the biting or grinding surfaces of the posterior teeth.

occlusion: the contact of the upper and lower teeth in a closed position. [from L. *occludere* to close]

-odont: (suffix) indicating types of teeth; toothed. [from Gr. *odon* tooth]

-odontics: (suffix) indicating a dental subject or discipline. [from -ODONT + Gr. *-ika* indicating a science or subject]

odonto- or **odont-:** (prefix) relating to teeth; indicating toothed.

odontoblast:
- the cell from which dentine is formed.
- the cells surrounding the dental pulp in the pulp chamber that are responsible for the deposition of secondary dentine. The nomenclature of odontoblast is misleading, as it implies that they form all the tissues of the tooth, which they do not. [from Gr. ODONTO- + -BLAST]

odontoclast: inflammatory, multinuclear giant cell formed from macrophages, identical in appearance to osteoclasts, responsible for the resorption of tooth substance, i.e. enamel, dentine and cementum. Descriptive term relating to the structure the cell resorbs. [from ODONTO- + Gr. *klastos* broken]

odontogenic: originating from a tooth or tooth germ. [from ODONTO- + *-genic* (suffix) in this context indicating generated, produced, from Gr. *genes* born]

-oma: (suffix) indicating a tumour. [Gr.]

open apex: See DILATED APEX.

open fracture: *Medicine.* a fracture where there is a breach in the overlying skin or mucous membrane.

oro-: (prefix) combining form indicating oral, mouth. [from L. *os* mouth]

ortho-: (prefix) straight. [from Gr. *orthos* straight, upright]

orthodontics: aspect of dentistry that deals with the study and treatment of irregular dentitions. [from ORTHO- + -ODONTICS]

orthograde: straight approach. In endodontics it indicates entry into the root canal from a coronal direction. [from ORTHO- + L. *gradus* step] Compare RETROGRADE.

osteo-: (prefix) indicating bone. [from Gr. *osteon* bone]

osteoblast: bone forming cell. [from OSTEO- + -BLAST]

osteoclast: large multinuclear cell that is associated with absorbing bone. [from OSTEO- + Gr. *klastos* broken] See ODONTOCLAST.

osteolysis: the pathological destruction or disappearance of bone. [from OSTEO- + *-lysis* (suffix) indicating a decomposition or breaking down, from Gr. *lusis* a loosening]

osteomyelitis: inflammation of the bone, which involves both the cortex and the marrow. Often implies an infectious cause. [from OSTEO- + Gr. *muelos* marrow + -ITIS]

osteopaenia: a decrease in the amount of bone due to an imbalance between its formation and resorption. [from OSTEO- + Gr. *penia* poverty]

osteotomy: surgical operation of cutting through a bone. [from OSTEO- + -TOMY]

overshot: See RETROGNATHISM.

palatal:
- of or pertaining to the roof of the mouth.
- indicating maxillary tooth surfaces and associated tissues that face the roof of the mouth. [from L. *palatum* roof of the mouth]

palato-occlusal angle: junction where the palatal and occlusal surfaces of a tooth meet.

palliative: treatment that alleviates the severity of pain or disease without curing it. [from L. *pallium* a cloak]

Palmer's dental notation: (also known as Zsigmondy/Palmer, angular, or grid system); a method of tooth charting, devised in 1891 by Dr Corydon Palmer (1820–1917), a dentist from Warren, Ohio, in which the quadrants of the mouth are illustrated diagrammatically. The vertical line of the + symbol represents the midline of the dental arches and the horizontal line indicates the occlusal plane. In dentistry the permanent teeth in each quadrant are identified numerically, from 1, which indicates each first incisor, to 8, the notation for the third molars.

paper point: miniature absorbent swabs, tapered in shape, used in endodontics for drying root canals.

papilla, gingival: gingiva lying in the interproximal space between adjacent teeth. [L. nipple]

partial coronal pulpectomy: procedure that involves amputating some of the exposed pulp in the pulp chamber and covering the remaining tissue with a material to maintain pulp vitality. In immature teeth it is used to encourage the deposition of a bridge of secondary dentine to wall off the contents of the root canal and allow for continued development of root anatomy to maturity. Usually inaccurately termed *pulpotomy*. See PULPECTOMY and TOTAL CORONAL PULPECTOMY.

paste filler: See ROTARY PASTE FILLER.

percutaneous: through the skin. [from L. *per-* (prefix) through + *cutis* skin]

peri-: (prefix) around. [Gr.]

periapical: indicating an area in the region of a root tip. [from PERI- + APICAL]

pericoronitis: acute inflammation of the soft tissues around a crown, usually associated with a partially erupted tooth. [from PERI- + CORONA +-ITIS]

periodontal: pertaining to the tissues that surround and support the teeth. [from PERI- + -ODONT]

periodontal ligament: fibrous tissue that acts as an attachment and support to the teeth through its insertion into the cementum of the roots and the lamina dura of the sockets.

periodontal membrane: See PERIODONTAL LIGAMENT.

periodontitis: inflammation of the supporting structures of the teeth that is usually characterised by destruction of the periodontal ligament and the alveolar bone. [from PERI- + -ODONT + -ITIS]

periodontium: the collective name for structures that surround and support the teeth; this usually includes the gingiva, the periodontal ligament and the alveolar bone.

periodontology or **periodontics:** area of dentistry concerned with the study and treatment of the diseases involving the gingivae and the supporting tissues of the teeth. [from PERI- + ODONTO- + *-logy* (suffix) the science of, from Gr. *logos* the word]

periodontosis or **juvenile periodontosis:** rapid destruction of the supporting tissues of the teeth, especially at a young age.

periosteum: fibrous membrane that covers bone, except for the articular surfaces of the joints. [from PERI- + OSTEO-]

phy-: (prefix) to generate. [from Gr. *phyein* to grow]

plaque: See BACTERIAL PLAQUE.

-plasia: (suffix) growth, development, change. [from Gr. *plassein* to mould]

plastic:
1. material capable of being moulded or shaped. When a change of consistency can be brought about it is through a chemical action or thermal changes.
2. made of a synthetic, usually organic, material. [from Gr. *plassein* to mould]

pleurodont: tooth that has no root but is attached to the lingual or palatal surface of the jaws. [from Gr. *pleura* side + -ODONT]

plexus: a complex network of nerves, blood vessels or lymphatics. [from L. *plectere* to braid]

pocket: an abnormally deep defect between the gingiva and the crown or root surface of the tooth. See FALSE POCKET and TRUE POCKET.

polymer: powdered, large molecular substance. In the manufacture of acrylic resins, polymethyl methacrylate, formed by the polymerisation of methyl methacrylate, constitutes the polymer ingredient. See MONOMER.

polyodontia: condition of having more than one supernumerary tooth.

polyphyodont: an animal which has a continuous succession of teeth throughout life. [from Gr. *polus* many + PHY- + -ODONT] Compare MONOPHYODONT and DIPHYODONT.

post: elongated cast, wrought, or screw structure, used in root canals to give support to a crown or large filling if insufficient supragingival tooth structure remains for the retention of the restoration.

posterior teeth: collective term for premolars and molars.

premaxilla or **incisive bone:**
- facial bone that lies rostral to the maxillae in most vertebrates and when present accommodates the upper incisor teeth.
- embryonic structure in humans that fuses with the maxillary bones.

prehensile: *Zoology.* adapted for grasping. [from L. *prehendere* to grasp]

premolars: teeth that lie distal to the canines and mesial to the molars.

primary dentine: dentine which is deposited to form the bulk of an anelodont tooth until the constriction of the apical foramen occurs. Compare SECONDARY DENTINE.

primary teeth: first, milk, deciduous or temporary teeth in diphyodont dentitions.

prognathism:
- anatomical relationship where the mandible lies in a rostral/protrusive position to the upper jaw.
- *Colloquial – Veterinary.* undershot. [from Gr. *pro-* (prefix) anterior/forward position + -GNATHISM] Compare RETROGNATHISM.

prosthesis:
- artificial device to replace missing natural part(s).
- *Dentistry.* crown, denture or bridge. [from Gr. *prostithenai* to add]

prosthodontics: branch of dentistry concerned with the restoration of damaged and missing teeth with fixed or removable appliances. [from PROSTHESIS + -ODONTICS]

proximal:
- *Dentistry.* see APPROXIMAL
- *Anatomy.* situated close to the centre of the body, the median plane, or the point of origin of an organ or limb. [from L. *proximus* nearest] Compare DISTAL.

pulp: vascular and innervated tissue occupying the innermost part of the tooth, the pulp chamber and root canals. [from L. *pulpa* flesh]

pulpal axis: plane in which the pulp lies from the root apex towards the direction of the incisal or occlusal surface, or coronal tusk tip.

pulp cavity: collective term for the pulp chamber and the root canals.

pulp chamber: anatomical cavity at the centre of the crown of the tooth that contains the bulk of the pulp tissue.

pulpectomy: the removal of pulp tissue from a tooth. [from PULP + -ECTOMY]

pulpitis: inflammation of the dental pulp. [from PULP + -ITIS]

pulpotomy: common but inaccurate term for the partial or total removal of pulp from the pulp chamber. [from PULP + -TOMY] See PARTIAL CORONAL PULPECTOMY and TOTAL CORONAL PULPECTOMY.

purulent: condition involving the presence of pus. [from L. *purulentus* festering]

pus: yellow, white or green fluid that is the product of inflammation, composed mainly of dead leucocytes, plasma and liquefied tissue cells. [from Gr. *puon* pus]

pyorrhoea (pyorrhoea alveolaris): a lay term denoting periodontal disease. [from Gr. *puon* pus + *rhoea* discharge, flow]

quadrant: one half of each of the dental arches forming the anatomical quarter of the full dentition. [from L. *quadrans* a quarter]

quidding: *Veterinary.* The dropping of clumps of semi-masticated food from the mouth, usually associated with herbivores (particularly horses) suffering with oral pain. [from Old Eng. *quid (related to cud),* piece of something, usually resin, suitable for holding in the mouth and chewing]

radiolucent: offering little or no resistance to the passage of X-rays. Compare RADIO-OPAQUE.

radio-opaque: offering resistance to the passage of X-rays. Compare RADIOLUCENT.

ramus of the mandible:
- *Anatomy.* part of the lower jaw that is devoid of teeth and from which the condyles and the coronoid processes originate.
- *Veterinary.* incorrect usage of the term for both of the main components of the lower jaw with prefix of its position (horizontal or vertical). [from L. *ramus* branch] See BODY OF THE MANDIBLE.

rarefaction: *Pathology.* loss of bone substance that creates an area of radio-opacity on radiographic examination. See RADIO-OPAQUE.

rasping: *Veterinary.* See FLOATING.

reamer: rotary hand- or engine-driven instrument, similar to twist drills, used to enlarge the diameter of pulp cavities.

repulsion: *Veterinary.* procedure whereby the cheek teeth of horses are extracted. A trephine hole is made in the jawbone from an extra-oral apical approach to the tooth to be removed. Through this the direct driving action of a punch is applied to the apex of the tooth root.

reserve crown: *Veterinary.* that part of the anatomical crown of a hypsodont tooth that is buried in the alveolus.

resorption:
- physiological absorption of alveolar bone after the extraction of teeth or the roots of primary teeth.
- pathological destruction of dentine through the action of odontoclasts. It can affect the wall of the root canal (internal resorption), or the external surface of the tooth (external resorption). [from L. *resorbere* to suck in, to absorb]

restorative dentistry: area of dentistry that is concerned with treatment, repair and conservation of teeth broken down through trauma or caries.

retro-: (prefix) from behind, backwards. [L.]

retrobulbar: indicating a position in the orbit behind the eyeball.

retrognathism:
- anatomical relationship where the mandible lies in an excessively caudal/retrusive position to the upper jaw.
- *Colloquial – Veterinary.* overshot. [from RETRO- + -GNATHISM] Compare PROGNATHISM.

retrograde: reverse approach; in endodontics indicates root filling from an apical approach. [from RETRO- + L. *gradus* step] Compare ORTHOGRADE.

rhinitis: inflammation of the mucous membrane lining the nasal passage. [from Gr. *rhis* nose + -ITIS]

root: part of an anelodont tooth that is covered with cementum and is devoid of enamel externally or internally. [from Old Eng. *wyrt* root]

root canal: channel at the centre of a root, from pulp chamber to apical foramen, that contains the pulp.

root canal sealer: biocompatible or sedative paste that sets hard and is usually used in conjunction with non-resorbable materials in the obturation of root canals.

root filling:
- process whereby the root canal is debrided, disinfected and obturated.
- material used in the obturation of the root canal in endodontic treatment.

rostral:
- *Anatomy usually Veterinary.* at or towards the nasal extremity of structures of the head. Compare CAUDAL.
- *Zoology.* of or like a beak or snout. [from L. *rostrum* beak]

rotary paste filler or **lentulo spiral filler:** an elongated, handpiece-driven instrument that has its twist in the reverse direction to reamers, and is used to spin paste, especially sealers, in an apical direction within root canals.

salivary mucocele: localised collection of saliva in tissues other than a salivary gland or duct.

scaler: instrument used to remove deposits, especially calculus, from the surfaces of the teeth. Its action may be through manual movements only, or the device is mechanically or ultrasonically driven.

scaling: the physical removal of deposits from the surfaces of the teeth.

secodont: teeth with sharp cutting edges that lie parallel to the line of the jaw and produce a shearing action (e.g. the carnassials of felids and canids). [from L. *secare* to cut + -ODONT]

secondary dentine: formed by:
- the slow physiological deposition of dentine inside the pulp cavity of an anelodont tooth throughout its life after the apical foramen has become constricted. Compare PRIMARY DENTINE.
- the physiological deposition of dentine throughout the life of an elodont tooth at the coronal extremity of its pulp chamber.

secondary dentine, reactive: the product of:
- the protective response by the pulp of an anelodont tooth to chronic irritants (e.g. attrition, abrasion, caries), through the accelerated deposition of dentine inside the pulp chamber in order to prevent an exposure.
- the accelerated deposition of dentine (or ivory pearls in the case of a tusk) inside the pulp chamber of an elodont tooth in an attempt to repair a pulp exposure.

sedation: drug-induced calmed state, diminished physical activity and a reduced response to stimuli, where pain is not eliminated and an effective swallowing reflex is maintained. [from L. *sedare* soothe, from *sedere* sit] Compare GENERAL ANAESTHETIC.

selenodont: teeth with crescent-shaped cusps (e.g. the molars of camelids and bovids). [from Gr. *selene* moon + -ODONT]

sequential eruption: method of tooth replacement where new teeth erupt horizontally from a distal/caudal direction (e.g. the molars of elephants, macropods and the manatee). [from L. *sequi* to follow] Compare GROUPED ERUPTION.

sequestrum: a detached piece of necrotic bone that is devoid of its blood supply. [from L. *sequestrare* to separate]

seroma: localised accumulation of serous exudate associated with a surgical dead space.

Sharpey's fibres: partly calcified portions of collagenous fibres of the periodontal ligament, embedded in the cementum covering the roots and the lamina dura of the alveolar bone.

shear-mouth: *Veterinary.* bilateral or unilateral malocclusion of the cheek teeth, especially in the horse, where there is an excessive anisognathism which results in severe enamel pointing. [The phrase is derived from the way the posterior teeth meet in these mouths. There is only a scissor-like action between the palato-occlusal angles of the maxillary and the bucco-occlusal angles of the mandibular cheek teeth.]

sialoadenectomy: removal of a salivary gland. [from Gr. *sialo-* (prefix) indicating salivary + *aden* gland + -ECTOMY]

silicone impression: See ELASTOMERS.

sinus:
- *Anatomy. Syn. antrum.* air cavity connected with the nose, e.g. *maxillary sinus.*
- *Medicine.* epithelially lined tract between an area of suppuration and a mucous membrane surface or the skin.
- hollow or cavity. [L. curve, bay] Compare FISTULA.

splint, intra-oral: a device, usually custom-made, that is used to immobilise a fractured jaw and/or mobile teeth during the healing phase.

Steinmann Pin: cylindrically shaped metal rod with threaded or trochar points used as an intramedullary splint in fracture repairs.

stomatitis: inflammation of the mouth. Often seen in cats, some of whom have a depressed immunological defence system. [from Gr. *stoma* mouth, orifice + -ITIS]

straight handpiece: instrument in which the burr is directed in line with the body of the instrument. Compare CONTRA-ANGLE HANDPIECE.

subgingival: a position or area apical to the gingival margin within the gingival sulcus or periodontal pocket.

subsonic scaler: mechanically operated scaling instrument that oscillates below 20, 000 cycles per second.

sulcular epithelium: a continuation of the gingival margin that forms the lining of the gingival sulcus.

superior: *Anatomy usually Human.* indicating the relative position of a structure that is higher than others specified when the body is in the anatomical position; often with reference to parts or organs of the same or a similar kind. [from L. *super* above] Compare INFERIOR.

supernumerary tooth: an extra tooth, in addition to the normal number found in the mouth of the species.

supra-: (prefix) above.
- *Anatomy.* indicating a position above that denoted by the qualified element.
- *Dentistry.* indicating a position coronal to that denoted by the qualified element. Compare INFRA-.

suppurate: to discharge pus. [from L. *suppurare*]

supragingival: signifying a position that is coronal to the gingival margin.

Susa fluid: a histological fixing solution containing mercuric chloride that enhances a tissue's capacity to be stained with only slight shrinkage of connective tissue.

symphysis: *Anatomy.* the central rostral point of the mandible where the two parts of the jaw join. This may remain a fibrous joint throughout life, or it may ossify at birth. [from Gr. *sun* fusion + -PHY]

synarthrosis: *Anatomy.* any immobile or fused joint that lacks a synovial capsule; it is usually formed by fibrous tissue, cartilage, or a mixture of both. [from Gr. *sun* fusion + *arthron* joint]

table, incisal or **occlusal:** the grinding surfaces of the teeth of herbivorous animals, especially that of the horse, that are flat and level. [from L. *tabula* a board]

teletherapy: radiation therapy using an external beam source. [from L. *tele* far + Gr. *therapeia* attendance]

temporomandibular joint: point of articulation between the mandible and the temporal bone of the skull.

teratoma: tumour or group of tumours composed of tissues that would not normally occur at that site. Derived from germ cells and often containing teeth or hair. [from Gr. *teras* monster + -OMA]

tetracycline stain: intrinsic grey, green, yellow or brown discolouration of the dentine and enamel caused by systemic treatment with a tetracycline-based antibiotic at the time of development of that part of the tooth.

thecodont: tooth attachment through socketing in the alveolus. [from Gr. *theke* sheath + -ODONT]

thermoplastic: materials that undergo a change in consistency with change in temperature without a change in composition. The term is usually used to describe impression and root-filling materials used in dentistry that are softened by heat and hardened by cold.

TMJ: See TEMPOROMANDIBULAR JOINT.

-tomy: (suffix) *Medicine.* surgical cutting of a part. [from Gr. *temnein* to cut]

tooth: a calcified structure containing dentine attached to the jaws of vertebrates occurring in or at the mouth; or in the alimentary canal of some invertebrates. [from Old Eng. *toth*]

tooth bud or **tooth germ:** the formative structure of a tooth in the dental follicle.

total coronal pulpectomy: the removal of all the pulp tissue from the pulp chamber, leaving the pulp undisturbed in the root canal(s) for conservative treatment. Usually inaccurately termed *pulpotomy*. See PARTIAL CORONAL PULPECTOMY.

trabecula: *Anatomy*. septum or lamella extending from the cortex of an organ, as in cancellous bone, and dividing it into chambers. [L. a litle beam]

traumatic occlusion: any form of abnormality in the way the teeth meet that causes damage to intra- or extra-oral structures. [from Gr. *trauma* a wound]

traumatogenic: condition caused by physical injury. [from Gr. *trauma* wound + *-genic* (suffix) in this context meaning generated, produced, from Gr. *genes* born]

trephine: cylindrical saw that is hand or motor driven to remove a circular section of bone. [from Gr. *trupan* to bore]

true pocket: an abnormal space occurring between the surface of the tooth and the gingiva caused by pathological apical migration of the epithelial attachment. Compare FALSE POCKET.

twitch: a loop of cord attached to a stick used to control horses during veterinary examination or treatment through pinching the upper lip by tightening the cord with the twisting action of the stick. [from Low Ger. *twikken* to pinch]

ulcer: break in the skin or mucous membrane resulting in the exposure of deeper structures. [from L. *ulcus* sore]

ulcerative gingivitis: See VINCENT'S INFECTION.

ultrasonic scaler: instrument which uses vibrations of frequencies beyond the limits of hearing of the human ear to aid in the removal of calculus from tooth surfaces. Instrument tips usually oscillate at frequencies between 20,000 and 45,000 cycles per second.

undercut:
- part of a cavity or structure that cannot be seen from a line of withdrawal (i.e. from a point that is directly above a structure and is viewed from an angle parallel to the majority of the walls of the structure).
- *Dentistry*. an area made below the general surface of a cavity for the mechanical retention of a filling.

undershot: See PROGNATHISM.

ventral: *Anatomy*.
- pertaining to, or indicating a position situated on, near or towards the abdominal wall or belly side of the body.
- indicating a relative position nearer the belly side of the body as opposed to one which is nearer the side of the spine. [from L. *venter* abdomen] Compare DORSAL.

Vincent's infection or **acute necrotising ulcerative gingivitis:** named after Jean Hyacinthe Vincent (1862–1950), a French Army physician and bacteriologist who in 1896 put forward the symbiotic infection theory, and in 1898 attributed the origin of ulceromembranous gingivitis/stomatitis to such an activity between organisms which were subsequently named *Fusobacterium plautivincenti* and the spirochaete *Borrelia vincenti*. It has been claimed that a German physician H.K. Plaut (1858–1928) also recognised the aetiology of the disease independently of Vincent as early as 1894.

Vincent's angina: acute ulcerative tonsillitis. [from Gr. *ankhone* strangling]

vital: *Dentistry*. tooth or pulp tissue with intact innervation and vascular supply. [from L. *vita* life]

Whitehead's Varnish: (Syn: Compound Paint of Iodoform BPC or Pigmentum Iodoform Compositum BPC) antiseptic used to impregnate packs in preventing the contamination of irreparable surgical defects and encouraging granulation infill. Contains Iodoform, Balsam of Tolu, Benzoin and Storax in a solvent Ether base.

wolf tooth or **wolf's tooth:** *Veterinary*. vestigial maxillary first premolar in horses. [Ger. *Wolfzahn*, derived from *Wolf*, implying something that is destructive or hurtful, as the wolf tooth is often blamed for damaging the labial mucosa or causing difficulty with the use of the bit.]

wry mouth: twisted, askew. Colloquial expression for a unilateral malocclusion. Often it implies that the mouth is twisted to one side. [from Old Ger. *wrich* bent]

INDEX

Numbers refer to pages.